AF413280

THE
GOOD-HEARTED
PHYSICIAN

VOLUME 2

THE GOOD-HEARTED PHYSICIAN

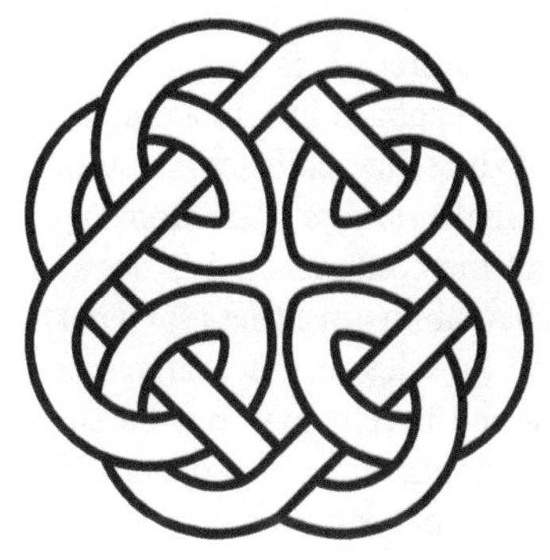

The Yoga of Medicine

JAMES D DUFFY

MD FANPA, FAAHPM, DABMA

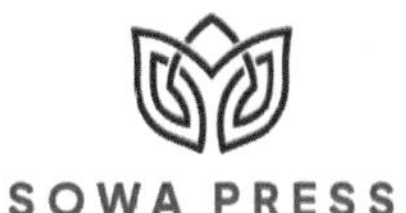

SOWA PRESS

SOWA PRESS

33 Laurel Rd, Essex, CT USA, 06426
Email: sowapress@gmail.com

Book cover design and typeset by www.raghavdesign.com

Hardcover ISBN 979-8-218-56963-1
Ebook ISBN 979-8-218-56964-8

The Summer Day

Who made the world?
Who made the swan, and the black bear?
Who made the grasshopper?
This grasshopper, I mean — the one who has flung herself
out of the grass, the one who is eating sugar out of my hand,
who is moving her jaws back and forth instead of up and down —
who is gazing around with her enormous and complicated eyes.
Now she lifts her pale forearms and thoroughly washes her face.
Now she snaps her wings open, and floats away.
I don't know exactly what a prayer is.
I do know how to pay attention, how to fall down into the grass,
how to kneel down in the grass, how to be idle and blessed, how to
stroll through the fields, which is what I have been doing all day.
Tell me, what else should I have done?
Doesn't everything die at last, and too soon?
Tell me, what is it you plan to do
with your one wild and precious life?
Mary Oliver

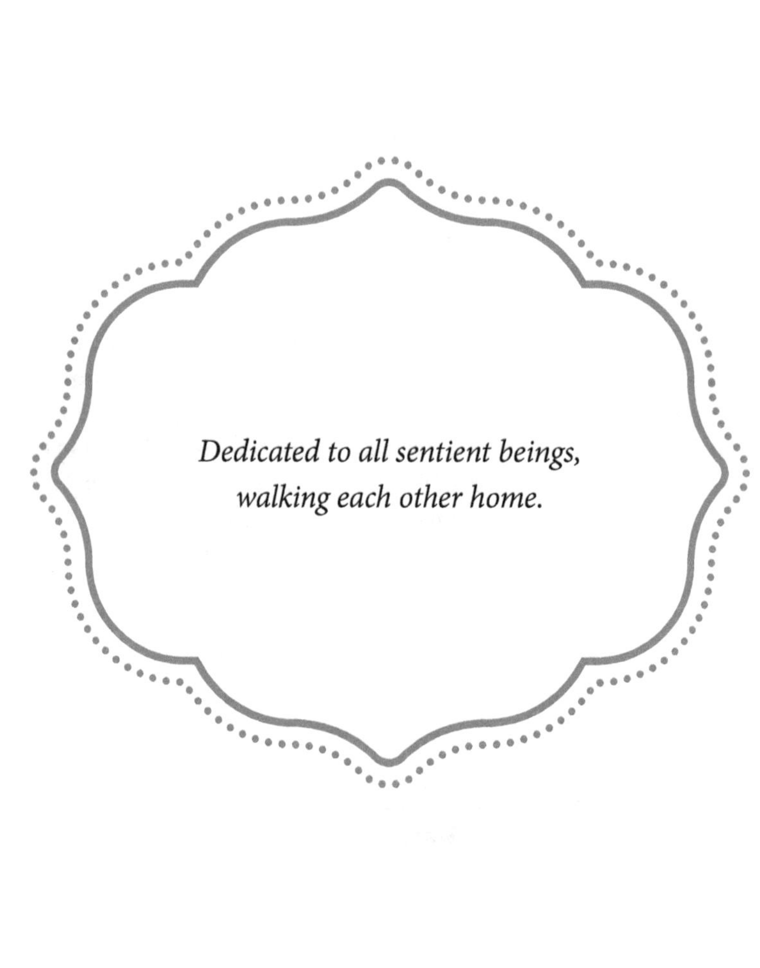

Dedicated to all sentient beings,
walking each other home.

Contents

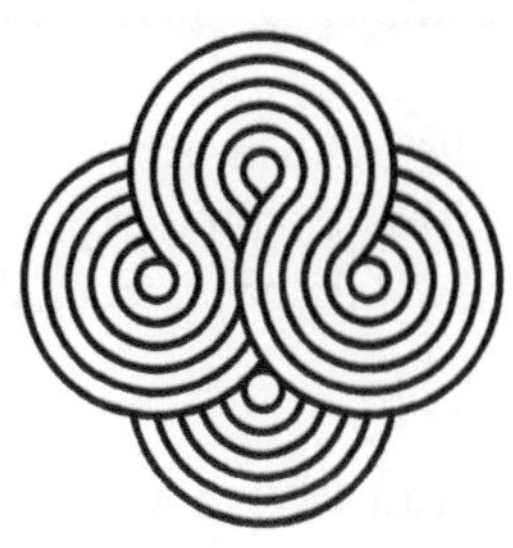

The Actions of the Healer

Character is what you do when no one is looking.
Henry Huffman

Volume One of "The Good-Hearted Physician" describes the personal attributes of a good-hearted physician. However, healers are ultimately defined by their actions. Healers must repeatedly engage with their patients as active participants in the dance of wholeness we call healing. Phronesis, wise action, requires more than theories. It demands practical guidelines that support the translation of theory into action, i.e., *theoria* to *praxis*. Volume Two of "The Good-Hearted Physician" aims to provide modern healers with practical ways of understanding the characteristics of their actions so that they can manifest phronesis in their healing work.

The first volume of "The Good-Hearted Physician" provided an overview of:

1. The characteristics of an "education of the heart" and education of a "good-hearted healer."
2. Integral Theory as a framework for understanding how we can understand and create synergy between our heart's wisdom and intellect's genius.

3. The developmental journey of the good-hearted healer, as represented by the story of Chiron, the Greek mythological "wounded healer."
4. The personal attributes of a good-hearted healer as described by the "Four Boundless Qualities" of compassion, lovingkindness, equanimity, and joy.

It can be challenging to distinguish between our personal attributes and the qualities of our actions. This chapter explores the distinction between these two frameworks and how this has practical implications for our work as healers.

The Four Immeasurables vs. The Twelve Actions
As we discussed in Section Four of Volume One, the "Four Immeasurables," also known as the "Four Divine Abodes" or "brahmaviharas" in Buddhist thought, refer to four boundless qualities that the healer cultivates as the very ground of their being[1]:

1. *Lovingkindness* (metta): An unconditional friendliness and goodwill towards all beings. As Thich Nhat Hanh describes, "Metta is the ability to embrace all parts of ourselves, as well as all parts of the world." [2]
2. *Compassion* (karuna): A heartfelt responsiveness to the suffering of others, coupled with a deep wish to alleviate that suffering. Buddhist scholar Christina Feldman writes, "Compassion is the trembling or the quivering of the heart in response to a being's pain." [3]
3. *Empathetic joy* (mudita): An ability to rejoice in the happiness and good fortune of others, free from envy or resentment. In Sharon Salzberg's words, it is "a natural ability to take delight in the happiness of others." [4]
4. *Equanimity* (upekkha): An evenness of mind, a spacious stillness that can embrace the full range of experiences with presence and poise. Joseph Goldstein describes equanimity as "a balance of mind, not being thrown off balance by the eight worldly winds of praise and blame, gain and loss, pleasure and pain, success and failure." [5]

These attributes are not merely fleeting or isolated sentiments but are the enduring characteristics of a healer that manifest in their interactions with all sentient beings - a fundamental orientation from which the healer engages the world. As the Taoist scholar and healer Jeffrey Yuen explains: "The Four Immeasurables are the expression of our true nature. They are not something we need to acquire from outside, but rather something we need to uncover from within." [6]

In contrast to the personal attributes described by the "Four Immeasurables," the "twelve characteristics of action" described in "The

Good-Hearted Physician" point to the healer's enlightened activities and conduct[7]. These twelve characteristics expand on the "Six Perfections (or Six Paramitas")" described in Buddhism, which include the first six characteristics described below.

Here are the brief definitions of the "twelve characteristics" of the healer's actions that will be discussed in much greater detail later in this section of the text.

1. *Generous*: Giving freely of one's time, energy, and resources for the benefit of others. This generosity includes not just material giving but also the gift of fearlessness, the gift of Dharma, and the gift of caring attention.
2. *Moral*: A commitment to non-harming and skillful action in one's conduct. This ethical behavior involves practicing restraint from harmful behaviors and actively cultivating virtuous ones.
3. *Patient*: Maintaining a spacious presence of mind in the face of provocation, frustration, or adversity. Patience allows us to respond to challenging situations with wisdom and care rather than reactivity.
4. *Vital*: Engaging one's activities with enthusiasm, delight, and wholehearted commitment. Manifesting vitality transforms our actions from a begrudging obligation into an inspired and joyous offering.
5. *Mindful*: Cultivating the ability to focus the mind single-pointedly and sustain an unwavering presence. This quality of deep attentiveness allows the healer to connect fully with self and others in each moment.
6. *Wise*: Seeing clearly the nature of things and responding to situations with intuitive appropriateness. In this sense, wisdom is not merely intellectual understanding but an embodied way of being and perceiving.
7. *Intelligent*: The healer's intelligence can be defined as "a multidimensional capacity, rooted in cognitive knowledge and skill but encompassing wisdom, insight, discernment, compassion, phronesis, intuition, and heart.
8. *Humble*: Humility is having a modest view of one's importance, recognizing one's limitations, being open to learning from others, and appreciating the value of all things and the contributions of others.
9. *Reverent*: Reverence is a deep feeling of respect, awe, and humility in the presence of something greater than oneself, whether it be the divine, nature, human life, or the mysteries of the universe. It involves recognizing all things' inherent worth and dignity and a willingness to subordinate one's ego and desires to something more significant than our agenda. Reverence is expressed through rituals and traditions; it is how one engages with the world, bringing meaning, purpose, and a sense of the sacred to life.

10. *Curious*: Curiosity is an eager desire to learn, explore, and understand. It involves questioning assumptions, remaining open to new experiences and perspectives, and embracing uncertainty. For healers, curiosity is a vital quality that drives the pursuit of knowledge, the desire to understand the root causes of disease, and the openness to explore new treatment approaches while recognizing each patient as unique.

11. *Creative*: Creativity generates novel and valuable ideas, solutions, or products that transcend traditional thinking or acting. It involves cognitive processes such as divergent thinking, mental flexibility, and openness to experience. For healers, creativity is crucial for finding innovative treatment approaches, connecting empathetically with patients, and promoting healing and well-being.

12. *Inspiring*: By embodying presence, compassion, and unwavering faith in human potential, the inspiring healer catalyzes their patients' innate healing capacities. They serve as a mirror, reflecting the wholeness and radiance that may have been obscured by suffering, and offer their patients a glimpse of their inherent capacity for flourishing.

If the Four Immeasurables are the soil, the "twelve actions" are the fruits - the tangible manifestation of those qualities in action.[8] The healer gives freely, behaves impeccably, meets adversity with patience, acts enthusiastically, rests in meditative poise, and responds with situational wisdom. Jeffrey Yuen notes, "The Six Perfections are the actualization of the Four Immeasurables. They are how we bring our innate enlightened qualities into the realm of human activity and relationship." [9]

The Nature of Action

Before we can begin a discussion on the qualities of action, we must clearly understand what we mean by the term "action." As with so many words that are part of our daily language, most of us have spent little or no time exploring the deeper meaning of what "action" represents. Action is central to our experience of our identity, and we typically experience ourselves as "human doings" rather than "human beings." The English word "action" derives from the Latin "action," meaning a doing, driving forward, or setting in motion.[10] An action is the exertion of power or influence to effect change.[11] When we act, we reach out from our being to engage and shape the world around us.

Our actions inevitably express our way of relating to the world, consciously and unconsciously. The Jungian psychologist James Hillman writes: "My behavior is the portrait of my soul, the visible aspect of my invisible psychic life, the mirror in which is reflected the quality of my consciousness." [12]

The philosopher Alva Noë develops this idea further with the concept of "enaction," suggesting that our cognition and consciousness are not merely brain processes but embodied activities of sense-making and world-shaping.[13] He writes: "Consciousness is not something that happens inside us. It is something we do or make better: it is something we achieve. Consciousness is more like dancing than it is like digestion." [14] From this view, the healer's consciousness - their way of being - is not separate from their actions but fundamentally intertwined. The healer knows and shapes the world through their engaged activity. As Jeffrey Yuen describes: "In Chinese medicine, we don't see the mind and body as separate. The Shen, or spirit, is expressed through our physical form and our actions in the world. Thus, the cultivation of the healer is simultaneously a cultivation of their consciousness and their conduct." [15]

Enaction, Autopoiesis, and the Co-Creation of Healing

Francisco Varela, Evan Thompson, and Eleanor Rosch originally developed the theory of enaction, which has profound implications for understanding the healing relationship.[16] From an enactive perspective, cognition is not the representation of a pre-ordered world by a pre-ordered mind but rather the vibrant enactment of a world and a mind based on a history of the variety of actions that a being in the world performs.

Autopoiesis is central to the enactive approach, initially developed by Humberto Maturana and Francisco Varela.[17] An autopoietic system continuously produces the components that specify it while simultaneously realizing it (the system) as a concrete unity in space and time, making the network of component production possible. *In other words, an autopoietic system is self-producing and self-organizing.* Therefore, the quality of our actions is crucial to any interaction's characteristics.

Applied to living systems, autopoiesis describes how organisms maintain their identity and organization amidst material and energetic exchanges with the environment. The critical insight is that living beings are not passive recipients of external stimuli but active agents that enact or "bring forth" their world through their structural coupling with the environment.[18]

In the context of the healing relationship, this suggests that both healer and patient are autopoietic systems engaged in a reciprocal process of mutual perturbation and response. The healer does not simply "fix" the patient but rather facilitates the conditions under which the patient's innate healing capacity can emerge. As Bradford Keeney, a pioneer in cybernetic psychology, explains: "The therapist does not 'do' therapy. Rather, the therapist dances with the client, participating in a co-creative process that brings forth new possibilities. The therapist's role is to help create a context in which the client's natural process of transformation can occur." [19]

This co-creative dance is not arbitrary or random but is guided by the healer's skillful means and therapeutic presence. The Four Immeasurables and "twelve characteristics of the healer" provide a map for this relational terrain, orienting the healer towards those qualities and actions most conducive to healing.

As Keeney notes, "The healer's job is not to make change happen, but to create a space where change can occur. This requires a deep trust in the wisdom of the system, a recognition that the seeds of healing are already present within the client." [20] The "twelve characteristics" define the ground in which the patient's innate capacity for healing can manifest.

The art of healing, then, is less about technique and more about attunement - the ability to sense and respond to each therapeutic encounter's unique rhythms and patterns. It is a kind of improvisation, a moment-by-moment adaptation to the unfolding process. Keeney likens it to a sailor's art: "A sailor can't change the wind, but he can adjust his sails. Similarly, a therapist can't control the client's process, but she can adjust her approach to create the optimal conditions for change." [21]

When seen through the lens of enaction and autopoiesis, healing is not done to the patient but emerges from the interaction between healer and patient. It is a co-creation, a mutual dance of transformation.

The Healing Relationship as Improvisational Jazz

Bradford Keeney offers a vivid metaphor for understanding the healing relationship through the lens of enaction, i.e., healing is like improvisational jazz.[22] In this analogy, the Four Immeasurables are the instruments, the foundation of the healer's art. Lovingkindness, compassion, empathetic joy, and equanimity are the trumpet, the saxophone, the piano, and the drums - the tools through which the healer expresses their therapeutic presence.

The "twelve characteristics" described in this book are the notes, the specific actions, and the interventions the healer offers in the relational space. They are the melodies, harmonies, and rhythms that the healer plays, shaping the unfolding of the therapeutic process.

But the music of healing is not a solo performance. It is a duet, a collaborative improvisation between healer and patient. Each listens attentively to the other, responds in the moment, and builds upon the emerging themes. The healer does not impose a pre-written score but works with the patient's unique context, capacities, and needs.

As the Taoist sage Zhuangzi says, "The perfection of action is like the dance of a master performer... the perfect man employs his mind as a mirror; it grasps nothing, it refuses nothing; it receives but does not keep." [23] Like the jazz musician, the healer enters the present moment with an open and responsive awareness, letting the music of the therapeutic encounter arise spontaneously.

The Chinese Character For Medicine And Healing As Improvisational Jazz

The Chinese character for medicine, 藥 (yào), offers a profound insight into the traditional Chinese understanding of health and healing. This character's composition and etymology provide a rich foundation for exploring the parallels between the healing process and improvisational jazz.

Character Composition
藥 (yào) is composed of two main parts:
The top part ⁺⁺ (cǎo), known as the "grass" radical, represents herbs or plants.
The bottom part 樂 (yuè) is the character for "music" or "happiness."
This combination suggests that medicine is fundamentally linked to the natural world (herbs) and the concept of harmony or joy (music) in the Chinese tradition.

Etymological Significance
The use of 樂 (yuè) in 藥 (yào) is particularly significant. 樂 itself is a visually evocative character, often interpreted as depicting:
A person (人, rén) with an instrument placed above or within a container, possibly representing the heart or mind.
This visual breakdown of 樂 implies that music—and, by extension, medicine—involves a harmonious interaction between the individual, their instrument (or healing modality), and their inner self.

Healing as Improvisational Jazz

The composition of 藥 (yào) aligns remarkably well with the concept of healing as a process akin to improvisational jazz:

Responsive Adaptation: Like jazz musicians who respond to each other in real-time, classical Chinese medicine emphasizes adapting treatments based on the patient's evolving condition and needs.
Harmony and Balance: Jazz seeks harmony within its apparent chaos, much like Chinese medicine aims to restore balance to the body's systems.
Individual Expression: Each jazz performance is unique, reflecting the musicians' styles. Similarly, healing in Chinese medicine is tailored to each individual's needs and constitution.
Integration of Elements: Jazz seamlessly blends various musical elements.

Likewise, Chinese medicine integrates therapeutic approaches (herbs, acupuncture, diet, exercise) to create a holistic treatment.

Rhythmic Flow: Jazz's rhythm mirrors the emphasis on the authentic flow of qi (life energy) in Classical Chinese medicine.

Intuition and Skill: Jazz musicians rely on both learned skills and intuition. Traditional Chinese healers combine rigorous knowledge with intuitively understanding of the patient's needs.

The character 藥 (yào) encapsulates a worldview where medicine is not just about treating symptoms but about creating harmony between various aspects of life—much like a jazz ensemble creates harmony from diverse musical elements. This perspective encourages us to see healing as a dynamic, creative process that responds to the unique "music," i.e., the healer's and patient's actions. [25]

Concluding Remarks

Seen through the lens of enaction, autopoiesis, and improvisational jazz, the "Four Immeasurables" and the "Twelve Characteristics" come alive as the instruments and notes of the healing relationship. They are not static techniques to be applied but dynamic qualities to be embodied and enacted in the present moment, in attunement to each patient's unique needs and capacities.

Jeffrey Yuen summarizes: "The path of the healer is a path of continuous cultivation and offering. We cultivate the Four Immeasurables as our instruments of being, and we offer the Six Perfections ("twelve characteristics" as our notes to the world. In this way, our actions become a form of music, co-creating the relational space in which healing can occur." [26]

In the dance of participatory sense-making, the healer and patient perform a spontaneous and emergent duet, co-composing the music of healing.

The poet Rumi invites us into this collaborative improvisation:

"Where there is ruin, there is hope for a treasure.
Why do you not seek the treasure of God in the wasted heart?
Your heart is the instrument, and you are its only player.
Let the wasteland bloom into a garden through your playing." [27]

Self-reflection questions

1. Consider your actions in the world, both personally and professionally. In what ways do you embody the Six Perfections - generosity, ethical discipline, patience, joyous effort, concentration, and wisdom? Where do you see room for growth and refinement?

2. Contemplate the relationship between your inner state of being and your outward actions. How does your way of relating to the world shape your behavior? How do your actions, in turn, influence your state of mind?

3. Reflect on a significant healing relationship in your life, either as a healer or a patient. In what ways was this relationship a co-creative process? How did you and the other person mutually influence and shape each other's experience?

4. Consider the idea that healing emerges from the interaction between healer and patient rather than being "done" by the healer. How does this perspective resonate with your own experience? What implications might it have for your approach to healing work?

5. Imagine yourself as a jazz musician, with the Four Immeasurables as your instrument and the "twelve characteristics" as your notes. What kind of music are you currently playing in your healing relationships? What new melodies, harmonies, or rhythms might you introduce?

6. Reflect on a challenging healing encounter in which you felt stuck or unsure how to proceed. How might the principles of enaction and autopoiesis—the ideas that we actively co-create our shared reality and that living systems are inherently self-organizing—offer a fresh perspective or approach?

7. Consider the Taoist idea of wu wei, or effortless action related to healing. How might you cultivate open, responsive awareness in your healing work rather than trying to force a particular outcome? What would it mean to "dance with" rather than "do to" your patients?

8. Reflect on the role of attunement and improvisation in the healing relationship. How do you currently sense and respond to each patient's unique needs and capacities? Where might you develop more flexibility, spontaneity, and creativity in your approach?

9. Contemplate the spiritual dimensions of healing, as represented by the Chinese characters for music (樂, a person with a musical instrument in their heart) and healing (愈, two dancing shamans above a person and the earth). How do you understand the relationship between your work's material and spiritual healing aspects? How might you deepen your attunement to these dimensions?

References

[1] Buddhaghosa, Bhadantacariya & Bhikkhu Nanamoli (2010). *The Path of Purification*. BPS Pariyatti Editions. p. 344.
[2] Thich Nhat Hanh (2017). *The Art of Living*. HarperCollins. p. 136.
[3] Feldman, Christina (2017). *Boundless Heart*. Shambhala Publications. p. 45.
[4] Salzberg, Sharon (2002). *Lovingkindness: The Revolutionary Art of Happiness*. Shambhala Publications. p. 121.
[5] Goldstein, Joseph (2013). *Mindfulness: A Practical Guide to Awakening*.

Sounds True. p. 287.

[6] Yuen, Jeffrey (2019). "The Spiritual Foundations of Chinese Medicine." New"England School of Acupuncture, Newton, MA, USA. September 21-22, 2019. Lecture.

[7] Shantideva & Padmakara Translation Group (2006). *The Way of the Bodhisattva*. Shambhala Publications. p. 111.

[8] Dalai Lama XIV (2017). *The Heart of Meditation*. Shambhala Publications. p. 13.

[9] Yuen, Jeffrey (2020). "Daoi"t Perspectives on the Six Perfections." Ame"ican University of Complementary Medicine, Beverly Hills, CA, USA. October 24-25, 2020. Lecture.

[10] Etymology Online. "Acti"n". ht" ps://www.etymonline.com/word/action

[11] Oxford English Dictionary. "Acti"n". ht" ps://www.oed.com/view/Entry/1938

[12] Hillman, James (2007). *Kinds of Power*. Crown Publishing Group. p. 66.

[13] Noë, Alva (2009). *Out of Our Heads*. Hill and Wang. p. 64.

[14] Noë, Alva (2009). *Out of Our Heads*. Hill and Wang. p. xii.

[15] Yuen, Jeffrey (2018). "Cultivating the HealeHealer's." New"England School of Acupuncture, Newton, MA, USA. November 17-18, 2018. Lecture.

[16] Varela, F., Thompson, E., & Rosch, E. (2016). *The Embodied Mind: Cognitive Science and Human Experience*. MIT Press.

[17] Maturana, H. R., & Varela, F. J. (1980). *Autopoiesis and Cognition: The Realization of the Living*. Springer Netherlands.

[18] Thompson, E. (2007). *Mind in Life: Biology, Phenomenology, and the Sciences of Mind*. Harvard University Press.

[19] Keeney, B. (2009). *The Creative Therapist: The Art of Awakening a Session*. Routledge. p. 18.

[20] Keeney, B. (1983). *Aesthetics of Change*. Guilford Press. p. 176.

[21] Keeney, B. (2005). *Circular Therapeutics: Giving Therapy a Healing Heart*. Zeig Tucker & Theisen Publishers. p. 48.

[22] Yuen, Jeffrey (2021). "The "ealer as Jazz Musician." Ame"ican University of Complementary Medicine, Beverly Hills, CA, USA. April 24-25, 2021. Lecture.

[23] Zhuangzi, & Merton, Thomas (2010). *The Way of Chuang Tzu*. New Directions Publishing. p. 74.

[24] Shuowen Jiezi (說文解字), entry on 樂 (yuè).

[25] [1] Unschuld, P. U. (2003). Huang Di Nei Jing Su Wen: Nature, Knowledge, Imagery in an Ancient Chinese Medical Text. University of California Press.

[26] Yuen, Jeffrey (2021). "The "heart of Healing." New"England School of Acupuncture, Newton, MA, USA. February 27-28, 2021. Lecture.

[27] Rumi, Jalal al-Din (1995). "The "music of Love." In "The Essential Rumi*, translated by Coleman Barks. HarperCollins. p. 102.

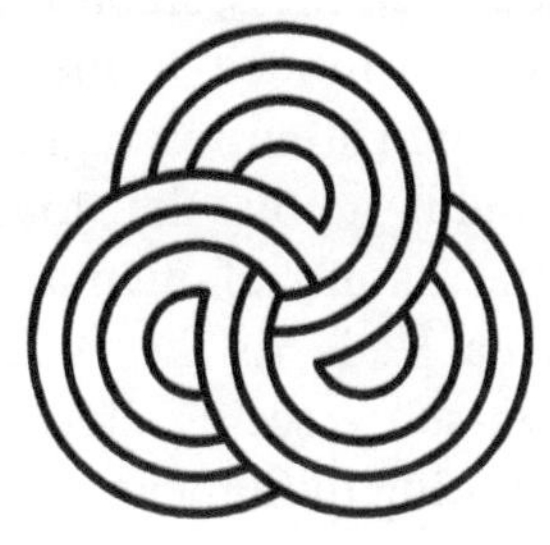

Being in the Flow

*"If we are hunting the highest version of ourselves, then we
need to turn work into play and not the other way round.
Unless we invert this equation, much of our capacity for
intrinsic motivation starts to shut down. We lose touch with
our passion and become less than what we could be
and that feeling never really goes away."*
Steven Kotler

The concept of "flow," as developed by psychologist Mihaly Csikszentmihalyi, has significant implications for our understanding of human well-being and flourishing, and our work as healers. Flow refers to a highly focused mental state of complete absorption in an activity, characterized by intense concentration, lost sense of self, distorted sense of time, and feelings of personal control or agency over the activity [1]. When in a flow state, individuals operate at full capacity, stretching their skills and rising to the challenges the activity presents.

This description of flow bears striking resemblance to certain aspects of contemplative experiences and practices. In particular, the intense concentration, present-moment awareness, and non-dual state of flow can be seen as parallel to stages of meditative absorption (dhyana) in Buddhist contemplative traditions like shamatha (calm abiding) and vipassana (insight) meditation.

In shamatha practice, the meditator aims to cultivate unwavering single-pointed concentration and mindfulness, leading to progressively deeper states of meditative absorption known as the dhyanas [2]. The pinnacle of shamatha is a state of profound stillness, stability and vividness of attention. Similarly, flow involves single-minded immersion in an activity to the exclusion of all distractions, with attention highly focused and stable.

Vipassana practice builds upon the foundation of shamatha to gain direct insight into the nature of mental and physical phenomena [3]. In particular, vipassana leads to the realization of impermanence, unsatisfactoriness, and non-self - seeing clearly how all experiences are fleeting, unable to provide lasting fulfillment, and empty of an inherent self. Absorbed in flow, the usual sense of self and duality between subject and object also dissolves. As Csikszentmihalyi writes, "In flow there is no room for self-scrutiny. Because enjoyable activities have clear goals, stable rules, and challenges well matched to skills, there is little opportunity for the self to be threatened." [4]

Some researchers have explicitly drawn comparisons between flow states and meditative absorption. For example, Yaden et al. [5] suggest that "flow states can be conceived of as a secular alternative to the self-transcendent mindset that is intentionally cultivated by contemplative practices." While flow may often arise unintentionally through immersion in worldly activities, certain spiritual practices like yoga, dance, music, calligraphy, and tea ceremony can also intentionally induce flow-like states as a form of active contemplative practice.

To be clear, flow is a psychological state, while contemplative practices like shamatha and vipassana are embedded in comprehensive spiritual paths aimed at deep self-transformation and wisdom. Brief moments of flow do not equate with the culmination of meditation practice as understood in contemplative traditions. Nevertheless, the parallels are evident and illustrate how flow can be a "gateway" contemplative experience accessible in everyday life. Cultivating flow can support the stabilization of attention and "thinning" of the self, which are foundations for contemplative insight. For those that connect with flow, practices that intentionally induce this state could provide a complementary contemplative discipline.

Flow and Human Flourishing

There are clear links between flow and human flourishing. Aristotle argued that eudaimonia (flourishing) results from the soul's rational activity in conformity with virtue [6]. Achieving flow requires the virtues of courage to tackle challenges, temperance to avoid distractions, and practical wisdom to find a balance between skill and difficulty. Furthermore, flow-inducing activities are often meaningful and purposeful, key elements of eudaimonic well-being.

Seligman's PERMA model of flourishing also aligns with key aspects of flow [7]. Flow fosters positive emotions like joy and exhilaration. Engaging in challenging flow activities builds accomplishment. The intense focus of flow exemplifies engagement and immersion. Meaningful activities that produce flow provide avenues for achievement, creativity, and self-expression.

The Gift that Keeps on Giving

One of the most striking features of flow is its autotelic nature - flow-producing activities are often desirable for their own sake rather than for some external reason or reward. As Csikszentmihalyi explains, "The key element of an optimal experience is that it is an end in itself. Even if initially undertaken for other reasons, the activity that consumes us becomes intrinsically rewarding." [8] This autotelicity is significant for human flourishing in several ways. Firstly, it enables the individual to "lose themselves" in the activity, quieting the ego and its anxieties. As Steven Kotler writes in The Rise of Superman, "In flow, there is no room for self-scrutiny. Self-scrutiny is replaced by self-optimization." [9] This loss of self-consciousness and transcendence of ego is often experienced as liberating and joyful.

Second, the autotelic nature of flow means that the activity is pursued for the inherent satisfaction and challenge it provides, not for external validation or reward. This intrinsic motivation is more sustainable and fulfilling than reliance on extrinsic motivators. It shifts the locus of control inwards, enhancing autonomy and self-determination, key elements of psychological wellbeing.

Third, flow's autotelicity means that the process of engaging in the activity becomes as important and rewarding as the end product. This mindset of growth and embracing challenge aligns with Carol Dweck's conception of the "growth mindset" [10], which is strongly associated with grit, resilience, and achievement. The journey becomes as significant as the destination.

Flow in Healing

The experience of flow is particularly relevant in medicine and healthcare, where practitioners regularly engage in highly challenging and absorbing activities with significant consequences. For surgeons, achieving a flow state during intense procedures can enhance concentration, dexterity, and stamina. As Kotler describes: "When a surgeon enters flow, error rates drop and efficiency increases. Situational awareness expands. Reaction times accelerate. For these reasons and more flow might just be the ultimate performance-enhancing drug." [9]

Surgeons in flow are totally immersed in the procedure, their awareness merging with their actions. Distractions and irrelevant stimuli recede from consciousness as the world shrinks to the immediate task. Time dilates - hours can feel like minutes. The ego falls away, yet the surgeon feels in complete control, able to respond almost automatically to the situation's demands.

In emergency medicine, flow allows physicians to cope with the intense pressures and fast pace. ER doctors must rapidly triage patients, absorb and integrate complex information, and make critical decisions, all while managing their own stress and fatigue. Accessing flow states enables them to stay focused, responsive and resilient in the face of repeated crises and challenges.

For psychiatrists and psychotherapists, entering flow during therapy sessions can facilitate deeper engagement and rapport with the patient. The therapist becomes intensely attuned to the patient, picking up on subtle cues and unconscious communication. Heightened empathy and intuition arise as the therapist's sense of self quiets. Creative insights and possibilities emerge spontaneously. The therapist is both fully present and strategically detached, guiding the process while allowing it to unfold naturally.

As psychiatrist Ned Hallowell describes: "I know I'm in flow when time disappears, my self-consciousness disappears, I feel one with the person I'm talking with and we're truly having a dialogue instead of two intersecting monologues. There's a feeling of timelessness, of connection, of being in a realm beyond the temporal." [11]

These flow states allow clinicians to provide higher-quality and more patient-centered care. The empathy, concentration, calmness, and confidence that flow provides enhance therapeutic efficacy and decision-making. Errors are reduced, insights magnified, and rapport deepened.

Flow as Improvisational Jazz
In the previous chapter, I discussed the similarities between healing and improvisational jazz. The experience of flow in medicine can be likened to the improvisational flow achieved by jazz musicians. In both cases, the individual must balance structure and spontaneity, planning and responsiveness, control and surrender. Jazz musicians use their deep knowledge of musical theory, forms and patterns as a launching pad for creative improvisation. They are guided by the underlying structure of the piece but are free to spontaneously explore, react, and innovate in the moment, stretching and recombining musical elements. As jazz great Charles Mingus put it, "You can't improvise on nothing; you've gotta improvise on something." [12]

Similarly, healthcare practitioners use their medical knowledge, clinical guidelines, and past experience as the underlying structure that supports their moment-to-moment responsiveness. Within the "chord changes" of best practices and protocols, there is space for intuition, spontaneity, and creativity in response to the patient's unique needs. Just as the jazz soloist must listen attentively to the other musicians, responding to and building off their musical offerings, the clinician in flow is exquisitely attuned to the patient, to the subtle verbal and nonverbal cues that guide the therapeutic interaction. Empathy and emotional resonance create a feedback loop of mutual attunement and co-regulation.

And like an improv performance, a clinical encounter has an element of risk and uncertainty - each is singular and unrepeatable, requiring both clinician and patient to tolerate ambiguity and vulnerability. But it is this very leap into the unknown that allows for growth and healing. In the words of Stephen Nachmanovitch: "In improvisation, there is only one time: This is what computer people would call real time. The time of inspiration, the time of technically structuring and realizing... the time of playing it, and the time of communicating with the audience, are all one." [13]

This merging of intention, action, and receptivity in the improvisational "flow space" enables what Csikszentmihalyi calls "the creative accomplishment of something that is new and meaningful," that is the essence of the flow experience and deep healing [1].

Flow as a Core Learnable Skill for Healthcare Providers
Given the performance-enhancing and stress-buffering effects of flow states, the capacity to access flow on demand should be a core skill for all healthcare providers. The ability to rapidly drop into a state of calm focused attention, and creative adaptation is crucial for optimal clinical decision-making, emotional regulation, and rapport-building. Research suggests that individuals can increase their likelihood of accessing flow states through deliberate practice and environmental design [14]. Here, we explore how each of the key flow triggers identified by Csikszentmihalyi and colleagues [1,8] can be applied in the context of modern healing:

A. *Clarity of goals and immediate feedback*
In medicine, goals exist on multiple levels, from the overarching aims of beneficence and non-maleficence to the specific objectives of a treatment plan and the micro-goals of moment-to-moment patient interaction. The modern healer can enhance flow by consciously aligning these goals and attending to real-time feedback.

For example, a surgeon may set the intention to execute a procedure safely and efficiently while closely monitoring physiological parameters and tissue responses, or a physician may determine a diagnosis and management plan while tracking the patient's understanding and agreement at each step.

Regularly defining proximal goals and tuning into multi-channel feedback keeps the clinician oriented and self-correcting, like a sailor adjusting sails and rudder to the wind and currents.

B. *Balance between perceived challenge and perceived skills*

The modern healer must consistently walk the edge between overwhelm and stagnation. This requires honestly appraising one's current skill level and seeking out appropriate challenges. An early career psychiatrist may find leading an inpatient therapy group to be the developmental sweet spot, whereas a more seasoned practitioner may need the challenge of working with a highly complex patient.

Skills can be further developed through deliberate practice, continuing education, and peer consultation. Challenges can be titrated by setting ambitious but achievable clinical targets, taking on leadership roles, or exploring new areas of practice. Striving at the limits of competence accelerates growth and maintains engagement. As Csikszentmihalyi notes, "Enjoyment appears at the boundary between boredom and anxiety, when the challenges are just balanced with the person's capacity to act." [8]

C. *Merging of action and awareness*

In the flow state, the usual divisions between self and activity dissolve. The surgeon becomes one with the scalpel, the deft movements an extension of embodied intention. The therapist experiences a wordless sense of union with the patient's inner world. This state of oneness arises when awareness becomes wholly absorbed in the present moment task. Distractions and self-consciousness dissolve in the intensity of focus. The modern healer can facilitate this merging by practicing mindfulness and presence. Techniques like focused breathing, body scans, and centering prayer train the mind to release mental chatter and align with the flow of experience. Rituals like donning scrubs or arranging one's clinical space can also serve as embodied signals to let go of outside concerns and merge with the healing role.

D. *Concentration on the task at hand*

Flow follows focus. The modern healer is challenged to maintain concentration amidst a barrage of distractions - electronic medical record alerts, phone calls, administrative demands, and personal preoccupations. Protecting time and space for uninterrupted clinical work is essential for accessing flow. This may require setting boundaries with colleagues, patients, and oneself. Strategies can include scheduling protected blocks for focused patient care, using "do not disturb" messaging, delegating non-clinical tasks, and practicing selective disengagement from personal devices and social media. Multitasking is anathema to flow. As Csikszentmihalyi warns, "When you are distracted, you literally cannot be creative." [15] The goal is to monotask—to give one's full attention to the patient and procedure at hand.

E. *Sense of control*
Flow is characterized by a feeling of effortless agency, of being in command even in challenging circumstances. The jazz musician in a solo, the rock climber negotiating a cliff, and the absorbed programmer coding late at night—all experience a sense of spontaneous mastery and intuitive decision-making. With modern healthcare's many regulatory, administrative, and resource constraints, clinicians often feel more like cogs in a machine than autonomous agents. Reclaiming a sense of control and efficacy is critical for accessing flow. This can be cultivated by identifying areas of discretion and impact, conscious ownership of clinical decisions, personalization of treatment plans, advocacy for patients' needs, and seeking leadership roles and opportunities to shape institutional policies and culture. Even in situations of limited external control, the clinician can always access an internal locus of control through mindset and meaning-making. Writing from a concentration camp, Viktor Frankl affirmed the ultimate human freedom to "choose one's attitude in any given set of circumstances." [16]

F. *Loss of self-consciousness, leading to self-transcendence*
In flow, the self disappears. The ego, with its anxieties, ambitions, and inhibitions, recedes into the background as awareness merges with action. There is a transcendence of self-referential thinking, a letting go of the autobiographical narrative. This dimension of flow can be both profoundly liberating and profoundly connecting. In losing oneself, one touches into a deeper mode of being. The boundaries between self and others become permeable, enabling genuine empathy, attunement, and presence. The modern healer can facilitate this self-transcendence by "bracketing" or setting aside personal concerns and preconceptions when entering the clinical encounter. Practices of self-emptying, such as meditation or prayer, create space for a more immediate and non-judgmental engagement. In seeing the patient as a "thou" rather than an "it," in Martin Buber's language [17], the clinician opens to the sacredness and mystery of the healing relationship. The self expands to include the other and, in this expansion, finds fulfillment.

G. *Transformation of the experience of time*
Flow alters the experience of time, typically compressing it so that hours pass by in minutes. But occasionally, time slows down, each moment

crystallizing in vivid detail. In both cases, there is a departure from the usual metric chronology, an immersion in what the Greeks called kairos, a time outside of time. The modern healer can leverage this temporal flexibility by strategically structuring clinical work. Matching the rhythm of practice to the ebb and flow of attention and energy. Intense procedures or therapy sessions requiring deep concentration can be scheduled for peak alertness and flow potential. Rote administrative tasks can be batched for low-energy periods. Weaving these focused periods of time dilation with restorative interludes of time expansion optimizes the "flow cycle" of struggle, release, flow, and recovery. [9] Pacing the tempo of clinical engagement enables the clinician to bring their full self to the moments that matter most.

H. *Autotelic experience*

As previously mentioned, flow states are autotelic - rewarding in and of themselves, regardless of outcomes. There is intrinsic motivation and satisfaction in meeting challenges with skills and in transcending the self in service of something larger. For the modern healer, tapping into this autotelic dimension is an antidote to burnout and nihilism. It affirms the inherent meaning and value of clinical work beyond external metrics and rewards. Cultivating a beginner's mind, a sense of wonder and curiosity about the human body and psyche. Approaching each patient as a unique being, each encounter as a creative act. Finding fulfillment in the process of diagnosis and discovery, the dance of empathy and insight. In the words of the 12th-century physician-philosopher Maimonides, "May I never see in the patient anything but a fellow creature in pain." [18] This spirit of compassion and service for its own sake lies at the heart of the healing vocation.

The Difference between Flow, Willpower, and Grit

While flow, willpower, and grit are all important for optimal performance and well-being, they represent distinct modes of motivational engagement. Understanding these differences can help the modern healer navigate the challenges of clinical practice with greater skill and sustainability.

Flow is an experiential state characterized by intense concentration, merging of action and awareness, altered sense of time, loss of self-consciousness, and intrinsic motivation. It arises when there is a dynamic balance between challenges and skills, immediate feedback, clarity of goals, and a sense of control. Flow is associated with peak performance, creativity, and enjoyment. It represents an ideal of spontaneous mastery and fluid, flexible response. However, it is difficult to sustain indefinitely and requires alternation with periods of struggle, release, and recovery.

Willpower, in contrast, is the ability to exert conscious control over one's thoughts, emotions, and behaviors in service of a goal. It is the deliberate overriding of impulses, habits, or distractions through choice and self-discipline. Baumeister and colleagues define willpower as "the capacity for altering one's own responses, especially to bring them into line with standards such as ideals, values, morals, and social expectations, and to support the pursuit of long-term goals." [19] It is the proverbial "triumph of mind over matter."

Willpower is a critical faculty for the modern healer, essential for everything from maintaining focus and composure in high-stress situations to resisting temptations and setting self-protective boundaries. The clinician must often subordinate personal needs and reactions to professional imperatives and the patient's welfare.

However, willpower is a limited resource that can be depleted through overuse. Baumeister's research shows that acts of self-control draw upon a finite "ego reservoir," leading to a state of "ego depletion" marked by the weakened ability to regulate thoughts, feelings, and behaviors. [20] Relying too heavily on sheer willpower to push through fatigue, frustration, or vicarious trauma is a risk factor for burnout. Baumeister warns, "Even people with excellent self-control may sometimes find themselves in circumstances that deplete their willpower to such an extent that they can no longer control themselves effectively." [21]

The modern healer must use willpower judiciously as a bridge rather than a crutch. Employing it to stay on track and override self-defeating impulses, but not as a substitute for adequate rest, emotional processing, and self-renewal. Willpower alone cannot indefinitely compel flow or override the body's natural rhythms.

Grit, as defined by Duckworth and colleagues, is "perseverance and passion for long-term goals." [22] It is the capacity to sustain effort and interest over prolonged periods despite setbacks, plateaus, and monotony. Where willpower is the ability to resist short-term distractions and temptations, grit is the tenacity to pursue an overarching aim over months or years.

Grit has been associated with achievement and success across diverse domains, from academics to athletics to the military. [23] It predicts retention and performance in challenging occupations like teaching and sales. For the modern healer, grit is essential for weathering the long years of training, the daily grind of clinical practice, and the inevitable disappointments and failures. However, grit is not just about dogged persistence. It also involves passion, the deep commitment to and abiding interest in one's chosen pursuit. This passion provides the meaning and intrinsic motivation to sustain effort over the long haul beyond external rewards or validation.

"Gritty individuals" have a "growth mindset," viewing setbacks as opportunities for learning and improvement rather than indictments of fixed abilities. [10] They embrace challenges, persist in the face of obstacles, and maintain effort and interest over the years.

For the modern healer, cultivating a growth mindset and sense of purpose is crucial for long-term resilience and fulfillment. It allows the clinician to find meaning in the day-to-day struggles and setbacks and to keep sight of the larger mission beyond the metrics.

At the same time, grit must be balanced with adaptability and self-compassion. Blind persistence in the face of futility or harm is not a virtue. The gritty clinician must know when to pivot, when to let go, and when to seek help. As Duckworth notes, "The gritty individual approaches achievement as a marathon; his or her advantage is stamina. But as in any race, a positive, unshakable belief that you can go the distance is an indispensable first step." [23]

Ultimately, flow, willpower, and grit are complementary capacities that enable the modern healer to bring their best selves to the challenges of clinical practice. Flow represents the ideal of effortless mastery and fluid performance, willpower, the capacity for conscious self-control and discipline, and grit, the long-term passion and perseverance for a meaningful mission. By developing all three capacities and using them judiciously and synergistically, the modern healer can optimize performance, resilience, and fulfillment over the long arc of a clinical career. In the words of positive psychologist Shane Lopez: "To do our best and be our best, we need the strength that comes from merging the forces of willpower, waypower [flow], and grit. Waypower alone won't be enough to get us through the tough times. Willpower provides [the] necessary pushing force. Grittiness supplies staying power." [24]

Flow as a Protective Factor Against Burnout

Burnout is a pervasive problem in modern society, characterized by emotional exhaustion, depersonalization, and reduced personal accomplishment resulting from chronic work stress [25]. It is particularly prevalent in high-stress occupations like healthcare, education, and social services, where the emotional demands of caring for others can lead to compassion fatigue and psychological depletion [26]. Given the significant personal and professional costs of burnout, there is a pressing need to identify protective factors that can mitigate its impact.

One promising line of research suggests that the experience of flow may serve as a buffer against burnout. Flow is a state of optimal experience characterized by total absorption in an activity, intrinsic motivation, and a sense of effortless mastery [1]. When in flow, individuals are fully immersed in the present moment, their attention focused on a clear goal, and their skills matched to the challenge at hand. Self-consciousness falls away, time becomes distorted, and the activity becomes autotelic - rewarding in itself, regardless of outcome [8].

A growing body of evidence indicates that regular flow experiences are associated with reduced burnout and enhanced well-being. For example, a study of nurses found that those who frequently experienced flow at work reported lower levels of burnout and higher levels of work engagement [27]. Similarly, a study of teachers found that flow was negatively correlated with emotional exhaustion and depersonalization, two key components of burnout [28].

These findings raise the question of how exactly flow might protect against burnout. Several mechanisms have been proposed:

1. *Flow provides a respite from self-conscious rumination and negative emotion.*
   When in flow, attention is fully absorbed in the present moment, leaving no room for worry, self-doubt, or other forms of negative self-focus. As Csikszentmihalyi explains, "In flow, there is no room for self-scrutiny. Because enjoyable activities have clear goals, stable rules, and challenges well matched to skills, there is little opportunity for the self to be threatened" [29]. This temporary freedom from self-concern may provide a much-needed break from the chronic stress and emotional labor that can lead to burnout.

2. *Flow enhances a sense of mastery and control.*
   Flow experiences arise when skills are optimally matched to challenges, leading to a sense of effortless control and mastery. This feeling of competence and efficacy can counteract the helplessness and futility that often accompany burnout. As Seligman and Csikszentmihalyi note, "The sense of personal control so central in flow leads to an experience of 'flow from within'" [30]. Repeated mastery experiences through flow can build self-efficacy and resilience in the face of stress.

3. *Flow provides intrinsic motivation and meaning.*
   Flow-producing activities are autotelic - they are inherently rewarding and meaningful, pursued for their own sake rather than external incentives. This intrinsic motivation can sustain engagement and buffer against the disillusionment and cynicism that characterize burnout. As McGonigal explains, "Intrinsic rewards, or the positive feelings associated with an activity, can serve as powerful motivators that help us muster the self-control and willpower to push through challenges" [31]. Flow allows individuals to reconnect with the inherent satisfactions of their work, renewing a sense of purpose and engagement.

4. *Flow facilitates social connection and support.*
    While flow is often studied as an individual phenomenon, it can also arise in social contexts, such as in collaborative work or play. Shared flow experiences can foster a sense of connection, trust, and mutual support among colleagues - protective factors against the isolation and alienation of burnout. As Walker notes, "Interpersonal flow, by promoting social bonds, could help to satisfy the basic need for relatedness. Feeling a sense of belonging has been linked to the reduction of burnout" [32].

5. *Flow promotes skill development and personal growth.*
    Regular flow experiences can lead to the progressive development of skills and personal growth over time. As individuals stretch to meet new challenges and expand their capacities, they build a sense of themselves as competent, adaptable, and resilient. This growth mindset is antithetical to the stagnation and depletion of burnout. In the words of Nakamura and Csikszentmihalyi, "Flow forces people to stretch themselves, to always take on another challenge, to improve on their abilities. To stay in flow, one must progress and learn" [33].

While these proposed mechanisms are compelling, it is important to note that the research on flow and burnout is still in its early stages. Most studies to date have been correlational, making it difficult to establish flow as a causal protective factor. It is possible that individuals who are less prone to burnout in the first place are more likely to experience flow. Longitudinal and intervention studies are needed to clarify the directionality of the flow-burnout relationship. Furthermore, flow is not a panacea for burnout. While it may provide temporary relief and gradual resilience, it is not a substitute for addressing the systemic causes of workplace stress, such as excessive workload, lack of autonomy, or inadequate support. As Maslach and Leiter caution, "The causes of burnout are fundamentally situated within the structures and functioning of the workplace... Individual solutions may help alleviate exhaustion, but they do not really address the root causes of the problem" [34]. Nevertheless, the available evidence suggests that cultivating flow can be a valuable part of a comprehensive approach to burnout prevention and mitigation. By providing a source of intrinsic motivation, meaning, mastery, and connection, flow experiences may help individuals build the psychological resources to withstand and bounce back from stress. As Seligman and Csikszentmihalyi argue, "Creating conditions that make flow experiences possible is a way to enhance individual well-being at the same time as it improves organizational performance" [30].

For individuals and organizations seeking to harness the power of flow, several strategies have been proposed. These include:

- Identifying and prioritizing flow-producing activities
- Setting clear goals and providing immediate feedback
- Optimizing challenge-skill balance through progressive difficulty
- Minimizing distractions and interruptions
- Providing autonomy and flexibility in work
- Fostering a sense of community and shared purpose
- Encouraging risk-taking, experimentation, and learning from failure
- Celebrating progress and accomplishments

By intentionally designing work and leisure to facilitate flow, individuals and organizations can tap into a powerful source of motivation, engagement and resilience. In the words of Csikszentmihalyi, "To counteract the entropy that inevitably follows prolonged engagement in a complex task, it is therefore crucial to create opportunities for regeneration, such as providing time off or encouraging regular participation in intrinsically rewarding activities" [35].

While more research is needed, the available evidence suggests that flow can serve as a protective factor against burnout by providing a respite from stress, enhancing mastery and control, providing intrinsic motivation and meaning, facilitating social connection, and promoting personal growth. By creating conditions conducive to flow, individuals and organizations can foster engagement, resilience, and well-being in the face of the challenges of modern work life. In the words of Csikszentmihalyi, "The best moments usually occur when a person's body or mind is stretched to its limits in a voluntary effort to accomplish something difficult and worthwhile. Optimal experience is thus something we can make happen" [8].

Concluding Remarks

The concept of flow offers a compelling framework for understanding and enhancing human flourishing in general and clinical excellence in particular. By cultivating the conditions for flow - clear goals, immediate feedback, balanced challenges, and minimal distractions - healthcare providers can access states of optimal performance, emotional regulation, and rapport-building.

The improvisational nature of flow, balancing structure and spontaneity, planning and responsiveness, control and creativity, allows clinicians to bring their whole selves to each unique patient encounter. Like a jazz musician riffing on a theme, the clinician in flow is able to draw on deep knowledge and skills while remaining open and attuned to the needs of the moment.

Regular immersion in flow enhances performance and may protect against burnout by providing a sense of mastery, meaning, and respite from self-conscious rumination. The grit and determination needed to persist through the challenges of medical practice is slowly transformed into a more easeful and absorbing engagement.

Flow, willpower, and grit are distinct but complementary capacities that enable the modern healer to navigate the challenges of clinical practice with optimal performance, resilience, and fulfillment. By using them strategically and synergistically, the clinician can bring their best self to each patient encounter while sustaining vitality over the long haul.

Ultimately, flow is about more than just performing well - it is about connecting with what is best and most vital within ourselves and bringing that forth in service of something larger. In the words of Csikszentmihalyi: "When we choose a goal and invest ourselves in it to the limits of our concentration, whatever we do will be enjoyable. And once we have tasted this joy, we will redouble our efforts to taste it again. This is the way the self grows." [8]

For healthcare providers, this growth of the self in service of relieving suffering and promoting health is the deepest form of professional fulfillment and personal flourishing available. By learning to find flow in their work, clinicians can discover a renewable source of passion, purpose, and well-being for themselves and for those they serve.

Self-Reflection Questions

1. How can you identify opportunities for flow in your clinical work? What are the key indicators that you are entering a flow state?

2. Reflect on a time when you experienced flow in a challenging clinical situation. What factors enabled you to access that state? How did it impact your performance and well-being?

3. Consider the balance between challenge and skill in your clinical practice. Are there areas where you need to develop your skills to meet the demands of the work? Are there challenges you could take on to stretch yourself and maintain engagement?

4. How can you structure your work environment and schedule to minimize distractions and interruptions that disrupt flow? What boundaries or rituals could you put in place to protect focused time?

5. Reflect on your sense of purpose and meaning in your work as a healer. What drew you to this profession? What sustains your commitment in the face of challenges? How can you stay connected to that intrinsic motivation?

6. Consider the interplay of flow, willpower, and grit in your own experience. When do you rely on each capacity? How can you develop and balance all three to optimize your resilience and performance?

7. How can you cultivate a "beginner's mind" and a sense of curiosity and wonder in your clinical practice? What practices or perspectives help you approach each patient and situation with fresh eyes and an open heart?

References

1. Csikszentmihalyi, M. (1990). Flow: The psychology of optimal experience. New York: Harper & Row.

2. Nakamura, J., & Csikszentmihalyi, M. (2009). Flow theory and research. In C. R. Snyder & S. J. Lopez (Eds.), Oxford Handbook of Positive Psychology (pp. 195-206). Oxford: Oxford University Press.

3. Vipassana Research Institute. (n.d.). What is vipassana? Retrieved from https://www.vridhamma.org/What-is-Vipassana

4. Csikszentmihalyi, M. (2004). Flow, the secret to happiness [TED Talk]. Retrieved from https://www.ted.com/talks/mihaly_csikszentmihalyi_flow_the_secret_to_happiness

5. Yaden, D. B., Haidt, J., Hood, R. W., Vago, D. R., & Newberg, A. B. (2017). The varieties of self-transcendent experience. Review of General Psychology, 21(2), 143-160. https://doi.org/10.1037/gpr0000102

6. Aristotle, ., Ross, W. D., & Brown, L. (2009). The Nicomachean ethics. Oxford: Oxford University Press.

7. Seligman, M. E. P. (2011). Flourish: A visionary new understanding of happiness and well-being. New York, NY: Free Press.

8. Csikszentmihalyi, M. (1998). Finding flow: The psychology of engagement with everyday life. New York: Harper Perennial.

9. Kotler, S. (2014). The rise of superman: Decoding the science of ultimate human performance. Boston: New Harvest.

10. Dweck, C. S. (2016). Mindset: The new psychology of success. New York: Random House.

11. Hallowell, E. (2014, August 8). Flow: A key to unlocking your greatest performances. Retrieved from https://drhallowell.com/flow-key-unlocking-greatest-performances/

12. Kernfeld, B. (1995). What to listen for in jazz. New Haven: Yale University Press.

13. Nachmanovitch, S. (1990). Free play: Improvisation in life and art. New York: J.P. Tarcher.

14. Ulrich, M., Keller, J., Hoenig, K., Waller, C., & Grön, G. (2014). Neural correlates of experimentally induced flow experiences. NeuroImage, 86, 194-202. doi:10.1016/j.neuroimage.2013.08.019

15. Csikszentmihalyi, M. (1996). Creativity: Flow and the psychology of discovery and invention. New York: Harper Collins.

16. Frankl, V. E. (2006). Man's search for meaning. Boston: Beacon Press.

17. Buber, M., & Smith, R. G. (2000). I and Thou. New York: Scribner18. Strauss, M. B. (1968). Familiar medical quotations. Boston: Little, Brown.

19. Baumeister, R. F., Vohs, K. D., & Tice, D. M. (2007). The strength model of self-control. Current Directions in Psychological Science, 16(6), 351-355. doi:10.1111/j.1467-8721.2007.00534.x

20. Baumeister, R. F. (2002). Ego depletion and self-control failure: An energy model of the self's executive function. Self and Identity, 1(2), 129-136. doi:10.1080/152988602317319302

21. Baumeister, R. F., & Tierney, J. (2012). Willpower: Rediscovering the greatest human strength. New York: Penguin Books.

22. Duckworth, A. L., Peterson, C., Matthews, M. D., & Kelly, D. R. (2007). Grit: Perseverance and passion for long-term goals. Journal of Personality and Social Psychology, 92(6), 1087-1101. doi:10.1037/0022-3514.92.6.1087

23. Duckworth, A. (2016). Grit: The power of passion and perseverance. New York: Scribner.

24. Lopez, S. J., & Ackerman, C. E. (2009). Clifton Strengths Finder 2.0. New York: Gallup Press.

25. Maslach, C., Jackson, S. E., & Leiter, M. P. (1996). Maslach Burnout Inventory Manual (3rd ed.). Palo Alto, CA: Consulting Psychologists Press.

26. Figley, C. R. (Ed.). (1995). Compassion fatigue: Coping with secondary traumatic stress disorder in those who treat the traumatized. New York: Brunner/Mazel.

27. Zito, M., Cortese, C. G., & Colombo, L. (2019). The role of resources and flow at work in well-being. SAGE Open, 9(2), 2158244019849732.

28. Salanova, M., Bakker, A. B., & Llorens, S. (2006). Flow at work: Evidence for an upward spiral of personal and organizational resources. Journal of Happiness Studies, 7(1), 1-22.

29. Csikszentmihalyi, M. (1997). Finding flow: The psychology of engagement with everyday life. New York: Basic Books.

30. Seligman, M. E. P., & Csikszentmihalyi, M. (2000). Positive psychology: An introduction. American Psychologist, 55(1), 5-14.

31. McGonigal, K. (2012). The willpower instinct: How self-control works, why it matters, and what you can do to get more of it. New York: Avery.

32. Walker, C. J. (2021). Battling burnout: Exploring the potential of interpersonal flow. Journal of Psychology in Africa, 31(4), 368-373.

33. Nakamura, J., & Csikszentmihalyi, M. (2002). The concept of flow. In C. R. Snyder & S. J. Lopez (Eds.), Handbook of positive psychology (pp. 89-105). Oxford: Oxford University Press.

34. Maslach, C., & Leiter, M. P. (1997). The truth about burnout: How organizations cause personal stress and what to do about it. San Francisco: Jossey-Bass.

35. Csikszentmihalyi, M. (2003). Good business: Leadership, flow, and the making of meaning. New York: Penguin.

SECTION ONE
The Heart-Based Actions of the Healer

CHAPTER 1

Generous

"That's what I consider true generosity: You give your all,
and yet you always feel as if it costs you nothing."
Simone de Beauvoir

"Generosity" and "charity" both refer to the quality of giving, but they have slightly different etymological roots and connotations. "Generosity" comes from the Latin "generosus," meaning "of noble birth," reflecting a magnanimous, freely giving spirit.[1] "Charity," on the other hand, derives from the Latin "caritas," which means "Christian love of fellow humans" and often implies giving to those in need.[2] In Buddhism, the Sanskrit term for generosity is "dana," which means giving or donation.[3, p.1] Generosity, therefore, describes the intention of the act rather than the act itself.

As we explore what cultivating generosity means as healers and human beings, it's worth remembering the Zen saying, "There are a hundred ways to kneel and kiss the ground."[4] This saying points to the countless ways in which life presents us with opportunities to give and receive and to appreciate the abundance that surrounds and sustains us. As healers, we have a truly precious and remarkable opportunity to practice generosity in every aspect of our work.

When we describe someone as generous or acting with generosity, we are experiencing a giving person. Synonyms of generous include liberality, magnanimity, abundance, amplitude, largesse, unselfishness, kindness, benevolence, and even hospitality. And yet, these definitions and synonyms can be confusing because they miss the fundamental truth of generosity—an openness that begins with letting go.

Generosity in the Interdependent Universe

Generosity is not just a human virtue but a vital characteristic of our interdependent universe. As physicist Fritjof Capra puts it, "The more we study the major problems of our time, the more we come to realize that they cannot be understood in isolation. They are systemic problems, which means that they are interconnected and interdependent."[5] In other words, generosity - the willingness to give and share - is woven into the very fabric of life.

Biologist Merlin Sheldrake echoes this sentiment, noting that "Organisms are not just collections of traits but also nexuses of relationships."[6] He points out that the mycelial networks of fungi, which permeate nearly all terrestrial ecosystems, serve as a kind of "wood wide web," facilitating the exchange of nutrients and information between plants. This underground economy of generosity enables the entire forest to thrive.

Authentic Generosity

Even more important than the generous act is the intention with which it is given. It is not genuine generosity if we give out of ego-clinging, self-aggrandizement, or the desire for recognition. In other words, making a gift to receive praise or recognition (e.g., a wealthy person giving money that they can afford in order to have their name on a building) is less valuable than a small, heartfelt gift that is made anonymously and without any expectation of recognition.

Shantideva, the great 8th-century Buddhist master, writes in his Guide to the Bodhisattva's Way of Life:

"Whatever generosity, discipline and other virtues
Are practiced by a bodhisattva who has the notion of self
Is like water in a leaky vase -
All the water runs out, leaving none inside."[3]

In other words, if our giving is tainted by self-cherishing and the illusion of separation, it doesn't liberate us or others. Tibetan teacher David Choepal clarifies, "When you're practicing generosity, the most important thing is the feeling you give with, not the object you're giving."[9]

But generosity, practiced with a pure heart, is the antidote to this sense of deficiency. When we give - truly give, without self-interest - we rupture the illusion of lack and open ourselves to the direct experience of life's boundless abundance. Author Peter Diamandis asserts, "Abundance is not about providing everyone on this planet with a life of luxury - rather, it's about providing all with a life of possibility."[11]

The Transformative Power of Generosity

Generosity is not just a virtue but a form of spiritual alchemy, transmuting our leaden ego-clinging into the gold of unconstrained sharing. Jampa Yonten, a monk and healer who works with the dying, reflects, "When I am giving, I try not to give from a place of sacrifice and heaviness, but from fullness and joy."[8] Mother Teresa would tell her nurses in Calcutta, "Find joy here, or go home." Their generosity, she knew, had to spring from a genuine fountain of compassion and care, not guilt or obligation.

There is no better exemplar of the transformative power of generosity than Chiron, the wounded healer of Greek mythology. Chiron was a centaur renowned for his wisdom and knowledge of medicine. Out of compassion, he agreed to take on the agonizing wounds of Prometheus and relinquish his immortality. Chiron himself transcended suffering by giving up what was most precious to him.[12]

This points to the most profound meaning of generosity - that in giving with an open heart, we discover nothing was ever ours to give. We are simply letting go, surrendering into the current of life's unceasing offering. As the writer Stephen Levine puts it, "Generosity is a living proof of our connectedness, a small price for the privilege of belonging to each other."[13]

The Three Types of Generosity

Buddhist philosophy describes three kinds of generosity. It is helpful for the healer to understand what kind of generosity they are providing in any particular situation.

1. *Outer generosity (Āmiṣa-Dāna)*: This involves giving material goods or services. This is perhaps the most common understanding of generosity - offering food, shelter, clothing, money, or our time and effort to help others in a tangible way. When we volunteer at a soup kitchen, donate to a charity, or hold the door open for a stranger, we practice outer generosity. In the medical context, this could involve providing free or discounted care to those who cannot afford it or going the extra mile to ensure a patient's comfort and well-being.

2. *Inner generosity (Dharma-Dāna)*: This is offering love, compassion, and spiritual counsel. This is a deeper form of giving that comes from the heart. When we listen with empathy to a friend in need, offer encouragement to someone struggling, or radiate kindness and goodwill, we engage in inner generosity. For healers, this might mean taking extra time to reassure an anxious patient, holding space for their emotional pain, or offering guidance to help them find meaning and purpose in the midst of illness. Sharing the teachings of the Buddha is considered the highest form of generosity. The dissemination of wisdom and spiritual guidance helps others on their path to enlightenment. As stated in the *Saddharmapuṇḍarīka Sūtra* (Lotus Sutra): "The gift of Dharma excels all gifts."

3. *Secret generosity (Abhaya-Dāna)*: This is sharing teachings that liberate beings from suffering. This is perhaps the most profound level of generosity, as it aims to address the root cause of suffering rather than just alleviating its symptoms. We practice secret generosity when we share wisdom, insights, or practices that have helped us find peace and freedom. In a medical setting, this could involve introducing patients to mindfulness meditation, discussing spiritual perspectives on healing, or simply embodying presence and compassion in a way that points to transcendence. Providing protection and comfort to those in fear is another vital aspect of Abhaya-Dāna. This can involve offering refuge, safety, or emotional support. By giving fearlessness, one helps to alleviate the anxieties and insecurities of others.

In the context of medicine, we can see all three levels of generosity at play. Healers offer their time, expertise, and physical care - often at great personal sacrifice, losing sleep and precious time with loved ones. At the inner level, they give emotional support, kindness, and encouragement to those suffering. In a more subtle but profound way, healers can provide what Joan Halifax calls "the gift of presence" - being fully there with a patient in a way that opens the door to spiritual solace and transcendence.[8]

Challenges to Generosity in the Modern World

Paradoxically, in our modern world of unprecedented material abundance, our culture is deeply rooted in a mindset of scarcity and lack. Despite all the wealth and productivity unleashed by science and capitalism, we fear there is not enough to go around. Psychologist Laurence Boldt observes, "The scarcity assumption has become such an integral part of our social consensus reality that any other way of looking at things seems hopelessly naive."[10, p.4]

Modern professional healers inhabit a competitive world. Simply gaining entry to a health professional school demands competitiveness. At each level of their professional training, students are measured in terms of their grade scores and class ranking. In this "only the fittest will survive" culture, the modern healer must inevitably become self-centered and experience fellow students as potential threats to their professional success. Following graduation, the contemporary healer continues to experience a world that rotates on an axis of fear shaped by their performance on "objective" outcome metrics and a hostile medico-legal culture. Most relationships in healthcare are brief, and it is challenging for modern healers to establish long-term relationships with their patients.

Furthermore, most modern healers have little or no control over the financial aspects of their practice, and any challenges patients may be experiencing in paying their medical bills are referred to a third party. These factors result in modern healers living in a "survival mode" that makes it challenging to experience an empathic connection with their colleagues and patients. Experiencing and manifesting generosity in this empathic blindness becomes almost antithetical to manifesting generosity.

The Benefits of Giving

Research suggests that generosity can have many benefits, including:

- Improved relationships: Generosity can help strengthen relationships with family, friends, and colleagues, both professionally and personally.
- Mental health: Generosity can reduce stress and depression and help build empathy and gratitude. It can also give you a more balanced perspective on yourself and others.
- Happiness: Neuroscience studies show that generosity can lead to lasting benefits for your happiness. You can feel better about yourself and life, not just when you give but also in the long term.
- Longer life: Some research suggests that generous people may live longer than those who don't give. Stress is a known risk factor for many chronic diseases, and generosity can help lower stress levels.

As Karl Menninger put it: "Love cures – both the ones who give it and the ones who receive it."

The Practice of Dāna

Practicing Dāna requires mindfulness and intention. It is not merely the act of giving but the cultivation of a generous spirit free from attachment and expectation. The Buddha emphasized the importance of the mental attitude behind giving. In the *Aṅguttara Nikāya*, he describes three types of givers:

1. "The inferior giver": who gives with reluctance and regrets the giving.
2. "The middling giver": who gives without reluctance but with the expectation of a reward.
3. "The superior giver": who gives spontaneously with joy and without expectation.

The superior giver exemplifies the ideal practice of Dāna, in which the act of giving expresses boundless compassion and wisdom.

The Significance of Dāna in the Six Pāramitās (Six Perfections)
As the first of the Six Pāramitās, Dāna is the entry point into the Bodhisattva's path. It prepares the practitioner for the subsequent perfections by fostering a mindset of selflessness and interconnectedness. The progression from Dāna to the other Pāramitās is natural and interdependent:

- Śīla (Morality): A generous heart leads to ethical behavior, as one naturally avoids actions that harm others.
- Kṣānti (Patience): The practice of generosity cultivates patience, as it often requires enduring personal discomfort for the benefit of others.
- Vīrya (Energy): The joy derived from giving energizes the practitioner and provides motivation to continue on the path.
- Dhyāna (Meditation): A mind free from attachment, cultivated through Dāna, finds it easier to settle into deep meditation.
- Prajñā (Wisdom): Ultimately, the practice of generosity leads to the realization of non-self and the interdependent nature of all beings, which is the essence of wisdom.

According to the *Prajñāpāramitā Sūtras*, a key Mahāyāna text:

- "The perfection of giving is accomplished when one recognizes the equality of self and others and does not cling to the idea of a gift, a giver, or a recipient."

This teaching underscores the Mahāyāna perspective that true generosity transcends the conventional notions of giver and recipient, leading to the realization of emptiness (Śūnyatā) and non-attachment.

Developing Generosity: The Mind of Letting Go
Eastern thinking offers some wisdom to clarify and deepen our notion of generosity. Dāna is a Sanskrit and Pali word that translates to "generosity." It connotes the virtue of offering or giving in Indian religions and philosophies. Giving and receiving require open hands—thus letting go.[14]

In Buddhist teachings, generosity cultivates giving freely without expecting anything in return, purely out of compassion, goodwill, or the desire to aid someone. It comes from open hands (material), an open heart (compassion), and an open mind (wisdom).[14]

The Bhavana Learning Group efficiently defines generosity as "an openness to giving and receiving freely." Developing generosity involves three key elements:[14]

1. *Letting Go and Openness:* Generosity begins with openness, a function of letting go. Letting go involves releasing control and clinging, an ongoing practice as we cling to attachments and judgments and continually identify with objects and concepts. When we practice letting go, we create a space for openness that offers the presence of mind and open hearts.
2. *Giving and Receiving:* Giving and receiving are part of an interdependent, free-flowing energy. The core of generosity is openness, which keeps the energy flowing freely without obstruction. Closed fists push others away and fix us in place, while open hands are receptive and invite flow. When we let go and are open to receiving life, we become a source of giving.
3. *Freely:* Perhaps the most challenging element of generosity involves this final point: "freely." Remember that the core of generosity is the openness that keeps energy flowing freely without any obstruction. Obstructions often involve a desire for virtue or decency out of an obligation to demonstrate generosity or to appear generous. "Freely" lacks any such desires, cravings, or expectations.

Generosity in Practice
Practicing generosity is done in our moment-to-moment existence. Given our exploration, this involves letting go for openness, developing appreciation, gratitude, and satisfaction for giving and receiving, and freely being with what arises.[14]

Applying generosity in life offers a different view of ourselves and reality. For instance, simply listening to someone else's problems is an act of generosity. A generous listener can do the following:[14]

- Let go of agendas, judgments, and expectations.
- Give time and complete attention to the person(s) they are with and fully receive their concerns and trust.
- Freely, without any attachments or hidden motivations, be with whatever arises.

Like listening, when we practice all three legs of generosity in any part of our lives, we develop the mind of letting go. We can access an inviting, expansive, and spacious free-flowing energy.[14]

Practicing cultivates an open-minded space—an openness to giving and receiving freely. It is perhaps why Dāna is both a principle and practice of Buddhism.[14]

When practiced, we become generous.[14]

A Definition of the Generous Healer

The generous healer is a healthcare professional who gives freely with an open heart and mind, offering their skills, compassion, and wisdom to alleviate suffering and inspire wholeness in others while cultivating their own path of awakening through the practice of generosity.

Concluding Remarks

In conclusion, the concept of Dāna, or generosity, in the Buddhist Six Pāramitās is a profound practice that transcends mere acts of giving. It is a fundamental virtue that nurtures selflessness, compassion, and wisdom. Through Dāna, practitioners lay the groundwork for developing the other eleven characteristics of a healer's actions, leading to the ultimate goal of enlightenment.

Moreover, as explored in the article "Generosity—The Mind of Letting Go," the true essence of generosity lies in the openness that begins with letting go. Cultivating generosity involves letting go of attachments and judgments, developing an appreciation for the abundance of life, and freely giving and receiving without expectation or obligation.

As healers and human beings, we have countless opportunities to practice generosity daily. Whether through outer acts of service, inner offerings of compassion, or secret sharing of liberating wisdom, generosity can transform both the giver and the receiver. By embracing the practice of Dāna and cultivating the mind of letting go, we progress steadily on the path to awakening, contributing to the well-being of all beings along the way.

As the Buddha taught, "Generosity brings happiness at every stage of its expression." May we all find the courage and openness to give and receive freely, discovering the boundless joy and connection that generosity unveils.

Self Reflections Questions
1. What are some recent examples of how I practiced outer, inner, and secret generosity in my work as a healer?
2. How often do I give with the pure intention of benefiting others without expecting anything in return? Are there times when my giving is motivated by ego, guilt, or obligation?
3. In what ways does my professional environment and training make it challenging for me to experience empathy and generosity? How can I work with these challenges skillfully?
4. How can I cultivate a genuine spirit of abundance and generosity amidst a culture of scarcity and competition? What practices or perspectives might support this?
5. What is one small act of generosity - outer, inner, or secret - that I can offer today to uplift myself and others?

References

1. "Generous." Online Etymology Dictionary. www.etymonline.com/word/generous. Accessed 8 June 2024.
2. "Charity." Online Etymology Dictionary. www.etymonline.com/word/charity. Accessed 8 June 2024.
3. Zopa, Lama. The Practice of Generosity. Lama Yeshe Wisdom Archive, 2003, pp. 1, 53.
4. Hanh, Thich Nhat. Peace Is Every Step: The Path of Mindfulness in Everyday Life. Bantam, 1992, p.178.
5. Capra, Fritjof. The Web of Life: A New Scientific Understanding of Living Systems. Anchor, 1996, p.3.
6. Sheldrake, Merlin. Entangled Life: How Fungi Make Our Worlds, Change Our Minds & Shape Our Futures. Random House, 2020, p.11.
7. Blake, William. "Auguries of Innocence." The Complete Poetry and Prose of William Blake, edited by David V. Erdman, Doubleday, 1988.
8. Halifax, Joan. "Dana Paramita: The Perfection of Generosity." Compassion as Remedy, edited by Nancy Kehoe and Elizabeth Olson, Paulist Press, 1997, pp. 30-42, 34, 66.
9. Choepal, David, and Anne Maiden. From Here to Enlightenment: Teachings on the Spiritual Path. Snow Lion Publications, 2002, p.22.
10. Boldt, Laurence G. The Tao of Abundance. Arkana, 1999, p.4.
11. Diamandis, Peter H., and Steven Kotler. Abundance: The Future Is Better Than You Think. Free Press, 2012, p.11.
12. Groesbeck, C. Jess. "The Archetypal Image of the Wounded Healer." Journal of Analytical Psychology, vol. 20, no. 2, 1975, pp. 122-145.
13. Levine, Stephen. A Year to Live: How to Live This Year As If It Were Your

Last. Bell Tower, 1997, p.18.
14. "Generosity—The Mind of Letting Go." Bhavana Learning Group, https://www.bhavanalearning.com/generosity-the-mind-of-letting-go/. Accessed 19 June 2024.

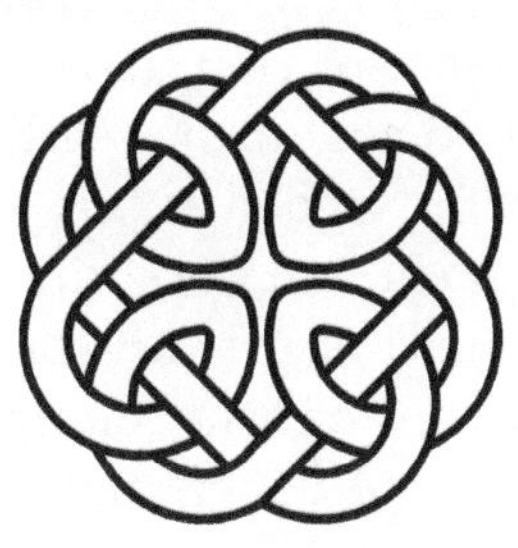

CHAPTER 2

Moral

"Integrity has no need of rules."
Albert Camus

*I*ntegrity, in its essence, is the unwavering adherence to moral and ethical principles, the commitment to honesty, and the consistency of character that inspires trust. In the context of the healing professions, integrity is the cornerstone upon which the patient-healer relationship is built. This foundation enables the healer to navigate the complex moral landscape of healthcare with compassion, wisdom, and a steadfast dedication to the well-being of those they serve.

The concept of integrity is deeply rooted in various healing traditions around the world, each offering unique insights into the nature of moral character and its role in the art of healing. In traditional Chinese medicine, integrity is closely tied to the Confucian concept of ren (仁), which encompasses qualities such as benevolence, humaneness, and compassion. As the Confucian philosopher Mencius states, "The great man is he who does not lose his child's heart" [1]. The healer of integrity, in this view, is one who maintains a sense of innocence, purity of intention, and unwavering commitment to the welfare of others.

In Tibetan Buddhist medicine, integrity is inseparable from the practice of compassion and the cultivation of wisdom. The healer's integrity is grounded in understanding the interconnectedness of all beings and recognizing the inherent dignity and worth of each individual. As the 14th Dalai Lama notes, "The essence of compassion is a desire to alleviate the suffering of others and to promote their well-being" [2, p.68]. The healer with integrity, in this tradition, embodies this compassion in every action, sees the humanity in each patient, and works tirelessly to ease their suffering.

In Ayurveda, the traditional Indian system of medicine, integrity is deeply intertwined with the concept of dharma, or righteous living. The healer's integrity is rooted in a profound understanding of the universe's natural order and the recognition of one's duty to uphold this order through ethical conduct. As the Charaka Samhita, one of the foundational texts of Ayurveda, states, "The physician who fails to enter into the body of a patient with the lamp of knowledge and understanding can never treat diseases. He should first study all the factors, including environment, which influence a patient's disease, and then prescribe treatment" [3]. The healer of integrity, in this view, approaches each patient with humility, attentiveness, and a deep commitment to understanding the unique factors that contribute to their suffering.

Across these diverse traditions, integrity is recognized as a manifestation of the healer's wisdom - the hard-earned fruit of self-reflection, moral cultivation, and a lifelong dedication to the service of others. As Rachel Remen notes, "Wisdom is a way of being - a way of being whole and fully open to each moment. It is a way of relating to life with compassion, humor, reverence, and humility. Wisdom is not knowing more but knowing with more of oneself, knowing deeper" [4]. The healer with integrity has learned to listen deeply, both to the needs of their patients and to the quiet voice of their conscience, and to act with compassion, courage, and a steadfast commitment to doing what is right.

Integrity versus Ethics versus Morality
While integrity, ethics, and morality are often used interchangeably, they represent distinct, albeit interconnected, concepts in moral philosophy and the healing professions. Understanding the nuances that distinguish these terms is essential for developing a more refined moral vocabulary and navigating modern healthcare's complex ethical landscape.

Ethics, in its broadest sense, refers to the philosophical study of morality, the systematic examination of moral principles, values, and norms that guide human behavior. As Tom Beauchamp and James Childress note in their seminal work, Principles of Biomedical Ethics, "Ethics is a generic term covering several different ways of examining and understanding the moral life" [5]. Ethics provides the conceptual framework and analytical tools for examining moral questions, evaluating the merits of different moral positions, and guiding moral decision-making.

Morality, on the other hand, refers to the actual norms, values, and beliefs that shape the moral life of individuals and communities. It is the lived experience of ethics, the embodiment of moral principles in everyday thoughts, words, and deeds. As Bernard Williams observes, "Morality is not a peculiar institution, but something that grows out of the practices of human life" [6]. Morality is deeply embedded in social and cultural contexts, reflecting the shared understandings and expectations of what constitutes right and wrong, good and bad, in a given community.

In contrast to ethics and morality, integrity refers to the consistency and coherence of an individual's moral character, the degree to which one's beliefs, values, and actions align. As Stephen Carter defines it, "Integrity, as I will use the term, requires three steps: discerning what is right and what is wrong; acting on what you have discerned, even at personal cost; and saying openly that you are acting on your understanding of right and wrong" [7]. Integrity is the bridge between ethical reflection and moral action, the quality of character that enables one to translate moral principles into lived realities.

In the context of the healing professions, these distinctions take on added significance. Ethics provides the intellectual foundation for examining healthcare's moral dimensions and analyzing the principles and values that should guide medical decision-making. Morality reflects the norms and expectations that shape the day-to-day practices of healthcare providers and the moral climate in which patient care unfolds. Integrity represents the moral compass of the individual healer, the inner sense of right and wrong that guides their actions and informs their relationships with patients, colleagues, and the broader community. Stated differently, ethics is an objectification, morality is an inter-subjective, and morality is a subjective perspective of "doing the right thing." One can quickly recognize how an integral framework can be helpful when he is attempting to determine what is the right action in any particular situation.

The Inadequacy of Modern Bioethics

While modern bioethics has made significant contributions to the moral discourse surrounding healthcare, providing valuable frameworks for analyzing ethical dilemmas and guiding medical decision-making, it has its limitations. As the pace of scientific and technological advancement continues to accelerate, the moral questions raised by modern medicine are becoming increasingly complex, often outstripping the capacity of traditional bioethical approaches to provide satisfactory answers.

One of the primary criticisms against modern bioethics is that it has become overly focused on the procedural aspects of ethical decision-making, on applying abstract principles and rules to specific cases, at the expense of a more holistic and contextual understanding of the moral dimensions of healthcare. As Arthur Kleinman argues, "Bioethics has become a method for the cognitive sanitation of anxiety-provoking clinical dilemmas, a way of containing moral messiness and providing a path, often in the form of a decision tree, to the 'right answer'" [8]. In this view, bioethics risks becoming a kind of moral algorithm, a mechanical process for resolving ethical quandaries that fails to capture the full complexity and nuance of real-world situations.

This procedural focus of modern bioethics is not wrong per se, but it is often inadequate, particularly when it comes to addressing the deeper existential and spiritual dimensions of illness, suffering, and healing. Christina Puchalski notes, "The spiritual dimension of healthcare is often overlooked in contemporary bioethics discourse, which tends to focus on issues of autonomy, beneficence, and justice. While these principles are certainly important, they do not fully capture the lived experience of illness and the search for meaning that often accompanies it" [9]. The healer of integrity, in this view, must be attuned not only to the biomedical aspects of patient care but also to the broader psychosocial, cultural, and spiritual factors that shape the illness experience.

Moreover, modern bioethics often fails to provide a robust foundation for cultivating phronesis, or practical wisdom, the kind of situated moral knowledge that enables healers to navigate the complex and often ambiguous terrain of clinical practice. As Hubert Dreyfus and Stuart Dreyfus argue, "Ethical expertise is not captured by any set of explicit rules, but consists in the ability to respond intuitively to the salient features of complex situations based on experience and training" [10]. Phronesis is not simply the application of general principles to specific cases but rather the capacity to discern the morally relevant features of a given situation and to respond with sensitivity, flexibility, and skill.

Cultivating phronesis requires more than just a mastery of bioethical principles and decision-making frameworks. It demands a certain kind of moral education, a process of character formation that enables healers to develop the virtues, habits of mind, and heart essential for navigating clinical practice challenges with integrity and compassion. As Edmund Pellegrino and David Thomasma argue, "The moral education of the physician is a lifelong process that must be integrated into all aspects of medical training and practice. It requires not only the acquisition of knowledge and skills but also the cultivation of moral wisdom, the capacity to discern the right course of action in complex and often uncertain circumstances" [11].

Integrity in Modern Healthcare

The integrity of the modern healer is often challenged by the complex realities of contemporary healthcare, a landscape shaped by rapid technological change, shifting societal expectations, and competing economic, political, and professional interests. In this context, maintaining a steadfast commitment to moral principles and navigating ethical dilemmas with wisdom and compassion can be daunting.

One of the primary challenges to the integrity of the healer in modern healthcare is the increasing bureaucratization and commercialization of medicine. As Arnold Relman warns, "The traditional ethos of medical professionalism, based on the primacy of patient welfare, scientific integrity, and self-regulation, is being gradually replaced by a business ethos that emphasizes profit maximization, competition, and customer satisfaction" [12]. In this market-driven environment, healers may face pressures to compromise their moral commitments in the name of efficiency, cost-effectiveness, or institutional loyalty.

Moreover, the sheer complexity of modern medical practice, with its ever-expanding array of diagnostic and therapeutic technologies, can make it difficult for healers to discern the right course of action in any given situation. As Eric Cassell observes, "The technological imperative in medicine - the felt need to do everything that can be done for a patient - creates a bias towards action, even when restraint might be the wiser choice" [13]. In this context, the integrity of the healer is often tested, requiring the moral courage to resist the pressure to intervene and the wisdom to know when enough is enough.

Despite these challenges, the integrity of the healer remains the cornerstone of ethical medical practice, the essential quality that enables healthcare providers to navigate complex decisions with moral clarity and compassion. As William Branch argues, "Integrity is the foundation of trustworthiness that makes possible the relationships clinicians need to do their work. It enables physicians to put patients' interests ahead of their own, to deal honestly with uncertainty and error, to keep confidences, and to practice medicine for the benefit of others rather than merely for personal gain" [14]. The healer with integrity remains true to their moral commitments, even in the face of competing pressures and demands, and approaches each patient with an unwavering dedication to their well-being.

The Foundations of Integrity in Healing

While the challenges to integrity in modern healthcare are significant, they are not insurmountable. Cultivating certain key attributes, rooted in the wisdom of ancient healing traditions and the insights of contemporary moral philosophy, can help support the healer's integrity and strengthen their capacity to navigate ethical dilemmas with skill and compassion.

One of the most essential attributes of the healer is equanimity, the capacity to maintain a balanced and composed state of mind in the face of the inevitable stresses and uncertainties of clinical practice. As described in Buddhist philosophy, equanimity is not a state of detachment or indifference but rather a quality of engaged and openhearted presence, a way of relating to the world with stability, clarity, and care. As the Dalai Lama explains, "Equanimity does not mean a neutral feeling toward others—that all are the same—it refers to the quality of composure that comes from recognizing that all beings experience happiness and suffering just as we do" [15]. The healer who cultivates equanimity is better able to respond to the challenges of medical practice with resilience, adaptability, and a clear sense of moral purpose.

Another critical attribute of the healer is compassion, the capacity to relate to the suffering of others with empathy, kindness, and a genuine desire to help. Compassion is not simply a feeling but an active commitment to alleviating suffering wherever it is found. Joan Halifax notes, "Compassion is the acknowledgment that not all pain can be 'fixed' or 'solved,' but all suffering is made more endurable through connection" [16, p.43]. The healer who embodies compassion can create a space of trust, understanding, and shared humanity, even in the most difficult and painful circumstances.

Closely related to compassion is the attribute of loving-kindness, or metta in Buddhist thought, a quality of unconditional goodwill and care extended to all beings. Loving-kindness is not a sentimental or superficial feeling but rather a deep and abiding commitment to the well-being of others, rooted in recognition of our shared vulnerability and interdependence. As Sharon Salzberg explains, "Loving-kindness is the ability to embrace all parts of ourselves, as well as all parts of the world. Practicing metta illuminates our inner integrity because it relieves us of the need to deny different aspects of ourselves" [17, p.29]. The healer who radiates loving-kindness is able to create a healing presence that touches the deepest levels of the human experience.

Finally, the attribute of joy, often overlooked in discussions of medical ethics, is essential for sustaining the integrity of the healer. In this context, joy does not refer to superficial or fleeting happiness but rather to a deep sense of meaning, purpose, and connection that arises from a life devoted to service and care. As Rachel Remen writes, "The pursuit of full humanity, of compassion and self-compassion, of meaning, and of the joy that arises from living a life of integrity and service is a lifelong challenge and an ongoing adventure. It is a journey of the heart" [18]. The healer who cultivates joy can draw strength and inspiration from the privilege of participating in the most profound and intimate aspects of human life.

Taken together, these attributes of equanimity, compassion, loving-kindness, and joy form a powerful foundation for the integrity of the healer. This moral compass can guide them through the complex landscape of modern healthcare. By cultivating these qualities through ongoing self-reflection, moral education, and a commitment to ethical practice, healers can strengthen their capacity to discern the right course of action in challenging situations and to respond with wisdom, skill, and care.

It is essential to recognize, however, that the cultivation of these attributes is not a purely individual or inward-looking process. The integrity of the healer is also shaped by the broader social, cultural, and institutional contexts in which they work, contexts that can either support or undermine their moral commitments. In particular, the intersection of capitalism and scientific materialism in modern healthcare creates a potential "morals-free" zone. Economic interests and narrow biomedical models of illness and health can eclipse broader considerations of meaning, values, and social justice in this space.

As Arthur Frank argues, "The medical story is increasingly a story of economics and a story of science. These stories are presented as morally neutral, as though they have no implications for values. But in fact, they are moral stories that differ radically from the moral stories ill people need to tell" [19]. The healer of integrity must be able to navigate these competing moral narratives and find ways of preserving the essential human dimensions of illness and healing within a system that often reduces them to economic and biomedical abstractions.

This requires not only individual moral courage but also collective efforts to create institutional and cultural environments that support ethical practice and moral discernment. As Larry Churchill argues, "The moral life of health professionals...is more a function of the moral ecology of their work setting than of the character and moral commitment that they bring to that work. The institutional arrangements for how medical work will be valued, structured, and rewarded profoundly shape the habits and mores of medical practice" [20]. Cultivating integrity in modern healthcare is not just a matter of individual virtue but also a matter of collective responsibility to create the conditions that enable healers to practice with moral clarity, compassion, and care.

Enhancing Integrity in Modern Healthcare

Given the challenges to integrity in modern healthcare and the essential role that moral character plays in shaping the quality and outcomes of patient care, it is crucial that healers have access to resources and strategies for cultivating and sustaining their moral commitments. While there is no single path to integrity, several approaches can help healers navigate modern medicine's complexities with greater skill, wisdom, and resilience.

One key strategy is cultivating mindfulness, a quality of present-moment awareness that enables healers to attend to their own experiences and their patients' experiences with greater clarity, compassion, and discernment. As Jon Kabat-Zinn defines it, "Mindfulness means paying attention in a particular way: on purpose, in the present moment, and non-judgmentally" [21]. Through practices like meditation, reflective writing, and contemplative dialogue, healers can develop the capacity to observe their own thoughts, feelings, and reactions with greater equanimity and respond to the needs of their patients with greater sensitivity and care.

Another important strategy is engagement with the arts and humanities, which can provide healers with new perspectives on their work's meaning and purpose and help them cultivate the moral imagination necessary for navigating complex ethical terrain. As Rita Charon argues, "The humanities offer health care professionals the means to understand the experiences of illness, disability, and caregiving and the means to reflect on the meaning of their own experiences in the care of the sick. Literature, film, drama, and the fine arts offer health care professionals a portal for reflection and self-awareness" [22]. By engaging with creative works that explore the depths of human experience, healers can expand their capacity for empathy, deepen their understanding of suffering, and find new sources of inspiration and resilience.

A third key strategy is participation in the moral community, the ongoing dialogue and shared reflection that enables healers to clarify their values, learn from the experience of their colleagues, and find support and guidance in navigating difficult ethical challenges. As William Branch and colleagues argue, "Participation in a moral community is essential for the development and maintenance of professional integrity. Moral communities provide the social support and guidance that enable individuals to uphold their moral commitments and to engage in ongoing moral learning" [23]. Through activities like ethics rounds, case conferences, and reflective practice groups, healers can create spaces for honest and open dialogue about the moral dimensions of their work and can cultivate the skills of moral discernment and action.

Cultivating integrity in modern healthcare requires a commitment to lifelong learning and growth and a willingness to engage in ongoing self-reflection and moral education. As Edmund Pellegrino argues, "The moral education of the physician is a continual process that must be integrated with the learning of medical science and clinical skills. It is a lifelong undertaking that requires the cultivation of habits of reflectiveness, self-knowledge, and self-discipline" [24]. By approaching their work with humility, curiosity, and a deep commitment to moral excellence, healers can continue to grow in wisdom and compassion and can serve as exemplars of integrity in a challenging and rapidly changing field.

A Definition of the Moral Healer

A moral healer is a healthcare provider who consistently adheres to moral integrity, demonstrates compassion and wisdom, and is committed to patient well-being. Through ongoing self-reflection and moral growth, a moral healer navigates the complexities of modern healthcare.

Self-Reflection Questions

1. What does integrity mean to me as a healer, and how do I embody this quality in my daily work?
2. How do I balance the competing demands of efficiency, cost-effectiveness, and patient welfare in my practice?
3. What are the greatest challenges to my integrity as a healer, and how do I navigate these challenges with moral courage and wisdom?
4. How do I cultivate equanimity, compassion, loving-kindness, and joy in my work, and what practices support my ongoing moral and spiritual growth?
5. How do I engage with the arts and humanities to deepen my understanding of the human experience and to expand my moral imagination?
6. How do I participate in a moral community, and what relationships and conversations support my ongoing ethical reflection and learning?
7. What institutional and cultural factors shape the moral ecology of my work environment, and how can I contribute to creating a culture of integrity and care?
8. How do I navigate the tensions between modern healthcare's economic and biomedical dimensions and the broader human and moral dimensions of illness and healing?
9. What is my vision of the good, and how does this shape my understanding of my role and responsibilities as a healer?

References

1. Mencius. (1970). The works of Mencius (J. Legge, Trans.). Dover Publications.
2. Gyatso, T. (1999). Ethics for the new millennium. Riverhead Books.
3. Sharma, P. V. (2003). Charaka samhita. Chaukhambha Orientalia.
4. Remen, R. N. (1996). Kitchen table wisdom: Stories that heal. Riverhead

Books.
5. Beauchamp, T. L., & Childress, J. F. (2019). Principles of biomedical ethics (8th ed.). Oxford University Press.
6. Williams, B. (1985). Ethics and the limits of philosophy. Harvard University Press.
7. Carter, S. L. (1996). Integrity. HarperCollins.
8. Kleinman, A. (1995). Writing at the margin: Discourse between anthropology and medicine. University of California Press.
9. Puchalski, C. M. (2008). Honoring the sacred in medicine: Spirituality as an essential element of patient-centered care. International Journal of Psychiatry in Medicine, 38(1), 113-117.
10. Dreyfus, H. L., & Dreyfus, S. E. (1991). Towards a phenomenology of ethical expertise. Human Studies, 14(4), 229-250.
11. Pellegrino, E. D., & Thomasma, D. C. (1993). The virtues in medical practice. Oxford University Press.
12. Relman, A. S. (1992). What market values are doing to medicine. Atlantic Monthly, 269(3), 98-106.
13. Cassell, E. J. (1991). The nature of suffering and the goals of medicine. Oxford University Press.
14. Branch, W. T. (2000). The ethics of caring and medical education. Academic Medicine, 75(2), 127-132.
15. Dalai Lama. (1999). Ethics for the new millennium. Riverhead Books.
16. Halifax, J. (2011). The precious necessity of compassion. Journal of Pain and Symptom Management, 41(1), 146-153.
17. Salzberg, S. (1995). Lovingkindness: The revolutionary art of happiness. Shambhala.
18. Remen, R. N. (2000). My grandfather's blessings: Stories of strength, refuge, and belonging. Riverhead Books.
19. Frank, A. W. (1995). The wounded storyteller: Body, illness, and ethics. University of Chicago Press.
20. Churchill, L. R. (1989). Ethics and the moral ecology of the professions. Southern Medical Journal, 82(12), 1522-1527.
21. Kabat-Zinn, J. (1994). Wherever you go, there you are: Mindfulness meditation in everyday life. Hyperion.
22. Charon, R. (2001). Narrative medicine: Form, function, and ethics. Annals of Internal Medicine, 134(1), 83-87.
23. Branch, W. T., et al. (1998). Teaching the human dimensions of care in clinical settings. JAMA, 280(11), 1001-1005.
24. Pellegrino, E. D. (1991). Character, virtue and self-interest in the ethics of the professions. Journal of Contemporary Health Law & Policy, 5(1), 53-73.

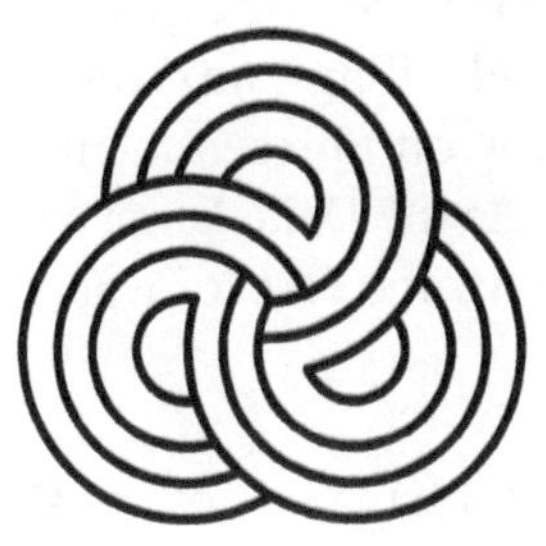

CHAPTER 3

Patient

"Be patient and tough; someday this pain will be useful to you."
Ovid

The English word "patience" derives from the Latin patientia, which comes from the verb patior, meaning "to suffer, endure, bear, experience." [1] This etymological root points to the close relationship between patience and the experience of being a patient. To be a patient is to suffer and endure pain, illness, or hardship. And to have patience is to bear with challenging circumstances without losing stability or reacting unskillfully.

In this way, patience is closely related to tolerance. As Dale Wright explains, "Tolerance is the capacity to continue in a valued practice or relationship even as one is exposed to that which is unwanted, discomfiting, or troublesome." [2] Just as a patient must tolerate physical and mental discomfort, we all must tolerate difficulties in our relationships, work, and communities. Patience allows us to bear with the imperfections of others and the frustrations of life without lashing out or shutting down.

However, it's essential to distinguish patience and tolerance from enabling co-dependent or harmful dynamics. As Wright notes, "Tolerance must be balanced by its complementary perfection, moral discipline (sila). Tolerance without moral discipline can turn into passivity, submissiveness, or indifference in the face of what should be opposed." [2] True patience springs from wisdom and discernment - it is not a boundless acceptance of anything and everything but a skillful engagement with life's ups and downs.

Patience is also interwoven with the quality of forgiveness. When we are patient with others' faults and failings, we create the conditions for forgiveness to arise. Rather than holding on to resentment or bitterness, patience allows us to let go and start anew. As the Dalai Lama writes, "Patience is the antidote to anger, a way to learn to love and care for whatever we meet on the path." [3]

Patience in Buddhism

In Buddhism, patience (kshanti) is one of the six paramitas or "perfections" practiced by bodhisattvas on the path to awakening. The Sanskrit word kshanti comes from the verb root kṣam, meaning "to be patient, endure, put up with." [4] In Tibetan, the word for patience is "sopa" (སྐྱོབ་པ་). As Lama Zopa explains, "Sopa means 'forebearance or bearing any problems' and pa means 'doing so'. Therefore, "sopa" describes 'willing to bear any problems.'" [5]

Lama Zopa points to the quality of being willing and able to face life's challenges with an open and courageous heart. It is the strength to remain present and engaged despite pain, provocation, or difficulty. In The Way of the Bodhisattva, Shantideva writes, "For unruly beings, long-accustomed to doing evil, there is no wrong that cannot be done. But for those who have perfectly tamed their minds, what can be done to disturb their serenity?" [6]

Patience and Equanimity

Patience is often compared to the quality of equanimity (upeksha). Like a vast ocean that remains undisturbed by the winds and waves on its surface, equanimity describes a quality of balance, composure, and evenness of mind. The Dalai Lama defines equanimity as "A balanced state of mind, free of the afflictive emotions of attachment and aversion." [4]

In many ways, equanimity is a prerequisite for true patience. Without a basis of inner stability and non-reactivity, life's provocations will continually throw us off balance. Equanimity is an inner anchor, allowing us to remain steady and grounded even in turbulent conditions.

At the same time, patience takes equanimity a step further. It is the active expression of calmness in challenging situations. Patience is stability in the trenches; the rubber meets the road. It is the choice to stay engaged and present even when everything in us wants to fight, flee, or freeze. As Chogyam Trungpa puts it, "Patience is the ultimate absence of neurosis... The neurotic state of mind says, 'If I have to stand any more of this, if I have to face this any longer, I can't stand it.' Patience says the complete opposite: 'That's fine.'" [7

Three Kinds of Patience

In The Profound Treasury of the Ocean of Dharma, Chogyam Trungpa describes three kinds of patience:

1. *Patience with external irritations* - The ability to remain unruffled under challenging people, situations, or environments. Rather than reacting with anger or frustration, we cultivate the capacity to stay present and engaged.
2. *Patience with one's meanness and limitations* - This is the ability to tolerate our faults, failings, and neuroses without beating ourselves up or falling into despair. It is the inner softening that comes from befriending and welcoming all parts of ourselves with kindness.
3. *Patience with the ultimate truth*—This is the willingness to remain open and wholeheartedly present to the fundamental nature of reality, even when it challenges our tightly held beliefs and conceptual frameworks. It is the courage to let go of our fixed reference points and allow the spaciousness of not knowing.

As we deepen in patience, we discover a profound inner freedom - the freedom to meet life as it is without getting hooked by hope and fear. Trungpa writes, "Patience is not learned in safety. It is not learned when everything is harmonious and going well... We can only learn patience through our irritations, our frustrations, our resistances... That is why patience involves letting be." [7]

Relationship to the Other Actions

Like all the actions of a healer, patience does not exist in isolation but is intimately connected with the other practices on the bodhisattva path.

Generosity and patience support each other in a dynamic balance. Generosity is the outward expression of letting go, while patience is the inner act of not holding on. As we practice generosity, we wear down the self-clinging that makes us lose patience. And as we cultivate patience, we find the inner spaciousness to keep giving, even when we feel we have nothing left.

Discipline and patience are two sides of the same coin. Discipline gives us the structure and containment to hold steady amid reactivity, while patience gives us the flexibility and openness to keep showing up with a tender heart. Together, they dance in a productive tension - strength balanced with suppleness, boundaries balanced with limitlessness.

Joyful effort and patience might seem like opposites, but they are essential partners. It takes tremendous energy and enthusiasm to keep opening our hearts in difficult moments. And it takes immense patience to sustain joyful effort over the long haul, to pick ourselves up repeatedly without losing heart.

Mindfulness and patience are intimately connected. Mindfulness is the quality of present-moment awareness, of paying attention to what is happening here and now without judgment or reactivity. As Jon Kabat-Zinn defines it, "Mindfulness means paying attention in a particular way: on purpose, in the present moment, and nonjudgmentally." [11]

Mindfulness supports patience by allowing us to catch our moments of impatience and frustration early before they spiral out of control. By becoming more aware of our mind states and bodily sensations, we can notice the first flickers of reactivity and choose to respond differently. Thich Nhat Hanh writes, "Mindfulness is like a light that shines upon our thoughts, words, and actions, and guides us to act in ways that will not create suffering." [12]

Patience is essential for the practice of mindfulness. It takes great patience to keep returning to the present moment, especially when it is uncomfortable or boring. Without patience, we may relinquish our mindfulness practice when it doesn't yield results or insights immediately. Jack Kornfield notes, "Mindfulness takes patience. We have to be willing to come back a hundred thousand times. We have to be able to sit quietly and listen, not knowing what will happen next." [13]

Wisdom and patience have an intimate relationship. We find the ultimate source of patience only by seeing clearly into the nature of reality—the impermanence of all things, the illusion of the self, and the truth of interdependence. When we let go of our attachment to outcomes and rest in the spaciousness of things as they are, patience becomes effortless.

Patience and courage are complementary qualities that support each other. Cultivating patience in a speedy, aggressive culture that wants us to react to every provocation takes courage. As the author Dani Dipirro writes, "Patience is the calm acceptance that things can happen in a different order than the one you have in mind. It's a kind of courage - the courage to trust, to wait, to not know yet." [14]

As the philosopher Bertrand Russell writes, "Men fear thought as they fear nothing else on earth - more than ruin, more even than death. Thought is subversive and revolutionary, destructive and terrible; thought is merciless to privilege, established institutions, and comfortable habits; thought is anarchic and lawless, indifferent to authority, careless of the well-tried wisdom of the ages.... But if thought is to become the possession of many, not the privilege of the few, we must have done with fear." [20]

Patience gives us the strength and stability to act courageously when needed. When we are grounded in patience, we are less likely to be paralyzed by fear or overwhelmed by the magnitude of the challenges we face. We can stay the course even when progress is slow or setbacks arise. Sharon Salzberg notes, "Patience doesn't mean passivity or resignation, but power. It's the power to accept fully what is, and to make our choice of response from the deepest place in ourselves." [15]

Patience and humility are closely connected. Humility is the recognition of our interdependence, our limitations, and our shared human vulnerability. When we are humble, we don't expect ourselves or others to be perfect or always in control. We accept that growth and change are gradual processes that require patience and perseverance.

At the same time, patience helps us cultivate humility by wearing down our selfish tendencies. When we practice patience, we learn to let go of our agendas and desire for quick results. We discover that we are not the center of the universe and that things don't always happen on our timeline. As the Zen teacher Shunryu Suzuki writes, "If your practice is good, you may become proud of it. What you do is good, but something more is added to it. Pride is something extra. Right effort is to get rid of something extra." [16]

Patience and reverence have a symbiotic relationship. Reverence is a deep respect and awe for the sacredness of life. When we approach the world with reverence, we are more likely to be patient with its imperfections and challenges. We recognize that everything is part of a larger unfolding that we cannot fully control or comprehend. As Rachel Naomi Remen writes, "Reverence is the sense of awe or profound respect for the person before you. Reverence is a way of honoring life, things, people, and places. It is a way of learning to see each thing in its own light." [17]

At the same time, patience allows us to cultivate a more profound reverence for life. When we are patient, we create space to appreciate the small miracles and sacred moments that are always available, even in difficulty. We find the capacity to be present with what is without rushing to fix, change, or judge it. As the poet Rainer Maria Rilke writes, "I want to beg you, as much as I can, dear sir, to be patient toward all that is unsolved in your heart and to try to love the questions themselves." [18]

Patience and curiosity are mutually reinforcing qualities. Curiosity is the desire to learn, explore, and understand. When we approach challenges with curiosity rather than frustration, we are more likely to stay engaged and open to new possibilities. Curiosity motivates us to keep showing up with patience, even when things are unclear or uncomfortable.

At the same time, patience creates the conditions for genuine curiosity to flourish. We often jump to conclusions or rely on habitual assumptions when we are impatient. But when we cultivate patience, we create space for fresh perceptions and insights to arise. We become more attentive to nuance and complexity and more willing to question our preconceptions. As the scientist

Stuart Firestein writes, "Patience is crucial because one must be ready to put aside even the most treasured ideas in the face of contradictory evidence." [19]

Patience and intelligence have an essential relationship. Our culture often associates intelligence with quick thinking, decisive action, and problem-solving prowess. However, accurate intelligence also requires the patience to sit with complexity, tolerate ambiguity, and let wisdom emerge in its own time.

Patience gives us the courage to engage in this kind of deep, unsettling thought. It allows us to question our assumptions, explore new paradigms, and expand our ways of knowing. At the same time, intelligence informs the practice of patience by helping us discern when to persevere, let go, push forward, and rest in not knowing. Together, patience and intelligence dance in a creative tension that is essential for growth and discovery.

Being Patient in the Modern World

Cultivating patience is a perennial challenge but especially difficult in our modern world. Life is faster than ever, and we are constantly bombarded with information and stimulation. We expect instant gratification and have little tolerance for discomfort or delay. In such a context, patience can seem like a quaint relic of a slower, simpler time.

This is especially true in healthcare, where time, technology, and bureaucracy pressures can erode the human connection at the heart of healing. In a system that privileges efficiency over empathy and procedure over presence, it takes great patience to carve out space for authentic listening and relationship. Joan Halifax writes, "Through patience, we develop equanimity and perseverance, the two essential qualities we need to work with suffering. Yet in our speeded-up world, patience is rarely supported or acknowledged. We're encouraged to multi-task, do everything faster, and ignore or suppress feelings of impatience. The bodhisattva, the compassionate one, has to learn to go against the stream to cultivate patience." [8]

The increasing polarization and reactivity of our public discourse also challenge patience. In a culture of outrage, where the echo chambers of social media amplify every provocation, it is easy to get swept up in cycles of anger and recrimination. Patience calls us to a different way of engaging—one rooted in deep listening, empathy, nuance, and a willingness to stay in dialogue even when we disagree.

Ultimately, patience is a radical act of resistance in a world that wants us to be endlessly productive, efficient, and on the go. It is a courageous choice to slow down, breathe, let go of our agendas, and be fully present in what is. As the Czech dissident Vaclav Havel writes, "Patience is strength. Patience is the foundation-stone of creative work; without patience, without being prepared to wait, no creative work is possible. Patience means sticking to the task in hand against all the odds; it means following the path you have chosen whatever comes your way." [9]

Patience

How do we cultivate this vital quality of patience in our lives and work? The Buddhist tradition offers a wealth of practices and perspectives to support us:

Meditative training: Formal sitting meditation is a powerful way to cultivate patient attention and practice returning to the present moment without judgment or resistance. As we become more familiar with our minds' restless, reactive nature, we find more space to breathe and respond skillfully.

Mindfulness in daily life: We can also bring patient awareness to our everyday activities and interactions. Whenever we notice ourselves getting hooked by impatience, we can pause, reconnect with our body, breathe, and choose a more skillful response. Over time, we build the muscle of stability amid life's provocations.

Recollection of impermanence: When we're stuck in reactivity, it can feel like our situation will never change. By reflecting on the transient nature of all things, we gain perspective and find the patience to ride out passing waves of pain or difficulty. Shantideva reminds us, "So, swept along by present pains, we lose all patience - unaware that all these fly away in but a moment's flash, just like the moment when, in sleep, our mind encounters some distress." [6]

Taking the long view: Patience springs from considering the bigger picture. When we remember our deepest values and aspirations and reaffirm our commitment to serving and awakening, we can more easily let go of immediate frustrations and keep our hearts open. As Lama Zopa writes, "If we think of the situation as training for our Dharma practice, for attaining higher realizations and enlightenment, then it is much easier to face." [5]

Self-compassion: One of the most significant challenges to patience is our self-judgment and perfectionism. By cultivating kindness and forgiveness toward ourselves, we create the inner conditions for true patience to blossom. As the Dalai Lama says, "If you don't love yourself, you cannot love others. You will not be able to love others. If you have no compassion for yourself then you are not able of developing compassion for others." [10]

Connecting with the community: Finally, we cannot cultivate patience alone. We need the support and inspiration of spiritual friends, mentors, and communities to keep us on track. By sharing our struggles and insights with others on the path, we tap into a deep well of collective wisdom and resilience.

A Definition of a Patient Healer

The patient healer cultivates equanimity and non-reactivity as the foundations of their practice. Equanimity allows the healer to maintain a balanced and stable presence in the face of life's challenges, while non-reactivity enables them to respond skillfully to difficult situations without being overwhelmed by emotions or impulses. By embodying these qualities, the patient healer creates a therapeutic space of safety, understanding, and acceptance, fostering healing and resilience in their patients. The patient healer recognizes that the ongoing practice of equanimity and non-reactivity is essential for navigating the complexities of the human condition with wisdom, compassion, and grace.

Concluding Remarks

In the words of Joan Halifax, "There is no more difficult and rewarding practice than patience... Patience reveals the face of compassion as a daily practice, in which we are willing to hold suffering and joy, to bear with the vicissitudes of the human condition without bitterness, recrimination, or expectation. The practice of patience shows us that we are all held in the infinite web of interconnectedness." [8]

Self-Assessment Reflections

1. In what situations do I most easily lose patience? What are my triggers and reactive patterns?
2. How do I treat myself when feeling impatient or frustrated? Can I be more kind and understanding of my struggles?
3. Who are the people in my life who embody patience? What can I learn from their example?
4. Where in my work as a healthcare provider am I called to deepen my capacity for patience? How might this benefit my patients and colleagues?
5. When I look at the larger systems and structures that shape healthcare, where is patience most needed? How can I contribute to creating a more compassionate and sustainable approach?
6. What daily practices can I commit to to cultivate patient awareness? How will I support myself in following through?

By continually reflecting on these questions, we deepen our understanding of patience as a lived practice, not just an abstract ideal. We learn to meet each moment with fresh eyes, to bring curiosity and care to the joys and sorrows of our world. And we discover that patience is not just something we have but something we are - a boundless capacity to embrace life in all its beauty and brokenness.

References:

1. Etymonline entry for "patience." Online Etymology Dictionary, https:// www.etymonline.com/word/patience

2. Wright, Dale S. The Six Perfections: Buddhism and the Cultivation of Character. Oxford University Press, USA, 2009, p.94-136.

3. Gyatso, Dalai Lama XIV. Transforming the Mind: Teachings on Generating Compassion. Thorsons, 2000, p.204.

4. Gyatso, Dalai Lama XIV. Dzogchen: Heart Essence of the Great Perfection. Snow Lion, 2004, p.147-148.

5. Lama Zopa Rinpoche. We are transforming Problems Into Happiness. Wisdom Publications, 2001, p.12-27.

6. Shantideva and Vesna Wallace. A Guide to the Bodhisattva Way of Life =: Bodhicaryāvatāra. Snow Lion, 1997. Chapter 6.

7. Trungpa, Chögyam. The Profound Treasury of the Ocean of Dharma, Volume 2: The Bodhisattva Path of Wisdom and Compassion. Shambhala Publications, 2013, p.232-237.

8. Halifax, Joan. Standing at the Edge: Finding Freedom Where Fear and Courage Meet. Flatiron Books, 2018, p.129-142.

9. Havel, Václav. Letters to Olga: June 1979-September 1982. Henry Holt, 1989, p.201.

10. Gyatso, Dalai Lama XIV. The Art of Happiness: A Handbook for Living. Riverhead Hardcover, 1998.

11. Kabat-Zinn, Jon. Wherever You Go, There You Are: Mindfulness Meditation in Everyday Life. Hyperion, 1994, p.4.

12. Hanh, Thich Nhat. The Heart of the Buddha's Teaching: Transforming Suffering into Peace, Joy, and Liberation. Broadway Books, 1998, p.37.

13. Kornfield, Jack. A Path with Heart: A Guide Through the Perils and Promises of Spiritual Life. Bantam, 1993, p.73.

14. Dipirro, Dani. The Positively Present Guide to Life: How to Make the Most of Every Moment. Watkins Publishing, 2015.

15. Salzberg, Sharon. Lovingkindness: The Revolutionary Art of Happiness. Shambhala, 1995.

16. Suzuki, Shunryu. Zen Mind, Beginner's Mind. Weatherhill, 1970, p.59.

17. Remen, Rachel Naomi. My Grandfather's Blessings: Stories of Strength, Refuge, and Belonging. Riverhead Books, 2000.

18. Rilke, Rainer Maria. Letters to a Young Poet. Norton, 1934.

19. Firestein, Stuart. Ignorance: How It Drives Science. Oxford University Press, 2012.

20. Russell, Bertrand. Principles of Social Reconstruction. George Allen & Unwin, 1916.

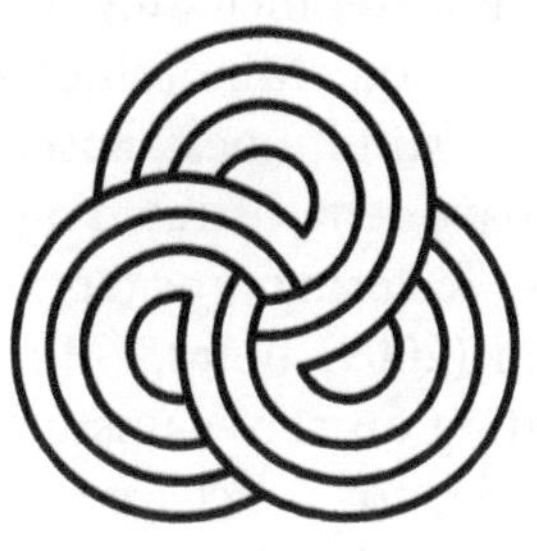

Chapter 4

Mindful

"The richness of present-moment experience is the richness of life itself. Too often we let our thinking and our beliefs about what we 'know' prevent us from seeing things as they really are."
Jon Kabat-Zinn

In recent decades, the concept of mindfulness has rapidly permeated nearly every facet of modern society, from education and business to psychology and healthcare. This widespread integration is mainly due to the pioneering work of Jon Kabat-Zinn, who first introduced mindfulness-based interventions (MBIs) into mainstream medicine in the late 1970s.

Kabat-Zinn's seminal program, Mindfulness-Based Stress Reduction (MBSR), was developed at the University of Massachusetts Medical Center to help patients with chronic pain and stress-related disorders. By repackaging traditional Buddhist contemplative practices in a secular, scientific framework, Kabat-Zinn made mindfulness accessible and relevant to modern Western audiences, particularly in healthcare settings.

As Kabat-Zinn (2003) describes, "MBSR was developed as one of a possibly infinite number of skillful means for bringing the dharma into mainstream settings . . . It becoming a vehicle for delivering the dharma that would be in harmony with the American mindset while at the same time honoring the universal dharma dimension." [1]

The success of MBSR paved the way for a wide range of mindfulness-based interventions in healthcare, including Mindfulness-Based Cognitive Therapy (MBCT) for depression, Mindfulness-Based Relapse Prevention (MBRP) for addiction, and Mindfulness-Based Childbirth and Parenting (MBCP). These programs have demonstrated significant benefits for patients and healthcare providers, fostering greater resilience, compassion, and well-being [2]. Kabat-Zinn (2009) notes, "Mindfulness provides a simple but powerful route for getting ourselves unstuck, back into touch with our wisdom and vitality. It is a way to take charge of the direction and quality of our own lives, including our relationships within the family, our relationship to work and to the larger world and planet, and most fundamentally, our relationship with ourselves as a person." [3]

The Rochester Zen Center has also been at the forefront of bringing mindfulness into healthcare through its Mindful Practice program for medical professionals. Founded by Dr. Ronald Epstein, a family medicine and psychiatry professor at the University of Rochester School of Medicine, the program integrates mindfulness, narrative medicine, and appreciative inquiry to help clinicians cultivate greater presence, self-awareness, and compassion. Epstein (2017) writes, "By stopping to consider how we think and how our minds and hearts work in caring for patients, we can begin to change how we practice medicine. The goal is not merely to take better care of our patients, but to take better care of ourselves as healers." [4] Epstein emphasizes the importance of cultivating a "beginner's mind" in medicine, approaching each patient encounter with fresh eyes and an open heart. He also highlights the value of "stopping amid chaos" to create a space for reflection and intentional action rather than simply reacting out of habit or stress.

Mindfulness as a Heuristic Umbrella
While the widespread adoption of mindfulness in healthcare has undoubtedly been beneficial, it has also created challenges and confusion. As "mindfulness" has become increasingly popular, it has often been used as a catch-all for various contemplative practices and approaches, each with unique characteristics and applications.

As the authors of "Beyond Mindfulness" point out, "The term 'mindfulness' has become so overused and watered-down in popular culture that it has lost much of its original meaning and power. It is often used interchangeably with 'awareness' or 'attention,' which can lead to a superficial understanding and practice" [5].

Andrew Holocek, a Buddhist teacher and author, echoes this concern: "The problem with the term 'mindfulness' is that it's very vague. It can mean anything from simple present-moment awareness to deep meditative insight. Without clarifying what we mean by mindfulness, there's a risk of diluting or misrepresenting the teachings" [6].

Healthcare professionals should develop a more rigorous understanding of the various contemplative practices available and their specific applications to address the confusion and potential misunderstandings arising from using a broad term like mindfulness. By utilizing these practices more specifically and skillfully, clinicians can tailor their approach to best suit the needs of their patients and themselves.

Three Foundational Mindfulness Practices

By examining and understanding specific practices such as Vipassana (insight), and Shamatha (calm abiding), and Samten (clear seeing) as well as their relationship to other key qualities like compassion and equanimity, we can develop a more comprehensive, nuanced, integrated, and practical approach to incorporating contemplative practices into healthcare.

Shamatha (Calm Abiding)

Shamatha, a foundational practice in Buddhist meditation, focuses on cultivating single-pointed concentration and mental stability. In its classical form, Shamatha involves developing sustained attention on a chosen object, traditionally the breath, a visual object, or a concept [7]. Through consistent practice, meditators progressively attain heightened stages of mental clarity, stability, and equanimity [8].

The essence of Shamatha lies in training the mind to remain focused on a single point, thereby quieting mental distractions and cultivating a deep sense of inner calm [9]. This practice is often compared to taming a wild horse - just as a skilled trainer patiently and persistently works with the horse to guide its energy in a constructive direction, the meditator gently and repeatedly brings the mind back to the chosen object whenever it wanders [10]. As their practice deepens, the meditator experiences a profound settling of the mind, characterized by a significant reduction in discursive thoughts and a heightened capacity for concentration [7]. This state of calm abiding provides a stable foundation for cultivating Vipassana, or insight meditation [11].

Modern Healing Applications of Shamatha

For contemporary healers, Shamatha offers essential skills for therapeutic presence and clinical effectiveness. The practice develops the sustained attention necessary for more attuned client observation, allowing practitioners to pick up on subtle nonverbal cues and unspoken emotional undertones [12]. Moreover, Shamatha enhances emotional regulation during challenging therapeutic encounters, enabling clinicians to maintain a grounded, centered presence even in the face of intense client distress [13]. This emotional stability is crucial for preventing burnout and maintaining the clarity of mind needed for effective diagnosis and treatment planning [14].

Research indicates that healthcare professionals who engage in regular Shamatha practice demonstrate improved clinical outcomes and higher patient satisfaction rates [12]. Maintaining focused attention while remaining emotionally present proves valuable in crisis intervention and trauma work, where clients' safety and well-being depend on the practitioner's capacity for grounded, compassionate engagement [13].

Vipassana (Insight Meditation)
Vipassana, often translated as insight meditation, aims to develop wisdom through direct, non-judgmental observation of present-moment experience [10]. Whereas Shamatha emphasizes concentration on a single object, Vipassana systematically expands awareness to encompass all aspects of experience, including physical sensations, emotions, thoughts, and mental patterns [15].

The practice of Vipassana is rooted in the Buddha's teaching on the Four Foundations of Mindfulness, which outlines a comprehensive system for investigating the nature of subjective experience [15]. By carefully attending to the ever-changing stream of sensations, feelings, mental states, and experiential phenomena, the meditator begins to discern the fundamental characteristics of existence, namely impermanence, unsatisfactoriness, and non-self [11]. As insight into these universal characteristics deepens, the meditator releases attachment to fixed views and conditioned reactivity patterns, developing greater cognitive flexibility, emotional balance, and psychological freedom [16]. This process of liberation through insight is the ultimate aim of Vipassana practice [10].

Modern Healing Applications of Vipassana
For contemporary healers, Vipassana offers powerful tools for self-development and clinical care. The practice enhances intuitive diagnostic abilities through refined somatic awareness and sharpened observational skills [12]. By attuning to their bodily sensations and mental states, clinicians develop a deeper understanding of mind-body interactions and psychosomatic processes [17]. This heightened self-awareness also facilitates early recognition of countertransference reactions and other emotional responses that may interfere with effective treatment [12]. By catching these reactions in real time,

practitioners can take steps to process their own experiences and maintain more explicit therapeutic boundaries [13].

Additionally, the non-judgmental awareness cultivated through Vipassana enables clinicians to hold a broader range of client experiences with greater equanimity and compassion [14]. This is particularly important when working with intense emotions, traumatic memories, or challenging behavioral patterns. By modeling an accepting, non-reactive presence, therapists create a safe space for clients to explore their inner world and develop new coping strategies [17].

Lhagthong (Samten – Clear Seeing)

Although most modern medical and scientific discussions of meditation limit themselves to Shamatha and Vipassana meditation, it is helpful to extend the discussion to include a brief review of Lhagthong meditative practice. This section provides a very brief overview of this profound, and radically simple contemplative tradition. Readers interested in exploring this practice are advised to seek an authentic teacher in this lineage.

Lhagthong is literally translated as "higher seeing" or "clear seeing" and describes a Tibetan Buddhist meditation practice emphasizing gaining insight into reality's true nature. It is considered an advanced meditative practice that is primarily associated with the Tibetan Buddhist Tantric Vajrayana schools, including Dzogchen and Mahamudra. While similar to Vipassana, Lhagthong expands insight to include the Mahayana understanding of *emptiness* (*shunyata*). This realization is not merely intellectual but a *direct* experience of the interdependent, illusory nature of all phenomena.

Key Characteristics of Lhagthong (Samten)

1. *Nature of Insight*: Lhagthong aims to penetrate the conceptual mind and experience *shunyata* (emptiness) — the ultimate nature of phenomena — while maintaining clarity and awareness. The "seeing" in Lhagthong refers not to ordinary perception but to a profound, direct insight into the true nature of mind and reality.
2. *Integration of Shamatha*: Unlike isolated Shamatha, where stability and calmness of mind are the goal, Lhagthong builds upon Shamatha by incorporating insight into impermanence, emptiness, and interdependence. Without Shamatha (calm abiding), Lhagthong cannot function fully, as a stable and focused mind is necessary for clear insight.
3. *Non-Dual Awareness*: Lhagthong often progresses toward non-dual awareness, where distinctions between subject and object dissolve. This is particularly emphasized in the Mahamudra and Dzogchen traditions.

Modern Healing Applications of Lhagthong (Samten)

1. *Seeing Beyond Conceptual Labels*
    Healers often rely on conceptual framework such as diagnoses, treatments, protocols—to address physical or mental suffering. While these tools are valuable, they can obscure the deeper reality of the human experience. Through the practice of Lhagthong, a healer cultivates insight into the "emptiness of phenomena," recognizing that a diagnosis or label, while helpful, is not inherently fixed or absolute. This enables the healer to see the whole person rather than reducing them to a collection of symptoms or pathologies.

2. *Calm, Clarity, and Compassion in Difficult Situations*
    Healers often face emotionally charged and high-stress environments, which can cloud judgment and evoke reactivity. Lhagthong supports both the calm abiding of Shamatha and the wise ("clear seeing") of insight. Calmness enables the healer to remain grounded amidst emotional or physical suffering. Clarity allows the healer to perceive reality clearly without being overwhelmed by attachment, aversion, or bias. Insight into inter-dependence naturally fosters deep compassion for patients, understanding that all beings share the desire to be free from suffering.

3. *Non-Attachment and Preventing Burnout*
    Healers are prone to burnout due to emotional attachment and over-identification with their patients' suffering. Lhagthong teaches the wisdom of non-attachment—engaging fully with compassion while recognizing the empty nature of suffering. This balance allows healers to provide care with an open heart without becoming overwhelmed or emotionally depleted. Compassion in this context is not rooted in self-sacrifice but in a deep understanding of the interconnected nature of all life.

4. *Skillful Action and Practical Wisdom*
    Drawing parallels with Aristotle's concept of phronesis, Lhagthong provides the healer with practical wisdom—the ability to respond skillfully and appropriately to ever-changing healing conditions. By directly perceiving the interdependent nature of phenomena, the healer moves beyond rigid thinking and applies solutions tailored to each patient's unique needs. This dynamic response is grounded in compassionate wisdom rather than mechanical or overly analytical reasoning.

Modern Research and Integration

In recent years, a growing body of scientific research has documented the benefits of Buddhist meditation practices for healthcare professionals and their clients [14]. Neuroscience, psychology, and medicine studies have found that regular meditation practice can significantly improve attention, emotional regulation, self-awareness, and overall well-being [16].

Research suggests that integrating meditation into clinical training and professional development for healthcare providers can help reduce burnout, improve decision-making, strengthen therapeutic alliances, and enhance job satisfaction [12]. Mindfulness-based interventions have also shown promise in treating a wide range of physical and mental health conditions, from chronic pain to depression and anxiety [14].

As the evidence base for meditation grows, many healthcare institutions are incorporating contemplative practices into their educational curricula and staff wellness programs [17]. Some pioneering medical schools, such as the University of Rochester and the University of Massachusetts, have even established dedicated centers for mindfulness research and training [14].

Practical Implementation for Healers
While the benefits of meditation for healthcare professionals are clear, integrating these practices into the demanding context of modern healthcare can be very challenging. Time constraints, competing priorities, and the need to adhere to evidence-based protocols inevitably hinder consistent practice [12]. However, with creativity and commitment, it is possible to weave contemplative practices into even the busiest clinical schedules. Here are some practical suggestions for incorporating Shamatha, and Vipassana into daily healing work:

1. *Pre-session preparation*: Before seeing clients, engage in a brief Shamatha practice to center attention and cultivate a calm, focused state of mind.
   - Use Vipassana-based body scans to increase somatic awareness and attune to one's physical and emotional state.
2. *During sessions*: Employ Shamatha-based attentional skills to maintain a stable, caring presence with clients, even amid distractions or intense emotions.
   - Practice Vipassana by tracking subtle changes in clients' facial expressions, tone of voice, and body language. Use these cues to guide therapeutic interventions.
3. *Post-session integration*: Take a few minutes after each session for Shamatha practice, allowing the mind to process and release any residual tension or preoccupation.
   - Reflect on key moments from the session through the lens of vipassana, noting insights into interpersonal dynamics, communication patterns, or therapeutic breakthroughs.

Integrating these practices into the rhythms of clinical work can transform healers' daily routines into opportunities for ongoing personal and professional development. Over time, the synergistic effects of Shamatha, Vipassana, (and Samten) can lead to profound growth in therapeutic skills, self-awareness, and compassionate action [13].

Challenges and Considerations

While integrating Buddhist meditation practices into modern healthcare holds great promise, it also raises significant challenges and considerations. One key issue is adapting ancient contemplative traditions to fit contemporary medical settings' cultural, ethical, and practical constraints [17].

For example, the traditional Buddhist framework of the Four Noble Truths and the Eightfold Path may only resonate with some clients or align with the evidence-based protocols mandated by many healthcare institutions [14]. Healers must find skillful ways to translate the essence of these teachings into a language and form accessible and relevant to modern patients [12].

Another challenge is the potential for meditation practices to blur the boundaries between personal and professional development [13]. As clinicians deepen their contemplative practice, they may grapple with intense emotions, existential questions, and shifts in worldview that can impact their therapeutic work [17]. Maintaining clear boundaries and seeking appropriate support is essential for navigating this terrain ethically and responsibly [12]. This highlights the crucial importance of having a skilled and experienced teacher of contemplative approaches, particularly in clinical settings. Hopefully, the importance and necessity for these teachers will become increasingly appreciated in the coming age of artificial intelligence that will actually provide more (and not less) opportunities to enhance the healer-patient relationship.

Additionally, the time demands of a consistent meditation practice can be challenging to reconcile with modern healthcare's fast-paced, high-pressure environment [14]. Clinicians may need to advocate for institutional support, such as protected time for contemplative practice or continuing education credits for meditation training [13].

Finally, it is essential to approach the integration of contemplative practices into healthcare with cultural humility and respect for diversity [12]. Not all clients or colleagues will share an interest in or affinity for meditation, and it is crucial to honor each individual's unique beliefs, values, and preferences [17]. By holding the teachings of shamatha, vipassana, and samten lightly as an invitation rather than an imposition, healers can create an inclusive, non-dogmatic atmosphere of exploration and growth [14].

Ultimately, integrating contemplative approaches into modern healing is a delicate dance requiring ongoing reflection, adaptation, and dialogue

[13]. By embracing both the challenges and the opportunities of this work, healthcare professionals can tap into a rich stream of wisdom and compassion, transforming their clinical practice into a profound path of service and awakening that will enliven their experience of themselves and their healing work [12].

It is also essential to distinguish authentic contemplative practices from the growing interest in entheogens, or psychedelic substances, as a means of inducing altered states of consciousness. While these substances may offer temporary experiences of inner peace, joy, or transcendence, they do not provide a sustainable path for personal and spiritual growth.

Andrew Holocek notes, "Entheogens can open doors to extraordinary experiences, but they cannot keep those doors open. True spiritual development requires a sober, disciplined approach to practice that transforms the mind and heart from the inside out." [19]

Furthermore, the use of entheogens outside of carefully controlled clinical settings can be hazardous, potentially leading to adverse psychological reactions, addiction, or other harmful consequences. As healthcare professionals, we are responsible for promoting safe, evidence-based approaches to healing and personal growth rather than encouraging the use of potentially dangerous substances.

The Importance of Guidance and the Potential for Harm

While contemplative practices offer tremendous potential for healing and transformation, they must be approached with care and discernment. Without proper guidance and support, they can sometimes lead to adverse effects or even harm.

As Willoughby Britton, a clinical psychologist and researcher at Brown University, has documented, a significant number of people who engage in contemplative practices like meditation can experience challenging or distressing experiences, such as anxiety, depression, or dissociation. These experiences are often referred to as "meditation-related difficulties" or "night" experiences [20]. Britton emphasizes the importance of working with an experienced teacher who can provide skillful guidance and support, particularly for those vulnerable to these experiences. She also highlights the need for a more balanced and realistic portrayal of contemplative practices in popular media and discourse. Britton notes, "The idealized, romanticized version of meditation that is often presented in the media and in many meditation communities can lead people to have unrealistic expectations and to feel like they are failing or doing something wrong when they encounter difficulties." [21]

To mitigate the potential for harm and maximize the benefits of contemplative practices, healthcare professionals must seek and learn from qualified teachers and approach them with a spirit of openness, curiosity, and self-compassion. By creating a supportive and inclusive environment for exploring these practices, clinicians can help ensure their safe and effective use.

Relationship of "Mindfulness" to the Other Heart-Based Actions

In the Buddhist tradition, mindfulness is considered one of the six perfections or qualities of the bodhisattva path. As discussed previously in this text, the other five perfections are generosity, discipline, patience, diligence, and wisdom. In the context of the healer, I have suggested expanding these to include the 12 actions of a healer. Mindfulness is the foundation for cultivating all these actions, providing the clarity and stability of mind necessary for their development.

As Reginald Ray explains, "The five perfections are grounded in the practice of mindfulness, which provides the basis for the cultivation of discipline, patience, diligence, generosity, and wisdom. Mindfulness allows us to see things as they are, without judgment or distortion, and to respond to life's challenges with equanimity and compassion." [22]

Without the clarity and stability of mindfulness, the other perfections can quickly become distorted or misguided. For example, generosity without mindfulness can become a form of people-pleasing or a way of avoiding discomfort rather than a genuine expression of care and compassion. Discipline without mindfulness can become rigid self-control or a way of punishing ourselves rather than a skillful means of cultivating wholesome qualities.

Chögyam Trungpa Rinpoche notes, "The practice of mindfulness is the foundation for the other paramitas. Without the practice of mindfulness, the other paramitas cannot be developed properly. Mindfulness provides the basic ground, the basic sanity, from which the other paramitas can be developed." [23]

Thich Nhat Hanh also emphasizes the central role of mindfulness in cultivating the other perfections: "Mindfulness is the base, the foundation of the other five paramitas. The practice of the other paramitas has to be based on the practice of mindfulness. If you practice generosity without mindfulness, your generosity will not be perfect. If you practice the precepts without mindfulness, your precepts will not be perfect. If you practice inclusiveness without mindfulness, your inclusiveness will not be perfect. If you practice diligence without mindfulness, your diligence will not be perfect. And if you have the desire to help other beings without mindfulness, your desire will not be perfect." [24]

By cultivating mindfulness as the ground of our being, we create the inner conditions for the natural unfolding of generosity, discipline, patience, diligence, wisdom, and the other six actions I describe in this text. As we learn to rest in the spaciousness and clarity of mindful awareness, we gradually dissolve the barriers of self-clinging, reactivity, and ignorance that prevent us from embodying these noble qualities in our lives and work.

Obstacles to an Effective Mindfulness Practice

Despite its many benefits, mindfulness practices are challenging. Chogyam Trungpa Rinpoche outlines eight main obstacles to mindfulness, each of which can manifest in unique ways within the context of modern healthcare [23]:

1. *Laziness*: In the fast-paced, high-stress environment of modern healthcare, it can be all too easy to succumb to feelings of fatigue, apathy, or procrastination. Clinicians may put off self-care practices like meditation or exercise, telling themselves they're too busy or exhausted to make time for these activities.
2. *Forgetting the instructions*: With the constant demands and distractions of clinical practice, healthcare professionals may need help remembering and applying mindfulness's core principles and techniques. They may get caught up in habitual patterns of thought and behavior, losing sight of the present moment and their intention to practice.
3. *Laxity and excitedness*: The stressful and unpredictable nature of healthcare work can lead to mental and physical agitation, making it difficult to settle into a calm and focused state of mind. At the same time, the long hours and demanding schedules can also result in feelings of dullness, sleepiness, or lack of energy, which can hinder the cultivation of explicit awareness.
4. *Non-application*: Even when healthcare professionals understand the value of mindfulness practices, they may need help applying them consistently in their daily lives and work. The pressures of time, workload, and competing priorities can make prioritizing self-care and contemplative practice challenging.
5. *Over-application*: To counteract stress and burnout, some clinicians may go to the other extreme, becoming rigid or perfectionistic in their approach to mindfulness practice. They may push themselves too hard, trying to force a state of calm or clarity rather than allowing their practice to unfold naturally with patience and self-compassion.
6. *Conflicting emotions*: The intense emotional demands of healthcare work can lead to a range of challenging feelings, from anxiety and frustration to sadness and despair. Navigating these emotions can be difficult, leading

to patterns of avoidance, suppression, or reactivity that undermine the cultivation of mindful awareness.

7. *Failing to apply the antidotes*: When faced with obstacles or difficulties in their practice, healthcare professionals may struggle to remember or apply the appropriate antidotes, such as reaffirming the intention to practice, cultivating joy and enthusiasm, or seeking support from a teacher or sangha.

8. *Applying them when they are no longer needed*: As clinicians develop greater skill and stability in their mindfulness practice, they may fall into the trap of clinging to particular techniques or approaches, even when they are no longer necessary or helpful. This can lead to stagnation or plateauing in one's practice rather than continuing to evolve and deepen.

By bringing awareness to these common obstacles and developing skillful means for working with them, healthcare professionals can gradually overcome the barriers to samten and cultivate a more consistent, nourishing, and transformative practice. This requires a spirit of patience, perseverance, and self-compassion, as well as a willingness to learn from one's challenges and seek support from others.

Defining the Mindful Healer

"A mindful healer is a healthcare professional who embodies presence, compassion, clarity, and equanimity in their work. They cultivate the ability to remain grounded in the present moment, attentive to their inner experiences and the needs of those they serve. Through mindfulness practices, they develop greater emotional regulation, resilience, and the capacity to respond skillfully to challenges. The mindful healer approaches their work as a path of awakening and service, dedicated to alleviating suffering and promoting well-being for all."

Concluding Remarks

Mindfulness offers healthcare professionals a powerful means of enhancing their well-being, resilience, and capacity to serve others. By drawing upon the wisdom of the ancient contemplative traditions and modern secular adaptations, healers can cultivate the qualities of insight, calm abiding, and compassionate presence essential for their work.

Ronald Epstein reminds us, "Mindfulness in medicine is a way of preserving our sense of humanity despite the often challenging circumstances of our work. It is a way of healing ourselves so that we can be of genuine service to others." [4]

Self-Reflection Questions

1. How can I integrate the practices of Shamatha, and Vipassana into my daily life and clinical work to cultivate greater presence, compassion, and equanimity?

2. In what ways have I experienced the confusion or dilution of mindfulness as a "heuristic umbrella" term, and how can I develop a more nuanced understanding of specific contemplative practices?

3. What obstacles to mindfulness do I most commonly encounter in my personal and professional life, and what strategies can I employ to work with these challenges skillfully?

4. How can I authentically and effectively balance the demands of evidence-based protocols and institutional constraints with the integration of contemplative practices?

5. In what ways might my contemplative practice blur the boundaries between personal and professional development, and how can I navigate this terrain with integrity and self-awareness?

6. How can I cultivate a beginner's mind and a spirit of curiosity in my clinical work, approaching each patient encounter with fresh eyes and an open heart?

7. What steps can I take to create a supportive environment for exploring contemplative practices safely and effectively within my healthcare setting?

8. How can I draw upon the wisdom of mindfulness to inform and enrich my understanding of the other essential actions of a healer, such as generosity, discipline, patience, diligence, and wisdom?

9. How can I discern between authentic contemplative practices and potentially harmful or misguided approaches, such as the ungrounded use of entheogens or the idealization of meditation in popular media?

10. What resources, relationships, and practices can I cultivate to support my ongoing commitment to mindfulness and compassion in the face of the challenges and demands of modern healthcare?

References

1. Kabat-Zinn, J. (2003). 'Mindfulness-Based Interventions in Context: Past, Present, and Future,' Clinical Psychology: Science and Practice, 10/2: 144-156.

2. Bauer, T. (2021). 'The State of Mindfulness Research: A Critical Review,' Journal of Psychosomatic Research, 147: 110503.

3. Kabat-Zinn, J. (2009). Full Catastrophe Living: Using the Wisdom of Your Body and Mind to Face Stress, Pain, and Illness. Random House, New York.

4. Epstein, R. M. (2017). Attending: Medicine, Mindfulness, and Humanity. Scribner, New York.

5. Dunn, D. & Swierski, J. (2020). Beyond Mindfulness: Buddhist and Taoist Practices for Awakening. Findhorn Press, Scotland.

6. Holocek, A. (2018). 'What Exactly Is Mindfulness? An Exploration of the Core Elements', Tricycle. <https://tricycle.org/trikedaily/what-is-mindfulness/>

7. Buddhaghosa, "Visuddhimagga" (The Path of Purification), 5th century CE

8. Dalai Lama, "Stages of Meditation," 2001

9. Wallace, B. Alan, "The Attention Revolution: Unlocking the Power of the Focused Mind," 2006

10. Gunaratana, Bhante H., "Mindfulness in Plain English," 1991

11. Bodhi, Bhikkhu, "The Noble Eightfold Path: Way to the End of Suffering," 1984

12. Siegel, Daniel J., "The Mindful Therapist," 2010

13. Halifax, Roshi Joan, "Standing at the Edge: Finding Freedom Where Fear and Courage Meet," 2018

14. Kabat-Zinn, Jon, "Full Catastrophe Living," 2013

15. "Satipatthana Sutta," Majjhima Nikaya 10

16. Goldstein, Joseph, "Mindfulness: A Practical Guide to Awakening," 2016

17. Epstein, Mark, "Thoughts Without a Thinker," 2013

18. Trungpa, Chögyam, "The Heart of the Buddha," 1991

19. Holocek, A. (2021). 'The Promises and Perils of Psychedelics in Buddhism', Tricycle.

20. Britton, W. et al. (2021). 'Meditation-Related Difficulties: A Taxonomy and Data from a Large Sample of Meditators', PLoS ONE, 16/5: e0250241.

21. Britton, W. (2019). 'Can Mindfulness Be Too Much of a Good Thing?', The Conversation.

22. Ray, R. A. (2021). The Practice of Pure Awareness: Somatic Meditation for Awakening the Sacred. Shambhala, Boulder.

23. Trungpa, C. (2013). The Profound Treasury of the Ocean of Dharma, Volume Two: The Bodhisattva Path of Wisdom and Compassion. Shambhala Publications, Boulder.

24. Hanh, T. N. (1998). The Heart of the Buddha's Teaching: Transforming Suffering into Peace, Joy, and Liberation. Harmony, New York.

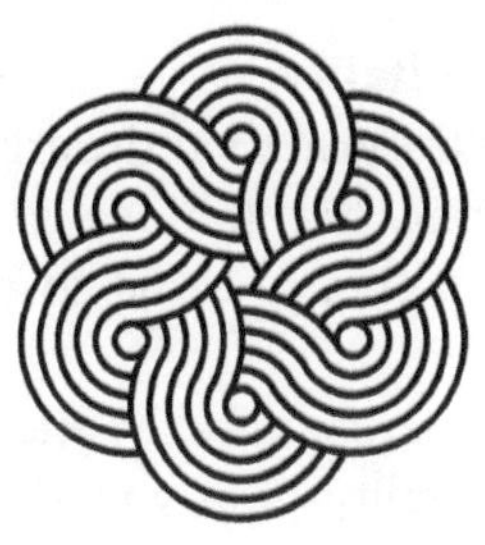

CHAPTER 5

Vital

"There is a vitality, a life force, an energy, a quickening,
that is translated through you into action, and because there is
only one of you in all time, this expression is unique."
Martha Graham

The path of the healer is demanding, requiring vast reserves of energy, compassion, and resilience. How can we cultivate the inner resources to sustain our vital presence in the face of unrelenting challenges and intense suffering? This chapter explores the Buddhist perfection of virya (energy/ diligence/perseverance), the psychological concept of grit, and awareness of common energy drains to offer valuable wisdom for the journey.

Indian yogi and spiritual teacher Sadhguru shares insights on the profound importance of cultivating vitality as a healer: "A healer is someone who has an abundance of energy. Without an exuberance of vitality, you cannot be of much help to others. Just as you cannot pour from an empty cup, you cannot give what you do not have within yourself. For any human being to function at their optimal capacity, a certain vitality is needed, but for the healer, it is absolutely essential." [1]

He further elaborates: "The fundamental ingredient for health is vitality. A healer is not just someone who fixes the body or mends the mind. A healer is someone who empowers another with vitality. When you are in touch with the vital energy within you, you can uplift people around you. This is the essence of healing." [2]

Etymology and Meaning of Vitality
The English word energy, on the other hand, derives from the Greek energeia, which means activity or work. It combines en, meaning "in," with ergon, meaning "work." Over time, energy came to refer to the force or power behind activity [3].

While sometimes used interchangeably, energy refers more to the power put into an activity, while vitality points to the vibrant, animating quality behind it. The Sanskrit term "virya" encompasses both meanings—the diligent effort and the inner life force propelling it. The Sanskrit word virya, often translated as energy or diligence, comes from the root vira, meaning hero or robust and courageous person. Related words include the Latin vir, meaning man, and virtue, meaning strength [4].

In Mahayana Buddhism, virya is one of the six paramitas or transcendent perfections, along with generosity (dana), moral discipline (sila), patience (kshanti), meditation (dhyana), and wisdom (prajna). As Dale S. Wright explains: "The final three perfections - energy, meditation, and wisdom - are connected with and in some sense undergird the first three: generosity, morality, and patience. At the very least, considerable energy, a great deal of meditative concentration, and penetrating wisdom are required to bring each of the first three to perfection." [5]

The Tibetan spiritual teacher, Lama Zopa Rinpoche, further emphasizes the importance of virya: "Virya, or enthusiastic perseverance, is the fuel that propels us to enlightenment. Without virya, the other perfections lack the strength to bear fruit. It is the locomotive that carries the other cars to their destination." [6]

The Two Types of Vitality (Virya)
Wright distinguishes two types of virya the bodhisattva must perfect:

1.   *Liberating energy* to free ourselves from afflictive states
2.   *Enlightening energy* to vigorously benefit others

Liberating energy fuels practices like meditation and self-reflection that transform our minds. Enlightening energy animates compassionate action like teaching, service, and activism that help liberate others.

Balancing Vitality (Virya)

Shantideva warns of the dangers of both overexertion and slacking: "The body is not made of wood or stone, while even they will fall apart. How much more this fragile form composed of four elements! Day after day, moment after moment, one must exercise a wealth of care. Not overexerting, not underexerting - discovering one's intended pace." [7] As we discussed in a previous chapter, equanimity describes this ability to stay centered and clear in the midst of oscillating energy - allows us to ride the inevitable waves, resting when depleted and offering our best when replenished.

Power and Peril of Grit

The psychological concept of grit, defined by pioneer researcher Angela Duckworth as "perseverance and passion for long-term goals" [8], provides another lens on the sustained effort required on the healing path.

Duckworth and her colleagues found that grit was a stronger predictor of success than IQ or conscientiousness in challenging domains like the National Spelling Bee, West Point cadet training, and sales jobs [9]. This has sparked immense interest in grit as a key to high achievement. However, some psychologists have cautioned against an overly simplistic interpretation of grit. Dr. Danielle Bassett points out potential pitfalls: "The discussion around grit often misses the importance of self-reflection and flexible adaptation. Grit without discernment can lead to burnout and inflexible persistence towards goals that may no longer serve us or others. Wise grit involves regularly reassessing whether our efforts are bearing good fruit and realigning as needed." [10]

For example, consider a doctor who keeps pushing herself to see more patients despite signs of burnout and deteriorating quality of care. Her single-minded drive, once an asset, has become a liability. A wiser approach would be to pause, reflect, and recalibrate her workload and self-care to restore balance.

Another risk is adopting a "grin and bear it" mentality in the face of genuine suffering and systemic issues. Dr. Lucy Hallam poignantly writes: "Many of us have been conditioned to stoically endure poor working conditions, excessive workloads, and even abuse as a testament to our grit and dedication. But this 'noble suffering' narrative can perpetuate harm and prevent much-needed change. True grit involves having the courage to set boundaries, speak up against injustice, and advocate for more humane and sustainable systems." [11]

So, while grit is a valuable quality, it must be balanced with self-awareness, discernment, and a willingness to question the status quo when it no longer serves. Grit in the service of liberating and enlightening aims is very different from grit in the service of ego or mere endurance of broken systems.

Characteristics of Grit

Despite failures and setbacks, grit involves commitment and consistency over long periods: "The gritty individual approaches achievement as a marathon; their advantage is stamina. Whereas disappointment or boredom signals to others that it is time to change trajectory and cut losses, the gritty individual stays the course." [8]

Potential Pitfalls of Grit

However, grit is not just about dogged persistence. Misapplied effort, even if energetic, can lead to burnout and poor outcomes. Psychologist Edy Greenblatt cautions: "Burnout occurs when the balance of deadlines, demands, working hours, and other stressors outstrips rewards, recognition, and relaxation. Overworking or working on non-valued projects sets the stage for disequilibrium and frustration." [12]

Harnessing Higher Energies

The key is to harness grit in a way that taps into our deepest sources of meaning and inspiration. As philosopher William James put it: "The capacity for 'higher energies' within each person must be awakened, activated through the call of an ideal. In becoming fired by their ideals, people gain a new level of power and energy. They are no longer limited by their habitual ways of thinking, feeling, and acting." [13]

Overcoming Energy/Vitality Drains

Even with the best intentions and a strong motivation to serve, every healer faces energy drains that can slowly erode their vitality and grit. Christopher Wallis identifies eleven common drains to watch out for [14]:

1. *Disorganization and Clutter*: A disorganized work environment or chaotic schedule can create constant low-grade stress and make it harder to focus. For healers dealing with complex cases and demanding administrative tasks, streamlining systems and creating order can free up significant energy.
2. *Incompletions and Unfinished Business*: The mental weight of looming undone tasks can be draining. Developing the habit of regularly reviewing and tying up loose ends can create a greater sense of clarity and control.
3. *Lack of Integrity and Inauthenticity*: Engaging in or enabling behavior that violates our core values creates inner dissonance that saps vitality. Healers face pressure to compromise in many ways, from over-prescribing to fit into rushed systems to staying silent about unethical

practices. Finding ways to align our actions with our principles, however imperfectly, is energizing.

4. *Toxicity in Body and Environment*: Many lifestyle and environmental factors, from processed foods to chronic stress to toxic workplace dynamics, can burden our systems. Making simple supportive shifts like improving nutrition, taking restorative breaks, and setting healthy relational boundaries can enhance overall resilience.

5. *Negative Thought Patterns and Self-Talk*: Our internal stories shape our experience. Catching and replacing self-defeating mental narratives like "I can't handle this" or "I have to be perfect" with more empowering ones is a powerful energy management tool.

6. *Unclear Priorities and Boundaries*: Without clear priorities, it's easy to get pulled in many directions and overextend ourselves. Clarifying what matters most and setting boundaries around our time, energy, and attention aligns our resources with our deepest values.

7. *Unresolved Conflict and Resentment*: Chronically unexpressed or unresolved tensions with others act as an ongoing drain. Developing skills to communicate constructively, repair ruptures, and release grievances-free energy for more positive aims.

8. *Resistance to Change and Growth*: While some stability is essential, resisting necessary change and growth can keep us stuck in draining patterns. Even through discomfort, cultivating an openness to learning and evolution keeps our vital energies flowing.

9. *Lack of Meaning and Purpose*: A sense of purpose is a profound source of vitality. Regularly reconnecting to our core mission and finding meaning even in mundane tasks grounds us in what matters most.

10. *Isolation and Disconnection*: Positive relationships and belonging are core human needs. Prioritizing time to connect meaningfully with others and to feel part of a caring community gives us a profound energetic boost.

11. *Neglect of Self-Care and Renewal*: Pushing ourselves relentlessly without proper rest, play, and nourishment is a recipe for depletion. Treating self-care as a sacred responsibility rather than a luxury is key to sustained vitality.

Each of these drains is very relevant to modern healers, given the intense pressures and complex systems they navigate. The invitation is to become mindful of what depletes us personally and take steps to reverse those patterns. Even small shifts can significantly affect our capacity to show up fully.

The Flywheel of Vitality

As we shore up our sources of vitality and release the drains, we set in motion a self-reinforcing flywheel of energy renewal. Psychologist Mihaly Csikszentmihalyi describes this beautifully in his pioneering research on flow states: "When we become fully absorbed in a pursuit that is challenging but within our skill level, we enter a flow state characterized by deep concentration, joy, and a sense of timelessness. In these moments, life becomes its own reward." [15]

Concepts from positive psychology offer further insight into this flywheel effect. Founder Dr. Martin Seligman identifies five key elements of flourishing summarized by the acronym PERMA [16]:

- *Positive emotions*: Regularly experiencing feelings like joy, gratitude, awe, and love
- *Engagement*: Fully immersing ourselves in activities that engage our strengths
- *Relationships*: Cultivating mutually nourishing connections with others
- *Meaning*: Belonging to and serving something greater than ourselves
- *Achievement*: Accomplishing goals that matter to us

When these five elements are vital, they work synergistically to create upward spirals of well-being and resilience. For instance, meaningful achievements fuel positive emotions, which make us more open to connection.

Researcher Barbara Fredrickson's "broaden-and-build" theory describes how positive emotions expand our awareness and thought-action repertoires at the moment while building enduring physical, intellectual, social, and psychological resources over time [17]. So, small boosts in mood can spark substantial ripple effects for overall vitality.

Sonja Lyubomirsky's work on the "happiness advantage" shows that happiness leads to success more than vice versa [18]. Contrary to the belief that we'll be happy when we're successful, raising our happiness baseline first makes us more productive, creative, and resilient.

But how do we raise that baseline? It's the cumulative effect of small practices and tweaks more than grand gestures. Some science-backed activities include [19]:

- Expressing gratitude
- Savoring positive experiences
- Practicing kindness
- Nurturing relationships

- Exercising and spending time in nature
- Learning new skills
- Contributing to meaningful causes

The more we can build these happiness habits into our daily routines as healers, the more resourced we'll be to sustain our grit and vitality for the marathon of our calling. This isn't about bypassing our natural stresses and sorrows but expanding our capacity to hold it all with grace.

As healers empowered with these tools, we can become what Seligman calls "constructive cavemen" - consciously evolving ourselves and our systems towards greater flourishing even as we grapple with the primal brain structures and instincts that can pull us into scarcity, reactivity and disconnection [20]. This is the hero's journey of our times - to wisely work with both shadow and light in service of a more whole and enlivened world.

The Challenges of Maintaining Vitality in Modern Healthcare

Wallis's energy drains are pervasive in modern healthcare settings, posing significant challenges to sustaining vitality for healers.

Systemic Pressures

Dr. Amitha Kalaichandran speaks to this in a poignant reflection on moral injury in healthcare: "The frenetic pace, the unending electronic health record demands, the pressure to see more patients in less time, and the 'conveyor belt' structure of medicine today are not what many of us imagined when we first aspired to be doctors." [21]

Moral Injury

Dr. Simon Talbot and Dr. Wendy Dean elaborate on the concept of moral injury: "Most physicians enter medicine following a calling rather than a career path. They go into the field with a desire to help people. Many approach it with almost religious zeal, enduring lost sleep, lost years of young adulthood, huge opportunity costs, family strain, financial instability, disregard for personal health, and a multitude of other challenges. Each hurdle offers a lesson in endurance in the service of one's goal, which, starting in the third year of medical school, is sharply focused on ensuring the best care for one's patients. Failing to meet patients' needs consistently profoundly impacts physician wellbeing — this is the crux of consequent moral injury." [22]

Self-Care Challenges

The relentless pressure and isolation many healers face can make finding time for self-care feel impossible. As Dr. Kalaichandran reflects: "Our medical education system frowns upon taking time off for self-care or for honoring familial commitments; the unspoken message being that we must sacrifice everything for our patients." [21]

Administrative Burdens
Rachel Naomi Remen observes: "Everyone in health care is stretched too thin, expected to do too much for too many with too few resources. Many feel frustrated, even defeated, by the need to limit the time and attention they give to others. The pressure to move quickly can cause us to lose touch with the essential human values which drew us to this work." [23]

Crisis of Meaning
Dr. Rana Awdish, author of In Shock, describes her crisis of meaning as a critical care doctor: "There was a time when I questioned whether I would be able to find my way back to this calling that had claimed my heart in childhood. Somehow I had lost my connection to purpose and to my belief in our collective ability to heal." [24]

Pandemic Pressures
Unpredictable but inevitable healthcare crises burden an already stressed healthcare system. The COVID-19 pandemic represents an obvious example of such a crisis. Dr. Victor Dzau, president of the National Academy of Medicine, and colleagues sounded the alarm: "Before the COVID-19 pandemic, the National Academy of Medicine (NAM) sounded the alarm on clinician burnout as a national crisis... Little did we know that the world would soon face a new crisis in COVID-19 that would stretch our health system and clinicians beyond anything we had anticipated." [25]

A Definition of the Vital Healer
The vital healer aligns their actions with a deep sense of purpose, finding sustenance in the sacredness of their calling. They cultivate inner resilience and abundant energy by connecting to the meaning behind their work and letting this fuel their efforts. The vital healer recognizes that true vitality arises not just from physical strength but from the coherence and conviction that come from serving something greater than oneself. By consistently orienting themselves toward their highest aspirations for compassionate service, they tap into a limitless source of grit and grace.

Concluding Remarks
While not always an easy path, dedicated cultivation of vitality, grit, and grace ultimately reconnects us with the sacredness of our calling. In staying true to

our deepest values and humanity, we gradually become, in the words of poet Mary Oliver "a bride married to amazement":

> "When it is over, I don't want to wonder
> if I have made of my life something particular, and real.
> I don't want to find myself sighing and frightened,
> or full of argument.
> I don't want to end up having simply visited this world.
> When it is over, I want to say: all my life
> I was a bride married to amazement." [24]

May we each find and sustain this sense of wonder and amazement as we walk the long and winding road of the bodhisattva healer, one brave and tender step at a time. May we draw strength from the bottomless well of virya to nourish us along the way.

Self-Reflection Questions

As we navigate the noble challenge of the healing path, some key questions can help us stay connected to our deepest source of vitality and grit:

1. What depletes my energy and vitality in my work as a healer? What restores and enhances it?

2. How might I balance both liberating and enlightening energy in my daily life and work?

3. What fears or attachments inhibit me from setting boundaries and caring for my vitality?

4. What courageous, vitality-enhancing actions am I being called to take in my professional life right now?

5. How can I leverage the other paramitas to support the cultivation of wise, compassionate, sustainable virya?

6. What is my deepest aspiration in cultivating virya? What would it mean to devote my life's energy to the welfare of all beings?

7. How can I practice discerning wise, skillful virya in my daily life and work? What does it feel like in my body, heart, and mind when I'm aligned with liberating effort?

References

1. Sadhguru. (2020). 'The Vital Role of a Healer', Isha Blog. .

2. Sadhguru. (2021). 'The Science of Vitality: Harnessing Life Energy', Isha Blog. <https://isha.sadhguru.org/us/en/wisdom/article/science-vitality-harnessing-life-energy> accessed 5 July 2024.

3. Drozdz, A. (2014). 'Greek and Latin Roots of the Word "Energy"', Energies,

7/9: 5888–5896.

4. Poupard, P. G. (ed.) (2005). Dictionary of Religions. Routledge, London.

5. Wright, D. S. (2009). The Six Perfections: Buddhism and the Cultivation of Character. Oxford University Press, Oxford.

6. Zopa, L. (2012). The Six Perfections. Wisdom Publications, Boston.

7. Shantideva. (2006). The Way of the Bodhisattva, P. Sherab and W. Samdup (trans.). Shambhala, Boston.

8. Duckworth, A. L., Peterson, C., Matthews, M. D., and Kelly, D. R. (2007). 'Grit: Perseverance and Passion for Long-Term Goals', Journal of Personality and Social Psychology, 92/6: 1087–1101.

9. Duckworth, A. (2016). Grit: The Power of Passion and Perseverance. Scribner, New York.

10. Bassett, D. (2022). 'The Wisdom of Grit: Balancing Persistence with Discernment', Mindful. <https://www.mindful.org/the-wisdom-of-grit/> accessed 5 July 2024.

11. Hallam, L. (2021). 'The Myth of Noble Suffering in Medicine', The BMJ Opinion. <https://blogs.bmj.com/bmj/2021/09/30/lucy-hallam-the-myth-of-noble-suffering-in-medicine/> accessed 5 July 2024.

12. Greenblatt, E. (2011). 'Stop Burnout: Teach Well', Education Week.

13. James, W. (1907). 'The Energies of Men', Science, 25/635: 321-332.

14. Wallis, C. D. (2021). 'How to Unleash Your Energy: Working with the 11 Blockages', Christopher Wallis. <https://hareesh.org/blog/2021/6/17

15. Csikszentmihalyi, M. (2008). Flow: The Psychology of Optimal Experience. Harper Perennial Modern Classics, New York.

16. Seligman, M. (2011). Flourish: A Visionary New Understanding of Happiness and Well-being. Atria Books, New York.

17. Fredrickson, B. (2001). 'The Role of Positive Emotions in Positive Psychology', The American psychologist, 56: 218-26.

18. Lyubomirsky, S. (2007). The How of Happiness: A New Approach to Getting the Life You Want. Penguin Books, New York.

19. Lyubomirsky, S., and Layous, K. (2013). 'How Do Simple Positive Activities Increase Well-Being?', Current Directions in Psychological Science, 22/1: 57–62.

20. Seligman, M. (2016). Homo Prospectus. Oxford University Press, New York.

21. Kalaichandran, A. (2020). 'Healing the Healers', The Healthscape. <

22. Talbot, S. G., and Dean, W. (2018). 'Physicians Aren't "Burning Out." They're Suffering from Moral Injury', Stat News. <

23. Remen, R. N. (2000). My Grandfather's Blessings: Stories of Strength, Refuge, and Belonging. Riverhead Books, New York.

24. Awdish, R. (2019). In Shock. Picador, New York.

25. Dzau, V. J., Kirch, D., and Nasca, T. (2020). 'Preventing a Parallel Pandemic — A National Strategy to Protect Clinicians' Well-Being', New England Journal of Medicine, 383/6: 513–515.
26. Oliver, M. (2004). 'When Death Comes'. In New and Selected Poems, Volume One. Beacon Press, Boston.

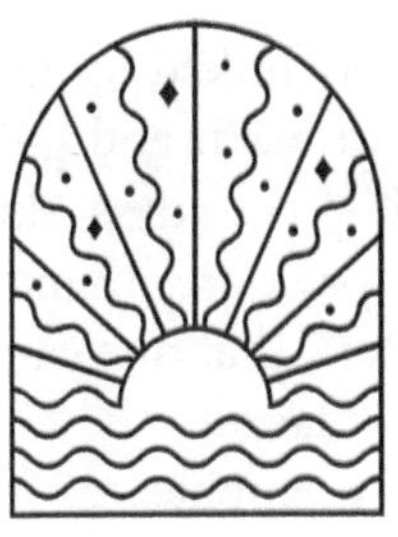

CHAPTER 6

Wise

"Where is the wisdom we have lost in knowledge?
Where is the knowledge we have lost in information?"
T.S. Eliot

Eliot's prescient words resonate deeply in modern medicine, where the explosion of scientific data and technological capability has not necessarily translated into wiser, more compassionate care. Amidst the marvels and hubris of biomedicine, we have perhaps lost sight of the essence of healing - the innate wisdom of the mind and heart.

In Buddhism, this primordial wisdom is known as prajna (Sanskrit) or sherab (Tibetan). Chogyam Trungpa describes sherab as "the knowledge of what is, transcending the object of knowledge as well as the act of knowing."[2] Prajna sees reality directly, without the distortions of conceptual thought. It is intrinsically selfless and panoramic, perceiving the interdependence of all things. And it is the very basis of compassion. As Shantideva wrote in the 8th century, "The perfection of wisdom is the unsurpassable skillful means" to liberate beings from suffering.[3]

Sherab has several key characteristics. It is non-conceptual, going beyond intellectual understanding to direct perception of the true nature of reality. As Trungpa explains, "The essence of sherap is that it is panoramic; it sees

93

the whole situation. It does not discriminate in terms of 'that's good' and 'that's bad.' It is just seeing what is."[2] Sherab is also intrinsically selfless and compassionate. With the wisdom of prajna, one acts skillfully to liberate beings from suffering.

In this way, prajna is closely linked to upaya or "skillful means." Upaya refers to the Buddha's ability to teach and guide beings in whatever way is most effective for them, using countless skillful strategies to lead them out of suffering. Prajna and upaya are inseparable - it is through the non-discriminating insight of wisdom that one can perceive the precise methods to benefit others in any given situation.

Zen teacher Joan Halifax emphasizes this connection: "Prajna is a liberating wisdom that supports compassion and actually allows compassion to be skillful and effective in the world...Upaya, skillful means, is informed by prajna. So there is an intimate relationship between the two - you could call them the two wings of the Dharma."[14]

This notion of wisdom as both insight and means finds its Western parallel in the ancient Greek concepts of sophia and phronesis. Sophia can be understood as the theoretical or intellectual apprehension of what is most valuable in life, while phronesis is the practical ability to apply this understanding to navigate complex real-world situations.[5]

In medicine, phronesis can be seen as clinical judgment guided by both scientific knowledge and an intuitive grasp of the patient's unique context and needs. It is the capacity to move deftly from general principles to the particular case at hand, interpreting data through the lens of human experience. Phronesis allows the clinician to tailor therapies not just to the disease but to the individual in all their messy complexity.

As Roger Walsh notes, "Phronesis involves the ability to see the whole situation with all its nuances. It perceives what is most relevant and important and how things are related."[6] This contextual discernment lies at the heart of medical phronesis. The wise clinician looks beyond symptoms and lab values to appreciate the full tapestry of biological, psychological, social, and existential factors shaping a patient's illness. They bring Sophia's theoretical frameworks into dynamic interplay with the patient's lived reality.

Such phronetic perception demands what Walsh calls "trans-perspectival awareness" and "integrative capacity."[6] The clinician must inhabit multiple vantage points at once—biomedical, personal, cultural, and spiritual— weaving them together to craft a coherent narrative. This cognitive suppleness and meta-perspective are hallmarks of post-conventional reasoning, allowing the practitioner to surf the ambiguities of the clinical encounter with grace.

Phronesis also entails moral skillfulness in promoting the patient's well-being amidst competing ethical claims. The "four principles" of biomedical ethics—autonomy, beneficence, non-maleficence, and justice—offer a valuable scaffold, but applying them wisely to a particular case requires phronetic discernment. Blind adherence to rules cannot substitute for a nuanced appraisal of the individual's values, relationships, and life.

It's important to distinguish prajna from mere knowledge or intellect. "Knowledge is regarded as something good, but it tends to block the way to wisdom...Wisdom allows you to see through knowledge," Trungpa notes.[2] Prajna is a direct, non-dual awareness, where the separation between subject and object falls away. The late Traleg Kyabgon Rinpoche described it as "a flashing forth of the mind, where dualistic thoughts are cut through...not by suppressing or stopping thoughts, but by seeing through them."[15]

This relates to the discriminating aspect of prajna, personified in the image of Manjushri's flaming sword that cuts through ignorance and wrong views. As Pema Chodron explains, "The sword that Manjushri holds is a sword of discriminating wisdom that cuts through delusion clean and sharp and definite..."[16] With prajna, one sees the illusory nature of the conceptual mind and the self, and can sever the root of the afflictive emotions (kleshas) - attachment, aversion, ignorance, pride and envy.

Buddhist teachings describe three levels of prajna:[2]

1. *Mundane wisdom*: This is the accurate perception of conventional reality, understanding the relative truth of how things appear and function. It includes the wisdom to live ethically and skillfully navigate worldly affairs. Trungpa explains, "The first level of sherap is dealing with conventional reality - how we conduct ourselves in the world and associate with people."[2]

2. *Wisdom that transcends worldliness*: At this level, one sees through the illusion of phenomena and realizes their empty, dreamlike nature. It is the wisdom of realizing shunyata (emptiness), going beyond dualistic perceptions. "The second level of wisdom is seeing the illusory nature of the world and transcending that by realizing emptiness, or shunyata," Trungpa writes. "It is seeing the transparency of things as they are. The process of birth, dwelling, and dying becomes transparent so that you begin to discover what is beyond that."[2]

3. *Ultimate wisdom beyond conceptual mind*: The third level of prajna transcends even the notion of dharma or any conceptual framework. It is the complete realization of non-duality, beyond subject and object, self and other. "The third level of wisdom is the realization of non-duality, transcending any kind of conceptualizations, seeing things as they are, beyond conceptions of this and that," describes Trungpa. "At this level, there is a sense of wisdom being so panoramic and so much beyond just

the act of knowing. It is wisdom being the self-arising quality of things as they are."[2, p.266]

The second and third levels of prajna are profoundly connected with compassion. With insight into emptiness and interdependence, one recognizes the non-separation between self and others, giving rise to boundless compassion for all beings. As the Dalai Lama often says, wisdom and compassion are the two wings of the dharma, equally essential for awakening.

"Just as a bird needs two wings to fly in the sky, the wings of wisdom and compassion must be spread to transcend the world of suffering," he explains. "From the perspective of emptiness, compassion arises as the heartfelt experience of the suffering of others. And from the perspective of compassion, emptiness arises as the heartfelt wish to free sentient beings of their suffering. In this way, wisdom and compassion are unified."[17]

Sherab is intimately connected to the other five paramitas - generosity, discipline, patience, exertion, and meditation. In fact, the perfection of wisdom is what infuses the other perfections with the insight and skillful means to truly liberate beings.

As Dilgo Khyentse Rinpoche explains, "True generosity is giving without any attachment or expectation...It is the wisdom of realizing that giver, gift and receiver are inherently empty, that enables us to give freely and purely."[18] With prajna, one sees through the illusion of a separate self who "owns" things, allowing for unconditional generosity.

Similarly, discipline and ethical conduct guided by prajna go beyond rote adherence to precepts. One acts from a place of intuitive wisdom, doing what is most beneficial without clinging to rigid rules. Patience and exertion are sustained by the profound understanding of karma and selflessness, seeing hardships as opportunities for practice rather than obstacles.

Most crucially, sherab develops through and enhances the practice of meditation. "Meditation, when joined with prajna, becomes transcendental wisdom - a state of awareness that can cut through delusion on the spot," writes Trungpa.[2] Deep shamatha (calm-abiding) practice builds the stability and clarity for vipassana (insight) to arise. And the insights of vipassana, in turn, fuel the diligence and inspiration to deepen shamatha.

As B. Alan Wallace notes, "The entire Buddhist tradition, all its various schools, agree that the culmination of the path to awakening is the perfection of wisdom...And what is the method by which this perfection of wisdom is achieved? It is none other than the practice of meditation."[9]

Wallace emphasizes the transformative potential of shamatha and vipashyana: "Shamatha is a contemplative technology for enhancing our attentional stability and vividness, and vipashyana is a means for experientially exploring the nature of the mind and its role in the creation of our experiential reality. Together, these two practices provide a means for achieving genuine wisdom."[10]

In this way, the six paramitas are not separate practices but facets of a unified path to awakening, with sherab as the guiding light that illuminates them all. As we cultivate generosity, discipline, patience, exertion, and meditation with the view of prajna, our actions become increasingly effortless, selfless, and attuned.

Trungpa beautifully summarizes this: "When we talk of the paramitas and the mahayana path, we are talking of the realization of wisdom as it applies to every activity of our life...Sherap is panoramic - the realization of wisdom and skillful means, prajna and upaya...It requires a sense of fearlessness, a sense of leaping, a sense of going forward without reference point."[2, p.269]

Cultivating prajna in modern healthcare settings organized around scientific materialism poses challenges. The Dalai Lama notes, "If science and technology are led by wisdom and compassion, they will be tools for humanity's peace and wellbeing. Without wisdom, they become a high-tech version of ego-gratification."[19] The values of efficiency and objectivity can overshadow care and connection. Phronesis is needed to unite technical knowledge with human insight.

As an example, consider a case where respecting a patient's autonomy by providing complete diagnostic information might cause terrible anxiety and despair, worsening their condition. A phronetic clinician would sensitively explore the patient's preferences around disclosure, their support system and coping resources, the likely trajectory of disease, and the potential for other therapeutic approaches. They would work to uphold the spirit of informed consent while finding skillful means to minimize harm - perhaps staging difficult conversations or enhancing the patient's resilience and sense of meaning first.

In another common scenario, the phronetic physician caring for a patient with a complex chronic illness must artfully balance the benefits and burdens of treatment. Simply following algorithms or fixating on disease markers is not enough; the clinician must enter the patient's world to understand their goals, fears, and tolerances. What are the daily activities and relationships that bring this person joy and purpose? What level of symptom control or functional status would allow them to meaningfully participate in these? How do their cultural and spiritual beliefs shape their experience of illness and the end of life? Guided by such insight, the practitioner can craft a care plan that aligns medical possibilities with the patient's own values and priorities.

A phronetic approach is also essential in delivering culturally competent and humble care. The practitioner must be aware of their own biases and knowledge limits while respectfully engaging with the patient's explanatory frameworks. In many traditional healing systems, illness signifies imbalance or disruption not just in the body but in the family and community. The phronetic clinician works to understand and address suffering at multiple levels, drawing on the patient's own resources of meaning and connection. This may involve flexibly integrating allopathic treatments with Indigenous or folk practices, or working with community leaders and healers to repair ruptured social bonds.

Ultimately, by wedding technical knowledge with contextual wisdom, phronesis allows the clinician to deploy their skills and tools not as end in themselves but in service of the patient's integral flourishing. It is an antidote to what Einstein warned was "the only thing more dangerous than ignorance" - arrogance.[7] In Tibetan Buddhist vision, the union of wisdom and compassion is symbolized by Avalokiteshvara's thousand arms, each bearing an eye in its palm.[8] Joined with prajna's clear-sight and fierce warmth, enlightened action flows forth spontaneously to meet suffering.

True phronesis in medicine thus demands cultivation of one's own wisdom and humanity - embarking on what Walsh calls the healer's journey "from expertise to wisdom."[6] This path of deepening insight and care has been followed by healers across cultures and ages. The "Bird Men" of the Andes, the Sangomas of Africa, the Daoist sages and Tibetan amchis all point to a perennial stream of wisdom as old as our species' capacity for compassion.

In their healing arts, proficiency in herbalism or bone-setting is indivisible from ethical and spiritual development. One becomes an "elder" or "medicine person" not just through technical training but through inner transformation - the progressive attenuation of ego, the ability to presence suffering, and communion with subtle forces of nature and spirit.[20] In apprenticing to these lineages, the modern clinician has an opportunity to reconnect medical science with its primordial roots in the sacred.

A Healer's Journey Into Wisdom

"To understand the phenomenal world, you must be initiated in higher sense-perception which is activated by meditation. Experiencing higher sense-perception in meditation, you find that everything is a reflection of the Absolute." - Swami Rama

My own journey on the healer's path began 20 years ago with a Kornfeld Fellowship that supported travel in search of medical wisdom. From sterilized academic towers to the Peruvian Amazon, from Chinese temples to the mountains of Dharamsala, I encountered profound repositories of "medicine earth" - embodied, relational, spiritual approaches to healing much older than modern biomedicine.

In the high Andes, I met the "Bird People" or Paq'os who practice a mystical art of transmuting sorcery into blessings through the power of their mesa - a portable altar crafted over many painstaking rituals.[21] The mesa becomes a map of inner and outer sacred landscapes, with kuyas (stones) carefully gathered from power places. By aligning these forces through song, invocation, and gestures, the paq'o helps restore balance between the patient, community, and cosmos.

Deep in the Amazon, an ayahuasquero shaman explained that illness was often due to damage to the animistic life energy or Sami shared by all beings. By entering non-ordinary states through the ayahuasca brew, he could journey to retrieve lost soul fragments dislodged by trauma or black magic. He taught me to see the body as a condensation of Spirit and healing as a process of remembering our fundamental unity with Source.

At the feet of a Tibetan lama-physician, I learned about the intricate correspondences between bodily humors and the five elements, the seasons, and the Buddha-dynamics of 'wholeness seeking itself.' Pulse and urine diagnosis were refined perceptual arts for detecting the play of these archetypal forces. Treatment aimed at restoring the innate equipoise or "gnostic balance" that reflects our awakened nature. "When the lamp of wisdom shines, even impure water appears as a Buddha realm," the lama would say, transmitting the view that our ultimate healing lies in recognizing the pure, intangible dimension of being.[22]

With a 30th-generation Daoist master, I studied the flow of qi through the "dragon paths" of the meridians. In qigong practice, one aligns body, breath, and mind in an unobstructed circuit, becoming a microcosmic reflection of primal forces of heaven and earth, yin and yang. Pathology arises from disconnection from the Dao - literally "the Way" - of dynamic harmony between organism and environment. The Daoist physician's role is to help the patient realign with natural rhythms and source in the generative ocean of qi.[23]

In the dusty villages of Africa, I took dream mushrooms and watched an igqirha or sangoma divine the ancestral origins of our maladies by casting bones, cowrie shells, and other "muti." Dancing and drumming into trance, possessed by helping spirits, they uprooted sickness by repairing our belonging to a living cosmology where "the dead are not under the earth, they are in the rustling tree," as Birago Diop's famous poem declared.[13]

As we begin incorporating these lived teachings into our clinical practice, we discover they recenter healing in the mysterious matrix of meaning, connection, and consciousness shared by patients, healers, and the world. Biomedical interventions become just one facet of a holistic response to suffering that also addresses psychospiritual, cultural, and existential dimensions. The healer's task was not just to "fix" but to "heal" in its etymological sense of "making whole" - helping restore intimacy with self, others, nature, and the numinous.

Such profound "re-membering" requires that clinicians risk vulnerability by bringing their whole selves into authentic therapeutic relationships. It asks us to expand our identities beyond white-coated experts to include the archetypes of wounded healer, mystic, shaman, and spiritual friend. By honoring illness as an initiation and healer as a fellow journeyer, we create sacred clinical spaces for deep inquiry, emotional processing, ritual, and meaning-making. Our medical technologies then find their place within the larger project of midwifing psychospiritual growth and transformation.

Ultimately, by marrying the genius of science with the wisdom of traditional healer lineages, we can craft an integral medicine that is truly adequate to the beauty, pathos, and mystery of the human condition. This perennial healing impulse, as old as our species, sees through dualistic illusions of separation to our fundamental interbeing. It knows that recognizing non-dual awareness is the ultimate medicine and that love and truth-telling are the enduring foundations of the healing arts. May we have the courage and humility to be worthy stewards of this precious inheritance.

Ultimately, prajna develops through practice - the experiential wisdom that comes from training the mind through meditation and integrating the teachings in life. "Prajna is not accomplished by thinking about it, but by directly undertaking the training that clear away the obstacles to panoramic awareness," writes Judy Lief.[24] With diligent effort in cultivating the paramitas and resting in non-dual awareness, the innate wisdom of the mind naturally shines forth.

Based on the insights of this essay, the wise healer can be defined as one who embodies the integration of scientific knowledge, contextual discernment, moral skillfulness, and transpersonal wisdom in service of the integral flourishing of those they serve. The wise healer sees through conceptual dualities to the fundamental interconnectedness and sacred nature of life, and works to catalyze wholeness and awakening through the vehicle of the therapeutic relationship.

A Definition of the Wise Healer

The wise healer maintains a clear, discerning awareness that sees beyond surface phenomena to the deeper reality of interconnectedness. With a flexible, open mind, they integrate diverse knowledge systems—scientific, cultural, and spiritual—to meet the unique needs of each patient. By embodying this integration of wisdom and skill in service of others, the wise healer becomes a catalyst for wholeness and a guide for navigating life's fundamental questions.

Self-Reflection Questions
1.When do I feel most connected to innate wisdom in my work? What supports that connection?
2. How can I balance knowledge and expertise with openness, not-knowing, and a "beginner's mind"?
3. How can I step back to see the bigger picture with clarity and compassion in challenging situations with patients or colleagues?
4. How can my work itself become a practice for cultivating wisdom - through mindful attention, caring presence, and letting go of ego?
5. What contemplative practices and self-care restore my balance and presence, allowing wisdom to surface?
6. What is the deeper meaning and purpose of my work as a healer? In what way am I serving the liberation and full flourishing of my patients?

References:
1. Eliot, T.S. (1934). The Rock.
2. Trungpa, C. (2013). The Profound Treasury of the Ocean of Dharma (Vol. 2). Shambhala Publications.
3. Shantideva. (2006). The Way of the Bodhisattva. Shambhala.
4. Halifax, J. (2018). Standing at the Edge: Finding Freedom Where Fear and Courage Meet. Flatiron Books.
5. Rooney, D., McKenna, B., & Liesch, P. (2010). Wisdom and Management in the Knowledge Economy. Routledge.
6. Walsh, R. (2015). "Wise Ways of Seeing: Wisdom and Perspectives." Integral Review, 11(2).
7. Isaacson, W. (2007). Einstein: His Life and Universe. Simon & Schuster.
8. Thurman, R. (1997). Essential Tibetan Buddhism. Castle Books.
9. Wallace, B. A. (2008). Embracing Mind: The Common Ground of Science and Spirituality. Shambhala.
10. Wallace, B. A. (2011). Minding Closely: The Four Applications of Mindfulness. Shambhala.
11. Abram, D. (1996). The Spell of the Sensuous: Perception and Language in a More-Than-Human World. Vintage.
12. Diop, B. (1960). "Souffles." Translated by Ulli Beier.
13. Wright, D. (2013). "Wisdom and Compassion as Medical Virtues." Handbook of Virtue Ethics in Business and Management.
14. Halifax, J. (2018). Standing at the Edge: Finding Freedom Where Fear and Courage Meet. Flatiron Books.
15. Kyabgon, T. (2003). The Benevolent Mind: A Manual in Mind Training. Zhyisil Chokyi Ghatsal Publications.
16. Chodron, P. (2010). The Three Commitments: Working with the Paramitas.

Shambhala Sun, Sept 2010.

17. Dalai Lama. (2019). The Heart of Meditation: Discovering Innermost Awareness. Shambhala.

18. Khyentse, D. (2007). The Heart of Compassion: The Thirty-seven Verses on the Practice of a Bodhisattva. Shambhala.

19. Dalai Lama. (2012). Our Human Potential: The Unassailable Path of Love, Compassion, and Wisdom. Shambhala.

20. Abram, D. (1996). The Spell of the Sensuous: Perception and Language in a More-Than-Human World. Vintage.

21. Wilcox, J. (2004). Masters of the Living Energy: The Mystical World of the Q'ero of Peru. Inner Traditions.

22. Clifford, T. (1994). Tibetan Buddhist Medicine and Psychiatry: The Diamond Healing. Motilal Banarsidass.

23. Ni, M. (1995). The Yellow Emperor's Classic of Medicine: A New Translation of the Neijing Suwen with Commentary. Shambhala.

24. Lief, J. (2014). What Is Prajna? Lion's Roar, June 2014.

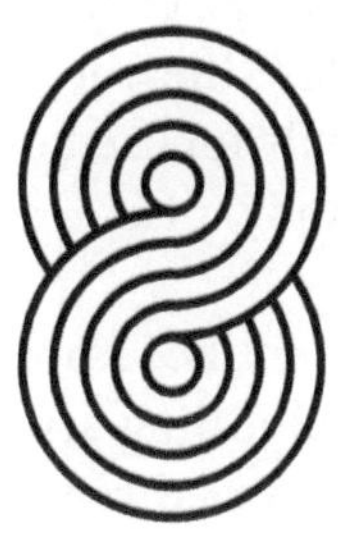

CHAPTER 7

Intelligent

"Man is so intelligent that he feels impelled to invent theories to
account for what happens in the world. Unfortunately,
he is not quite intelligent enough, in most cases, to find correct
explanations. So that when he acts on his theories,
he behaves very often like a lunatic."
Aldous Huxley

*M*odern healers are typically considered to be very "intelligent". Indeed, since their lives are literally in the hands of their healers, patients are eager to experience their healers as being intelligent. Although the word "intelligence" is used very frequently, the concept of intelligence has long been debated and defined in different ways. The term "intelligence" derives from the Latin verb intelligere, meaning "to understand". In modern times, intelligence is often defined as the capacity for logic, understanding, self-awareness, learning, emotional knowledge, reasoning, planning, creativity, critical thinking, and problem-solving. [1]

Traditional Views of Healer Intelligence
In the healing professions, intelligence is traditionally associated with cognitive abilities and the mastery of a large body of factual knowledge. Entry

into professional healthcare schools is usually determined by applicants demonstrating their intelligence through strong academic performance and high scores on standardized tests like the MCAT, which assesses logical reasoning, problem-solving, critical thinking, and knowledge of scientific concepts and principles. The curricula of medical and healthcare training programs are then heavily focused on learning extensive fact-based knowledge about the human body, diseases, pharmacology, clinical skills, and procedures. [2]

While this fact-based scientific knowledge provides an essential foundation for medicine and the healing arts, it represents only one facet of the healer's intelligence. The renowned physician William Osler recognized the limitations of a solely fact-based education, stating: "Man cannot live on facts alone, and after all, the real problems are human - those of a man's relation to his family, his profession, and his community - and for these facts alone do not suffice. He must learn wisdom. For wisdom is the knowledge of how to use knowledge." [3]

A broader context and additional intellectual capacities are needed to understand and treat human suffering effectively. As [reference] discusses, medicine's emphasis on "educating the head" needs to be balanced and augmented with "educating the heart and the hand." Factual knowledge alone, no matter how extensive, is insufficient. The intelligence of the master healer must encompass other aptitudes and understandings beyond cognitive brilliance in order to compassionately and intuitively care for the whole person in body, mind, and spirit.

Intelligence and Ancient Healing Traditions
Ancient wisdom traditions have long described a more expansive view of the healer's intelligence. The Tibetan knowledge holder Jampa Yonten explains: "Intelligence in Tibetan medicine does not mean being clever in an academic sense, but refers to a quality of open and unobstructed clarity that is able to engage any situation in a fresh way. Although learning is important, true intelligence comes down to an innate ability to see what needs to be done in any situation." [4]

Jampa Yonten further elaborates: "The first chapter of the Gyurmed (Blue Beryl) outlines the ten special qualities of the physician, the first being intelligence. It states: 'Examine very well the physician who possesses intelligence. If you wonder how the intelligent physician should be, the physician who has heard much, contemplated much, and has much experience is described as intelligent. Moreover, a physician needs intelligence that realizes how to proceed when treating a patient.'" [4]

In the Tibetan medical tradition, the physician's intelligence arises from deep study, contemplation, and extensive clinical experience. But beyond that, it is an innate capacity to see clearly, without obstruction or preconception, and to directly know the right way to proceed in treating each individual patient in their unique situation. This is a more vast and intuitive intelligence that transcends the merely conceptual or procedural. The essential Tibetan medical text, the Four Tantras (Gyurmed), portrays the ideal qualities of the physician, emphasizing intuition, compassion, and perceptiveness in addition to knowledge and technical skills. Translators describe it as outlining "the special intelligence and insight of the physician who sees the patient as an integral entity, an understanding that integrates analytical knowledge and intuitive wisdom." [5]

Similarly, the foundational Chinese medical classic, the Huangdi Neijing (Yellow Emperor's Inner Classic), portrays the exemplary physician as possessing unique wisdom and insight into the deepest principles of nature and the human condition. The great physician Sun Simiao wrote extensively about the importance of the doctor's "virtue" and their medical insight. Translator Sabine Wilms explains:

"All of Sūn Sīmiǎo's writings exhibit a concern with the moral requirements for being a good physician that goes far beyond the mere perfunctory statement... At the very foundation of his vision lies a sincere commitment to being a good person and thereby earning the moral authority to effectively practice medicine." [6]

In the Ayurvedic tradition of India, the true vaidya (physician) is portrayed as a great seer and knower of reality. Beyond just mastering the medical texts and techniques, the vaidya must possess prajna (higher wisdom and insight), karuna (compassion), and sadhana (dedicated spiritual practice). As author Robert Svoboda describes: "The wisdom that the Ayurvedic doctor requires is that which gives insight into the whole of life, which reveals the physician's kinship with the patient as a fellow human being, as well as his or her unique clinical situation." [7]

Phronesis and Practical Wisdom

This concept of practical wisdom that integrates knowledge, experience and intuitive insight has been termed "phronesis." Phronesis was a core concept in ancient Greek philosophy, with Aristotle describing it as the virtue of practical thought and the ability to discern modes of action regarding things that are good or bad for humans.

In healthcare, phronesis has been defined as "the ability to discern the right thing to do in the right way at the right time, balancing knowledge, skill, and intuition in the care of each unique patient and clinical situation." [8] It requires not just factual knowledge but perceptiveness, sound judgment, and situational awareness. Philosopher Ian Kerridge describes phronesis as "the accumulated wisdom of the clinician that can be used to reach conclusions, make decisions and take actions in the context-specific circumstances of each clinical interaction." [9]

Integral Theory and Multiple Intelligences
Modern Integral theory, as developed by philosopher Ken Wilber, posits that human intelligence is not a single general capacity but involves multiple interdependent aptitudes or "lines of intelligence." [10] In addition to the cognitive line that IQ tests attempt to measure, these include:

- *Emotional intelligence*: The ability to recognize and regulate emotions in oneself and others
- *Moral intelligence*: The capacity to discern right from wrong and act ethically
- *Intuitive intelligence*: Access to inner knowing and guidance beyond the rational mind
- *Kinesthetic intelligence*: Skillful use of the body and refined sensory awareness
- *Interpersonal intelligence*: Relational skills, empathy, and ability to communicate effectively
- *Spiritual intelligence*: Awareness of ultimate meanings, values, and transcendent realities

Cognitive intelligence alone is insufficient for the healer. Emotional and interpersonal intelligence are vital for empathy, attunement, and therapeutic rapport. Moral and spiritual intelligence provide an ethical foundation, intuitive wisdom, and access to transpersonal resources. Kinesthetic intelligence allows for the skillful use of the hands and body in diagnosis and treatment.

Psychologist Robert Sternberg has proposed a "triarchic theory" of intelligence encompassing three main aspects: [11]

1. *Analytical intelligence* - the ability to complete academic, problem-solving tasks, such as those used in traditional intelligence tests. This corresponds to cognitive or rational intelligence.
2. *Creative intelligence* - the ability to deal with new situations using past experiences and current skills. This aspect of intelligence is related to intuition, imagination and innovation.
3. *Practical intelligence* - the ability that individuals use to solve real-world problems. Practical intelligence involves adapting to, shaping,

and selecting environments in order to accomplish goals and handle challenges. This relates to phronesis or practical wisdom.

For the healer, cultivating and integrating all three of these intelligences - analytical, creative, and practical - is key to therapeutic mastery and effective care.

Limitations of Cognitive Intelligence
While cognitive intelligence and factual knowledge provide an essential foundation for the healer, an overemphasis on this type of intelligence has significant limitations. A solely fact-based education does not adequately prepare clinicians for the real-world complexities and ambiguities of clinical practice. As physician and educator Rachel Remen states:

"Fact-based curricula emphasize the acquisition of information and skill...but provide little opportunity to use this information in the care of sick people. These curricula focus on mastery of the science and technology of medicine but give limited attention to the paradoxical mix of technical and humanistic demands inherent in the actual practice of medicine. They... largely ignore the issues that result from genuine connection to sick people and their families: issues of meaning, perspective, relationship, responsibility, commitment and service." [12]

Cognitive intelligence, for all its importance, can also promote a detached, objectifying stance that neglects the subjective experience of the patient. Overvaluing analytical intelligence can lead to a reductionistic view that fails to apprehend the whole person. As author Victoria Sweet cautions, "Doctors can get so caught up in the details of the body that they forget the person who inhabits it." [13] A more holistic, multidimensional intelligence is needed to truly see and respond to the unique individual seeking care.

An excess of information without the wisdom to apply it appropriately can also result in problems of overdiagnosis and overtreatment. Physician and epidemiologist H. Gilbert Welch warns that modern medicine's ever-expanding knowledge base and sophisticated technologies have led us to detect and treat "abnormalities" of unclear significance, sometimes causing more harm than good. [14] Discernment and good judgment, born of experience and sound reasoning, are needed to utilize medical knowledge judiciously.

"Artificial" Intelligence and the Future of Medicine
The increasing use of artificial intelligence and machine learning in healthcare is likely to further highlight the limitations of cognitive intelligence alone. AI systems are already able to rapidly process and analyze vast amounts of medical data, assist in diagnosis, and guide evidence-based treatment decisions. [15]

In the future, much of the fact-based knowledge that has traditionally defined the physician's expertise may be readily accessible through AI.

While AI may augment and even surpass human cognitive intelligence in medicine, it is unlikely to replace the other vital intelligences of the healer in the foreseeable future. AI lacks the emotional and relational intelligence to provide true empathy, compassion, and human connection. It does not possess the moral intelligence and ethical reasoning to navigate complex dilemmas and value-based decisions. It has no access to the intuitive wisdom and insights that often guide master clinicians. It cannot match the dexterity, embodied awareness and "touch" of human hands.

As AI assumes more of the cognitive load in medicine, the other intelligences of the healer will become increasingly important and differentiating. Healers will need to cultivate their uniquely human capacities - their emotional, relational, intuitive, somatic and spiritual intelligences. They must grow in the phronesis and practical wisdom born of experience, reflection, and sound judgment. While embracing the power of artificial intelligence, they must remember that "No healing system that has endured over millennia was based on anything but the healing power of love in action." [16] In an age of AI, it is the healer's Heart that will matter most.

A Definition of "The Intelligent Healer"
"The intelligent healer embodies a multidimensional intelligence that integrates cognitive, emotional, intuitive, relational, somatic, moral, and spiritual capacities to understand and alleviate human suffering. Beyond mastering an extensive base of medical knowledge and technical skills, the truly intelligent healer cultivates wisdom, insight, discernment, compassion, presence, and heart."

Concluding Remarks
In summary, the intelligence of the healer can ultimately be defined as a multidimensional capacity, rooted in cognitive knowledge and skill but encompassing wisdom, insight, discernment, compassion, phronesis, intuition and heart. It is an expansive understanding that weds the knowledge of the head with the wisdom of the heart and the skillful action of the hands to relieve suffering and enhance wholeness. This fuller spectrum of the healer's intelligence has been recognized across time and culture as essential for mastering and effectively practicing the healing arts.

As Paracelsus, the great 16th-century physician and alchemist, declared: "Medicine is not only a science; it is also an art. It does not consist of compounding pills and plasters; it deals with the very processes of life, which must be understood before they may be guided." [17]

To guide the processes of life and death, to minister to body and being in all their intricacy, the healer must bring the whole of their humanity - mind, heart, and hands. They must be, in the words of Hippocrates, "philosophers in medicine," [18] wedding rigorous study to seasoned wisdom, precision to compassion, expertise to humility, competence to caring. For it is in this union of science and art, knowledge and wisdom, head and heart, that true healing intelligence resides.

Self-Reflection Questions

1. How do I balance my cognitive intelligence with other forms of intelligence in my healing practice?

2. How do I cultivate and utilize intuition in my clinical decision-making process?

3. How do I integrate analytical, creative, and practical intelligence into my patient care approach?

4. To what extent do I recognize and develop my interpersonal and intrapersonal intelligence in my healing work?

5. How do I incorporate bodily-kinesthetic intelligence and embodied awareness in my practice?

6. In what ways do I nurture my moral and spiritual intelligence to support my role as a healer?

7. How do I reconcile the emphasis on factual knowledge in my training with the need for wisdom and practical judgment (phronesis) in clinical situations?

8. To what extent do I embody the qualities of intelligence described in traditional healing systems (e.g., Tibetan, Chinese, or Ayurvedic medicine)?

9. How do I cultivate the ability to see each patient as unique and respond with fresh, unobstructed clarity?

10. How can I further develop my capacity for compassion, insight, and perceptiveness to complement my technical skills and knowledge?

References

1. Legg, S., & Hutter, M. (2007). A collection of definitions of intelligence. Frontiers in Artificial Intelligence and Applications, 157, 17.

2. Cooke, M., Irby, D. M., Sullivan, W., & Ludmerer, K. M. (2006). American medical education 100 years after the Flexner report. New England Journal of Medicine, 355(13), 1339-1344.

3. Osler, W. (1907). The reserves of life. St Mary's Hospital Gazette 13:95-8

4. Weaner, K. (2019). The Gift of Jampa Yonten. Lion's Roar, July 2019.

5. Desi, Y. (2017). Foreword. In Desi Sangye Gyatso, Mirror of Beryl. Boston: Simon & Schuster.

6. Wilms, S. (2014). Introduction. In Sūn Sīmiǎo, Bei Ji Qian Jin Yao Fang

(Vol. 2). NY: Happy Goat Productions.

7. Svoboda, R. (2004). Ayurveda: Life, Health and Longevity. London: Penguin.

8. Kaldjian, L. C. (2014). Practicing medicine and ethics: integrating wisdom, conscience, and goals of care. Cambridge University Press.

9. Kerridge, I. (2011). Ethics and EBM: acknowledging bias, accepting difference and embracing politics. Journal of evaluation in clinical practice, 17(5), 939-940.

10. Wilber, K. (2000). Integral Psychology. Boston: Shambhala.

11. Sternberg, R. J. (1997). The triarchic theory of intelligence. In D. P. Flanagan, J. L. Genshaft, & P. L. Harrison (Eds.), Contemporary intellectual assessment: Theories, tests, and issues (pp. 92–104). New York: Guilford Press

12. Remen, R. N. (2001). Recapturing the soul of medicine: physicians need to reclaim meaning in their working lives. Western Journal of Medicine, 174(1), 4.

13. Sweet, V. (2012). God's hotel: a doctor, a hospital, and a pilgrimage to the heart of medicine. Penguin.

14. Welch, H. G., Schwartz, L., & Woloshin, S. (2011). Overdiagnosed: making people sick in the pursuit of health. Beacon Press.

15. Topol, E. J.15. Topol, E. J. (2019). High-performance medicine: the convergence of human and artificial intelligence. Nature Medicine, 25(1), 44-56.

16. Chopra, D. (2015). The Future of God: A practical approach to spirituality for our times. Harmony.

17. Pachter, H. M. (1951). Magic into Science: The Story of Paracelsus. Henry Schuman.

18. Marketos, S. G., & Skiadas, P. (1999). The modern Hippocratic tradition. Some messages for contemporary medicine. Spine, 24(11), 1159.

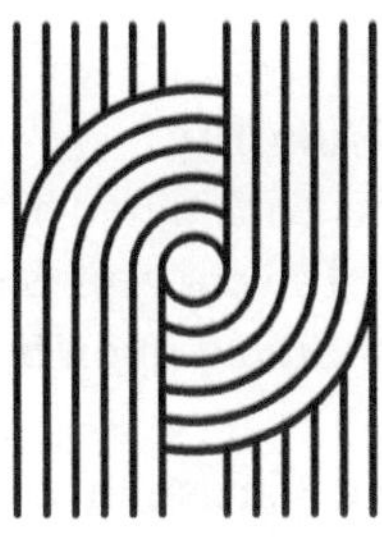

CHAPTER 8

Humble

"Do you wish to rise? Begin by descending.
You plan a tower that will pierce the clouds?
Lay first the foundation of humility."
Saint Augustine

The word "humility" has its roots in the Latin word "humilitas," which itself is derived from "humus," meaning "ground" or "earth" [1]. This etymology provides a profound insight into the nature of humility, suggesting that it is about being grounded, down-to-earth, and connected to our foundational nature.

Humility can be defined as having a modest view of one's importance, acknowledging one's limitations and imperfections, and being open to learning from others and experiences [2]. It involves a realistic appraisal of our abilities and achievements without undervaluing or overvaluing them.

In psychological literature, humility is often described as a multi-faceted construct that includes:

a. An accurate assessment of one's abilities and achievements
b. The ability to acknowledge one's mistakes and limitations
c. Openness to new ideas, contradictory information, and advice

111

d.   Keeping one's abilities and accomplishments in perspective
e.   A relatively low self-focus or an ability to "forget the self."
f.   An appreciation of the value of all things, including the contributions of others [3]

Judeo-Christian Concepts of Humility

In Christian theology, humility is considered a central virtue, often seen as the foundation for all other virtues. The concept is deeply rooted in the teachings of Jesus Christ and has been elaborated upon by numerous Christian thinkers throughout history.

One of the most profound Christian concepts related to humility is kenosis. Derived from the Greek word κένωσις, meaning "emptying," kenosis refers to the self-emptying of one's own will and becoming entirely receptive to God's divine will [31]. This concept is exemplified in Philippians 2:5-8, which describes Christ's humility in becoming human: "Have this mind among yourselves, which is yours in Christ Jesus, who, though he was in the form of God, did not count equality with God a thing to be grasped, but emptied himself, by taking the form of a servant, being born in the likeness of men." [32]

Mother Teresa, known for her humble service to the poor, often spoke about the importance of humility in Christian life: "If you are humble nothing will touch you, neither praise nor disgrace, because you know what you are. If you are blamed you will not be discouraged. If they call you a saint, you will not put yourself on a pedestal." [33]

Thomas Merton, a Trappist monk and influential spiritual writer, emphasized the transformative power of humility: "Pride makes us artificial and humility makes us real." [34] He further elaborated: "A humble man is not afraid of failure. In fact, he is not afraid of anything, even of himself, since perfect humility implies perfect confidence in the power of God before Whom no other power has any meaning and for Whom there is no such thing as an obstacle." [35]

The biblical story of Job provides a profound exploration of humility in the face of suffering. Despite losing everything - his wealth, children, and health - Job maintains faith and humility before God. His story illustrates that true humility involves accepting both blessings and hardships with grace, recognizing that our understanding is limited compared to God's wisdom [36].

Job's humility is powerfully expressed in his response to God: "I know that you can do all things, and that no purpose of yours can be thwarted. 'Who is this that hides counsel without knowledge?' Therefore I have uttered what I did not understand, things too wonderful for me, which I did not know." (Job 42:2-3) [37]

Job's humility ultimately shapes his experience of suffering, allowing him to find meaning and growth through his trials rather than being consumed by bitterness or despair.

The Concept of Humility in Daoism and Buddhism

In Eastern philosophies such as Daoism and Buddhism, humility is regarded as a fundamental virtue and a path to enlightenment. These traditions emphasize the importance of releasing ego attachments and recognizing the interconnectedness of all beings.

In Daoism, humility is closely tied to the concept of wu wei, or "non-action." This doesn't mean inertia but rather acting in accordance with the natural flow of the Dao without forcing or striving [4]. Jason Gregory, author of "Fasting the Mind," explains, "In Daoism, humility is seen as a natural expression of living in harmony with the Dao. It's about recognizing that we are part of a greater whole, rather than separate, superior entities" [5].

The Daoist classic, Tao Te Ching, frequently emphasizes humility:
"The highest virtue is like water.
Water benefits all things and does not compete.
It stays in lowly places that others reject.
This is why it is so similar to the Dao." [6]

In Buddhism, humility is considered essential for spiritual growth. The Buddhist concept of anatta, or "non-self," teaches that there is no permanent, unchanging self, which naturally leads to a humble perspective [7]. The Dalai Lama often speaks about the importance of humility in Buddhist practice: "The whole purpose of religion is to facilitate love and compassion, patience, tolerance, humility, and forgiveness" [8].

Jack Kornfield, a prominent Buddhist teacher, emphasizes the transformative power of humility: "True humility is not thinking less of yourself; it is thinking of yourself less" [9]. This perspective aligns with the Buddhist practice of cultivating bodhicitta, or the altruistic intention to attain enlightenment for the benefit of all beings [10].

The Nature of Arrogance and Pride

Arrogance, derived from the Latin "arrogare," meaning "to claim for oneself," is characterized by an exaggerated sense of one's importance or abilities [11]. Pride, from the Old English "pryde," related to "proud," similarly involves an inflated self-perception [12].

Arrogance can be seen as a form of ignorance because it prevents individuals from recognizing their limitations and learning from others. It creates a closed mindset that hinders personal growth and understanding. Albert Einstein wisely noted, "The more I learn, the more I realize how much I don't know" [13].

An anonymous quote aptly captures the relationship between confidence, compassion, and humility: "Self-confidence is very important. But without compassion and humility, it's just arrogance" [14]. This highlights the fine line between healthy self-esteem and arrogance, emphasizing the importance of balancing self-confidence with humility and compassion.

It's crucial to distinguish between humility and shame. While shame involves a negative self-perception and often leads to withdrawal and self-doubt, humility is about having an accurate and balanced view of oneself [15]. Humility is not disempowering; instead, it empowers individuals to grow and learn continuously.

Respect and reverence are closely linked to humility. When we approach life with humility, we naturally develop a more profound respect for others and reverence for the mysteries of existence [16]. This attitude fosters better relationships, deeper understanding, and a more harmonious society.

Unfortunately, humility is often misconstrued as a weakness in many competitive educational environments, including those for healthcare professionals. This misconception can lead to a culture that values individual achievement over collaborative learning and growth [17]. Such environments may inadvertently promote arrogance and hinder the development of essential qualities like empathy and teamwork.

In contrast, the Japanese concept of "Kenkyo" emphasizes modesty and humility to support social cohesion [18]. This cultural value recognizes that true strength acknowledges our interconnectedness and mutual dependence. Kenkyo encourages individuals to consider the collective good and interact with others to maintain harmony and respect.

Modern Education and the Risk of Arrogance

Modern education systems prioritizing the acquisition of facts over the development of wisdom can inadvertently foster arrogance. When knowledge is treated as a commodity to be possessed rather than a journey to be undertaken, it can lead to a false sense of mastery and superiority [19]. This issue is particularly prevalent in fields that require extensive memorization of facts, such as medicine. Students may develop a sense of superiority based on their ability to recall large amounts of information without necessarily developing the wisdom to apply this knowledge effectively or the humility to recognize the limits of their understanding [20].

A crucial shift in educational philosophy is needed to counteract this tendency towards arrogance. Instead of focusing solely on having the correct answers, education should emphasize the importance of asking good questions. As the philosopher Karl Popper stated, "The more we learn about the world, and the deeper our learning, the more conscious, specific, and articulate will be our knowledge of what we do not know, our knowledge of our ignorance" [46]. This approach aligns with the Socratic method, emphasizing inquiry and dialogue over rote learning. We can foster a sense of intellectual humility by encouraging students to question their assumptions, explore different perspectives, and engage in critical thinking [47].

Moreover, embracing uncertainty and acknowledging the limits of human knowledge can paradoxically lead to greater wisdom. As the physicist Richard Feynman famously said, "I think it's much more interesting to live not knowing than to have answers which might be wrong" [48].

To counter the risk of arrogance, educational systems should incorporate:

a. Critical thinking skills that encourage students to question their assumptions and biases
b. Experiential learning that exposes students to real-world complexities and uncertainties
c. Reflective practices that promote self-awareness and personal growth
d. Collaborative learning environments that emphasize teamwork and mutual respect
e. Exposure to diverse perspectives and cultures to broaden understanding and foster empathy [21]
f. An emphasis on the process of inquiry rather than just the acquisition of facts
g. Recognition and celebration of intellectual humility as a strength rather than a weakness

By fostering an educational culture that values curiosity, open-mindedness, and intellectual humility, we can better prepare students to navigate the complexities of the modern world and approach their roles as professionals and citizens with wisdom and compassion.

The Psychology of Humility

From a psychological perspective, humility is a complex construct that has gained increasing attention in recent years, particularly within the field of positive psychology.

June Price Tangney, a leading researcher in this area, defines humility as a multifaceted construct involving:

a.   An accurate assessment of one's abilities and achievements
b.   The ability to acknowledge one's mistakes and limitations
c.   Openness to new ideas, contradictory information, and advice
d.   Keeping one's abilities and accomplishments in perspective
e.   A relatively low self-focus
f.   An appreciation of the value of all things, including the contributions of others [38]

Positive psychology, which focuses on the strengths that enable individuals and communities to thrive, has identified humility as a key character strength. In their seminal work "Character Strengths and Virtues," Christopher Peterson and Martin Seligman classify humility under the virtue of temperance, describing it as a protective factor against excess [39].

Research in positive psychology has shown that humility is associated with numerous psychological and social benefits. For instance, a study by Kruse et al. found that humble individuals tend to have better relationships, higher self-esteem, and greater well-being [40]. Another study by Exline and Hill found that humility was positively associated with helpfulness, generosity, and gratitude [41].

Sonja Lyubomirsky, a prominent positive psychology researcher, emphasizes the importance of humility in achieving lasting happiness: "Humble people are more likely to be grateful for what they have and to appreciate the contributions of others, both of which are key components of happiness." [42]

Moreover, humility has been linked to better leadership outcomes. A study by Bradley Owens and David Hekman found that leaders who exhibit humility - by admitting mistakes, spotlighting follower strengths, and modeling teachability - are more effective and inspire higher levels of team commitment and engagement [43].

Research has shown that physician humility is associated with improved patient satisfaction and outcomes in healthcare. A study by Ruberton et al. found that patients of physicians who demonstrated greater humility reported better health-related outcomes and were more likely to follow their doctor's recommendations [44].

It's important to note that psychological research distinguishes between genuine humility and false modesty or low self-esteem. True humility involves an accurate self-assessment and a balanced perspective on one's strengths and weaknesses rather than an undervaluation of one's worth or abilities [45].

Humility and Learning from Mistakes

Humility is essential for learning from our mistakes. As Mahatma Gandhi wisely stated, "I claim to be a simple individual liable to err like any other fellow mortal. I own, however, that I have humility enough to confess my errors and to retrace my steps" [22].

This quality is particularly crucial for healers. Acknowledging mistakes, learning from them, and continuously improving are fundamental to providing effective and compassionate care. Research has shown that healthcare professionals who exhibit humility are more likely to:

a.   Seek feedback and advice from colleagues and patients
b.   Engage in continuous learning and professional development
c.   Admit to and learn from errors, leading to improved patient safety
d.   Collaborate effectively in interdisciplinary teams
e.   Build trust and rapport with patients, leading to better health outcomes [23]

Humility in Higher Levels of Healing

In advanced healing practices, there's a recognition that healing occurs "through" the practitioner, not "by" them. This perspective requires a deep sense of humility, acknowledging that we are channels for healing rather than its source [24].

This concept is present in various healing traditions:

a.   In energy healing practices like Reiki, practitioners are taught to see themselves as conduits for universal life energy rather than the source of healing power [25].
b.   In shamanic traditions, healers work with spirit guides and natural forces, recognizing their power is limited [26].
c.   In psychotherapy, Carl Rogers' concept of "unconditional positive regard" emphasizes the therapist's role as a facilitator of the client's inherent capacity for growth and healing [27].

By embracing this humble approach, healers can avoid the pitfalls of ego and burnout while remaining open to the mystery and power of the healing process.

Humility as the Foundation of Presence

Humility is the cornerstone of genuine presence. When we approach others with humility, we create an open space for authentic connection. As Thomas Merton beautifully expressed, "Pride makes us artificial and humility makes us real" [28].

In healthcare settings, humility allows practitioners to be fully present with patients, free from the barriers created by ego or presumed superiority. This presence is essential for building trust, understanding patients' needs, and facilitating true healing [29].

Research has shown that healthcare providers who exhibit humility:

a. Are better able to establish rapport with patients
b. Demonstrate improved listening skills and empathy
c. Are more likely to involve patients in shared decision-making
d. Show greater cultural competence and sensitivity
e. Experience higher job satisfaction and lower burnout rates [30]

A Definition of a Humble Healer

The humble healer understands that healing is a collaborative process and recognizes that their role is to facilitate and support the patient's innate healing capacity rather than control or dictate the outcome. They prioritize building authentic, empathetic relationships with their patients, colleagues, and community and strive to create a safe and inclusive healing environment. The humble healer recognizes the limitations of their knowledge and expertise and is open to learning from the wisdom of other healing traditions and disciplines. They approach their work with curiosity, flexibility, and adaptability and are willing to question their assumptions and biases.

Concluding Remarks

Humility is not a weakness but a strength. It allows us to remain open, to learn continuously, and to connect deeply with others. In the realm of healing, it enables practitioners to serve as effective channels for healing energy and to provide compassionate, patient-centered care.

By cultivating humility, we enhance our growth and well-being and contribute to a more harmonious and compassionate world. As we face the complex challenges of modern healthcare and society, humility offers a path to greater wisdom, empathy, and effective healing.

Self-Reflection Questions

1. How do I understand and define humility in my own life? Does my understanding align with the definitions and concepts discussed in this chapter?
2. In what areas of my life do I find it most challenging to practice humility? What barriers or fears prevent me from embracing humility in these situations?
3. Reflect on a time when I experienced or witnessed genuine humility. What

impact did this have on me and others involved? What can I learn from this experience?

4. How does my cultural, religious, or philosophical background influence my perception and practice of humility? Do I need to re-examine any beliefs or attitudes in light of this chapter?

5. In my role as a healer or healthcare professional, how can I cultivate greater humility in my interactions with patients, colleagues, and myself? What specific actions can I take to embody humility in my work?

6. Reflect on a time when I made a mistake or faced a setback. How did I respond to this situation? Did I approach it with humility, and if not, how could I have done so? What did I learn from this experience?

7. How do I distinguish between genuine humility, false modesty, or low self-esteem? What are the signs that my humility is authentic and grounded in a healthy sense of self-worth?

8. In what ways might I be contributing to or perpetuating a culture of arrogance or ego-driven behavior in my personal or professional life? What steps can I take to become more humble and compassionate?

9. Reflect on the connection between humility and presence. How does cultivating humility enhance my ability to be fully present with others and myself? What practices or reminders can I use to maintain this connection?

10. What role does humility play in my healing and growth? How can I use the insights from this chapter to deepen my self-awareness, resilience, and capacity for transformation?

11. Consider the relationship between humility and leadership. How can I model and promote a culture of humility in my personal and professional spheres of influence? What qualities or actions define a humble leader?

12. Reflect on humility as a foundation for lasting happiness and well-being. In what ways does this align with or challenge my current beliefs and priorities? What shifts can I make to prioritize humility as a pathway to a more fulfilling life?

References

[1] Harper, D. (2022). Online Etymology Dictionary. Retrieved from https://www.etymonline.com/word/humility

[2] Tangney, J. P. (2000). Humility: Theoretical perspectives, empirical findings and directions for future research. Journal of Social and Clinical Psychology, 19(1), 70-82.

[3] Davis, D. E., Hook, J. N., Worthington Jr, E. L., Van Tongeren, D. R., Gartner, A. L., Jennings, D. J., & Emmons, R. A. (2011). Relational humility: Conceptualizing and measuring humility as a personality judgment. Journal of Personality Assessment, 93(3), 225-234.

[4] Slingerland, E. (2003). Effortless Action: Wu-wei As Conceptual Metaphor and Spiritual Ideal in Early China. Oxford University Press.

[5] Gregory, J. (2017). Fasting the Mind: Spiritual Exercises for Psychic Detox. Inner Traditions.

[6] Lao Tzu. (n.d.). Tao Te Ching. (S. Mitchell, Trans.). Retrieved from https://www.poetryintranslation.com/PITBR/Chinese/TaoTeChing.php

[7] Harvey, P. (2012). An Introduction to Buddhism: Teachings, History and Practices. Cambridge University Press.

[8] Dalai Lama. (1999). Ethics for the New Millennium. Riverhead Books.

[9] Kornfield, J. (2008). The Wise Heart: A Guide to the Universal Teachings of Buddhist Psychology. Bantam.

[10] Shantideva. (2006). The Way of the Bodhisattva. (Padmakara Translation Group, Trans.). Shambhala.

[11] Harper, D. (2022). Online Etymology Dictionary. Retrieved from https://www.etymonline.com/word/arrogance

[12] Harper, D. (2022). Online Etymology Dictionary. Retrieved from https://www.etymonline.com/word/pride

[13] Calaprice, A. (2011). The Ultimate Quotable Einstein. Princeton University Press.

[14] Anonymous. (n.d.). Quote on self-confidence, compassion, and humility.

[15] Brown, B. (2012). Daring Greatly: How the Courage to Be Vulnerable Transforms the Way We Live, Love, Parent, and Lead. Gotham Books.

[16] Woodruff, P. (2001). Reverence: Renewing a Forgotten Virtue. Oxford University Press.

[17] Coulehan, J. (2010). On humility. Annals of Internal Medicine, 153(3), 200-201.

[18] Davies, R. J., & Ikeno, O. (2002). The Japanese Mind: Understanding Contemporary Japanese Culture. Tuttle Publishing.

[19] Freire, P. (2000). Pedagogy of the Oppressed. Continuum.

[20] Berger, A. S. (2002). Arrogance among physicians. Academic Medicine, 77(2), 145-147.

[21] Mezirow, J. (1997). Transformative learning: Theory to practice. New Directions for Adult and Continuing Education, 1997(74), 5-12.

[22] Gandhi, M. K. (1940). An Autobiography: The Story of My Experiments with Truth. Navajivan Publishing House.

[23] Watling, C., LaDonna, K. A., Lingard, L., Voyer, S., & Hatala, R. (2016). 'Sometimes the work just needs to be done': socio-cultural influences on direct observation in medical training. Medical Education, 50(10), 1054-1064.

[24] Dossey, L. (1993). Healing Words: The Power of Prayer and the Practice of Medicine. HarperOne.

[25] Miles, P., & True, G. (2003). Reiki--review of a biofield therapy history,

theory, practice, and research. Alternative Therapies in Health and Medicine, 9(2), 62-72.

[26] Harner, M. (1990). The Way of the Shaman. HarperOne.

[27] Rogers, C. R. (1957). The necessary and sufficient conditions of therapeutic personality change. Journal of Consulting Psychology, 21(2), 95-103.

[28] Merton, T. (1961). New Seeds of Contemplation. New Directions.

[29] Krasner, M. S., Epstein, R. M., Beckman, H., Suchman, A. L., Chapman, B., Mooney, C. J., & Quill, T. E. (2009). Association of an educational program in mindful communication with burnout, empathy, and attitudes among primary care physicians. JAMA, 302(12), 1284-1293.

[30] Ruberton, P. M., Huynh, H. P., Miller, T. A., Kruse, E., Chancellor, J., & Lyubomirsky, S. (2016). The relationship between physician humility, physician–patient communication, and patient health. Patient Education and Counseling, 99(7), 1138-1145.

[31] Kreider, K. E. (2019). Kenosis. In Encyclopedia of Psychology and Religion (pp. 1-3). Springer, Berlin, Heidelberg.

[32] The Holy Bible, New International Version. (2011). Biblica, Inc.

[33] Teresa, M. (1997). No Greater Love. New World Library.

[34] Merton, T. (1955). No Man Is an Island. Harcourt Brace Jovanovich.

[35] Merton, T. (1972). New Seeds of Contemplation. New Directions.

[36] Kushner, H. S. (2012). The Book of Job: When Bad Things Happened to a Good Person. Schocken.

[37] The Holy Bible, New International Version. (2011). Biblica, Inc.

[38] Tangney, J. P. (2000). Humility: Theoretical perspectives, empirical findings, and directions for future research. Journal of Social and Clinical Psychology, 19(1), 70-82.

[39] Peterson, C., & Seligman, M. E. (2004). Character strengths and virtues: A handbook and classification (Vol. 1). Oxford University Press.

[40] Kruse, E., Chancellor, J., Ruberton, P. M., & Lyubomirsky, S. (2014). An upward spiral between gratitude and humility. Social Psychological and Personality Science, 5(7), 805-814.

[41] Exline, J. J., & Hill, P. C. (2012). Humility: A consistent and robust predictor of generosity. The Journal of Positive Psychology, 7(3), 208-218.

[42] Lyubomirsky, S. (2008). The How of Happiness: A Scientific Approach to Getting the Life You Want. Penguin.

[43] Owens, B. P., & Hekman, D. R. (2012). Modeling how to grow: An inductive examination of humble leader behaviors, contingencies, and outcomes. Academy of Management Journal, 55(4), 787-818.

[44] Ruberton, P. M., Huynh, H. P., Miller, T. A., Kruse, E., Chancellor, J., & Lyubomirsky, S. (2016). The relationship between physician humility, physician–patient communication, and patient health. Patient Education and

Counseling, 99(7), 1138-1145.
[45] Tangney, J. P. (2009). Humility. In S. J. Lopez & C. R. Snyder (Eds.), Oxford Handbook of Positive Psychology (pp. 483-490). Oxford University Press.
[46] Popper, K. R. (2002). The Logic of Scientific Discovery. Routledge.
[47] Paul, R., & Elder, L. (2006). The Thinker's Guide to the Art of Socratic Questioning. Foundation for Critical Thinking.
[48] Feynman, R. P. (1999). The Pleasure of Finding Things Out: The Best Short Works of Richard P. Feynman. Perseus Books.

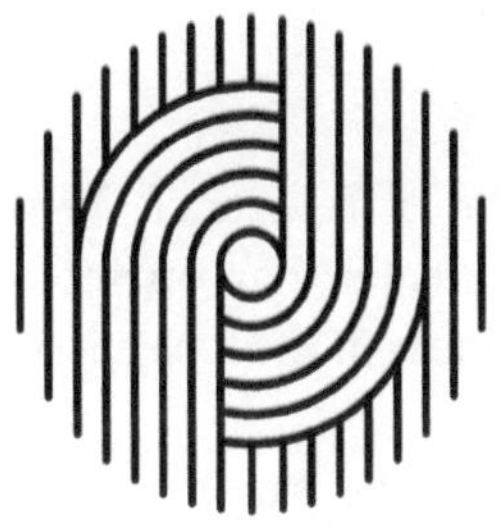

CHAPTER 9

Reverent

"When we approach with reverence, great things decide to approach us. Our real life comes to the surface and its light awakens the concealed beauty in things. When we walk on the earth with reverence, beauty will decide to trust us."
John O'Donohue

Reverence is a term seldom used in contemporary conversations, particularly in the setting of modern healthcare. However, reverence and devotion are essential characteristics of our work as healers. One can argue that reverence is critical if we are to experience our work as a calling and not simply mundane work.

Etymology and General Definition of Reverence
The word "reverence" derives from the Latin "reverentia," which means "awe, respect, or fear" [6]. It is closely related to the verb "revere," which means "to regard with deep respect, love, and awe" [8]. Reverence is a profound feeling of respect and admiration for someone or something, often tinged with a sense of awe or even fear.

Reverence and respect are closely related concepts, but reverence goes beyond mere respect. As Paul Woodruff writes in his book "Reverence:

Renewing a Forgotten Virtue," "Reverence is more than just respect. It is an ancient virtue that survives among us in half-forgotten patterns of civility, in moments of inarticulate awe, and in nostalgia for the lost ways of traditional cultures" [11].

Humility and Reverence

Humility is a key component of reverence. When we experience reverence, we acknowledge something greater than ourselves, inspiring awe and wonder. This recognition of our smallness in the face of something vast and magnificent is the essence of humility.

However, humility is not the same as reverence. One can be humble without feeling reverence, but true reverence always involves a degree of humility. As Woodruff notes, "Reverence begins in a deep understanding of human limitations; from this grows the capacity to be in awe of whatever we believe lies outside our control" [11].

Reverence as a Lost Virtue

In our modern world, with its emphasis on scientific progress and individual achievement, reverence has become a somewhat lost virtue. We are often so focused on pushing the boundaries of knowledge and technology that we forget to step back and marvel at the mysteries of the universe.

Albert Einstein once said, "The most beautiful thing we can experience is the mysterious. It is the source of all true art and science. He to whom this emotion is a stranger, who can no longer pause to wonder and stand rapt in awe, is as good as dead: his eyes are closed" [5].

Reverence for All Aspects of Life

Reverence is not limited to the realm of religion or spirituality. It has applicability to all aspects of life, from our relationships with others to our engagement with the natural world. As the philosopher Abraham Joshua Heschel wrote, "Awe is an intuition for the dignity of all things, a realization that things not only are what they are but also stand, however remotely, for something supreme" [7].

Reverence and Rituals

Section Five of this text extensively reviews the vital importance of rituals. Rituals are often a way of expressing and cultivating reverence. Whether it's a religious ceremony, a cultural tradition, or a personal practice, rituals can help us step out of our ordinary, mundane experiences and connect with something deeper and more meaningful.

As Woodruff writes, "Rituals are the outward signs of reverence, and they are a good place to start in bringing reverence back into our lives. But rituals are empty unless they are based on deep feelings of reverence" [11].

Reverence in Classical Chinse Medicine: Li

In Chinese culture, reverence is closely tied to the concept of "li," which can be translated as "ritual propriety" or "ceremonial correctness." Li is not just about following rules or going through the motions; it's about cultivating a deep respect and reverence for the social and cosmic order.

As Confucius said, "If you do not study the rites, you will not have a firm standing" [3]. For Confucius and his followers, li was essential for creating a harmonious society and aligning oneself with the Way of Heaven.

Reverence in the Greek Classics

The ancient Greeks also valued reverence. In the Homeric epics, heroes are often described as showing reverence for the gods, their elders, and the sacred bonds of hospitality. In the Odyssey, for example, Odysseus shows reverence for the gods by making offerings and sacrifices and for his hosts by following the proper rituals of guest friendship.

In the "Euthyphro," Plato has Socrates say that "reverence is that part of justice which attends to the gods" [9]. For Plato, reverence was a feeling and a moral obligation to honor and respect the divine.

Reverence in Japan: The Significance of the Bow

In Japanese culture, reverence is often expressed through the act of bowing. Bowing is not just a physical gesture but a way of showing respect, gratitude, and humility. The depth and duration of the bow can vary depending on the social context and the relationship between the people involved.

Anthropologist Ruth Benedict wrote in her classic study "The Chrysanthemum and the Sword," "The bow is an expression of reverence and respect. It is no mere formality. It is an integral part of the code of behavior" [1].

Reverence for Lineage and Elders

Reverence for lineage and elders is a common theme across many cultures. In traditional societies, elders are often seen as repositories of wisdom and experience and are treated with great respect and deference.

As the African proverb says, "When an elder dies, a library burns to the ground." This proverb reminds us of the value of elders' knowledge and stories and the importance of treating them with reverence and respect.

The Six Characteristics of Reverence
Woodruff identifies several key characteristics of reverence:

1. A sense of awe or wonder in the presence of something greater than oneself
2. A feeling of humility and the recognition of one's limitations
3. A willingness to subordinate oneself to something larger or higher
4. A capacity for shame and the desire to avoid transgressing against what is revered
5. A sense of the sacred or the holy
6. A recognition of the inherent dignity and worth of all things

Reverence in Craftsmanship and Work as a Calling
Reverence is a feeling and a way of engaging with the world. In the realm of craftsmanship, reverence involves a deep respect for the materials, tools, and traditions of one's craft. As the philosopher and auto mechanic Matthew Crawford writes in his book "Shop Class as Soulcraft," "The craftsman's reverence for the material he works with, and for its limits, is in stark contrast to the mentality that regards the world as something to be manipulated and 'processed' according to human will" [4].

Similarly, when we approach our work as a calling rather than just a job, we bring a sense of reverence to it. As the theologian Frederick Buechner writes, "The place God calls you to is the place where your deep gladness and the world's deep hunger meet" [2].

The Reverent Healer
Reverence, for the healer, is a deep feeling of respect, awe, humility, and devotion in the presence of the sacred mystery of life and the inherent worth and dignity of every human being. It is a recognition that in the context of healing, one is in the presence of something greater than oneself, whether it be the divine spark within each person, the profound wisdom of nature and the body's capacity for healing, or the ineffable mysteries of human existence.

The reverent healer approaches their work humbly, recognizing their knowledge and control limitations. They cultivate a willingness to subordinate their ego and desires to serve the larger mission of healing and wholeness. For the reverent healer, practicing medicine or healing arts is not merely a job or a set of technical skills but a sacred calling and a way of being in the world.

The reverent healer expresses this depth of respect and devotion through how they engage with their patients or clients - listening deeply, being fully present, honoring the autonomy and uniqueness of each individual, and creating a safe and sacred space for healing to unfold. They also honor the lineages of wisdom, both scientific and spiritual, that have shaped their understanding and practice of healing.

Ultimately, reverence allows the healer to tap into a more profound sense of meaning, purpose, and connectedness that can be a wellspring of resilience, compassion, and healing presence. By approaching their work with reverence, the healer becomes a conduit for the profound mysteries of healing and transformation.

Reverence in Healing

Reverence and devotion are essential in the context of healing. As healers, we are called to honor the inherent worth and dignity of every person we serve and approach our work with a deep sense of respect and humility.

This means cultivating reverence for the human spirit – the inner essence of each person that is whole, complete, and worthy of love and care. It means seeing beyond labels, diagnoses, and surface appearances to the sacred humanity within.

It also means cultivating reverence for the healing process – the mysterious and often miraculous journey of growth, transformation, and wholeness that is possible for every person. As the physician Rachel Naomi Remen writes, "Healing may not be so much about getting better, as about letting go of everything that isn't you – all of the expectations, all of the beliefs – and becoming who you are" [10].

Finally, cultivating reverence as healers means honoring the lineage of teachers, mentors, and wisdom traditions that have shaped our understanding and practice of healing. It means recognizing that we are part of something much larger than ourselves and that our work is a sacred trust passed down through generations.

As Woodruff writes, "Reverence is the virtue that keeps people from trying to act like gods. It reminds us that we are human, and it protects us from the kind of arrogance that comes from thinking that the world is something we can control" [11].

Reverence and devotion are closely connected concepts involving a deep sense of respect, awe, and dedication towards something greater than oneself. Devotion builds upon the foundation of reverence. If reverence opens our eyes to the sacred, devotion is the active choice to orient our lives around it. Devotion involves wholehearted dedication, loyalty, and love for the object of our reverence. It is a commitment to serving, honoring, and aligning ourselves with what we revere. As Buechner writes, "The place God calls you to is the place where your deep gladness and the world's deep hunger meet" [2]. Devotion is the bridge that connects our inner reverence to outer service in the world.

In the realm of healing, reverence alone is not enough. Healers must also have devotion - an unwavering commitment to serving the healing and flourishing of those they treat. Devotion fuels the hard work, presence, and dedication required to walk alongside someone in their healing journey. It transforms the practice of healing from a mere job to a sacred calling. As Woodruff notes, "Reverence is the virtue that allows us to see beyond our own desires and fears to something greater than ourselves. It is the foundation of civilization, and it is essential to the good life" [11].

Reverence and devotion are expressed and strengthened through rituals, traditions, and how we engage with the world. Rituals of reverence, such as bowing, prayer, or offerings, attune us to the sacred and cultivate an inner posture of humility and respect. In Japanese culture, for example, the act of bowing is a powerful expression of reverence [1]. Devotional practices, such as service, prayer, or dedicating one's work, consecrate our lives to what we revere.

However, as Woodruff cautions, "Rituals are empty unless they are based on deep feelings of reverence" [11]. True reverence and devotion flow from an authentic experience of the sacred, not mere blind obedience to tradition. Rituals rooted in deep reverence and devotion connect us to a lineage of wisdom and infuse our lives with meaning and purpose. As Heschel writes, "Awe is an intuition for the dignity of all things, a realization that things not only are what they are but also stand, however remotely, for something supreme" [7].

Ultimately, reverence and devotion invite us to radically re-envision our place in the world. Rather than seeing ourselves as isolated individuals pursuing our interests, reverence awakens us to our interconnectedness with all of life. As Einstein said, "The most beautiful thing we can experience is the mysterious. It is the source of all true art and science. He to whom this emotion is a stranger, who can no longer pause to wonder and stand rapt in awe, is as good as dead: his eyes are closed" [5]. Devotion calls us to offer our gifts to serve the greater whole humbly.

As healers and as human beings, we are invited to cultivate reverence and devotion - to open our eyes to the sacred within and around us and to dedicate our lives to serving and honoring it. In doing so, we tap into a deep well of meaning, connection, and purpose that can sustain us through life's challenges. As Woodruff eloquently puts it, "Reverence is the virtue that allows us to live in peace with the permanent human condition of ignorance and vulnerability. It is the foundation of civility and the compass that can guide us in the darkness" [11].

In a world that often feels fragmented and adrift, the intertwined virtues of reverence and devotion offer a path back to wholeness. They remind us of our smallness, while at the same time elevating our lives by connecting us to that which is greater. They challenge us to look beyond surface appearances to the inherent dignity of all life. And they call us to a life of humble service, dedicated to the healing and flourishing of all. As Heschel writes, "Our goal should be to live life in radical amazement...get up in the morning and look at the world in a way that takes nothing for granted. Everything is phenomenal; everything is incredible; never treat life casually. To be spiritual is to be amazed" [7].

A Definition of the Reverent Healer

The reverent healer approaches their work with a deep sense of respect, awe, humility, and devotion. They recognize the inherent worth and dignity of every person they serve and the sacred nature of the healing process. The reverent healer understands that they are in the presence of something greater than themselves and seeks to cultivate a healing presence through deep listening, compassion, and a commitment to service. They honor the wisdom of both scientific and spiritual lineages and approach their work as a sacred calling rather than merely a technical skill. By embodying reverence, the reverent healer becomes a conduit for the profound mysteries of healing and transformation.

Self-Reflection Questions

1. How do you understand the difference between respect and reverence? In what areas of your life do you experience reverence?

2. Reflect on a time when you felt a sense of awe or wonder in the presence of something greater than yourself. How did this experience affect you?

3. How do you practice humility in your personal and professional life? How does humility relate to your understanding of reverence?

4. Do you agree that reverence has become a "lost virtue" in our modern world? If so, what factors do you think have contributed to this loss?

5. How can you cultivate a sense of reverence in your daily life beyond religion or spirituality?

6. What rituals or practices help you connect with a sense of reverence? How can you incorporate more of these practices into your life?

7. Reflect on the concept of "li" in Chinese culture. How does this idea of "ritual propriety" relate to your understanding of reverence?

8. In what ways do you show reverence for your elders, mentors, or teachers? How has their wisdom and experience influenced your growth and development?

9. When you engage in your work or creative pursuits, do you approach them with reverence? How might cultivating reverence enhance your experience of work or creativity?

10. Reflecting on the characteristics of reverence outlined in this chapter, which ones resonate most strongly with you? Which ones do you find most challenging to embody?

11. As a healer (or in your role as a caregiver, teacher, or helper), how do you cultivate reverence for the people you serve? How does this reverence influence your approach to your work?

12. Moving forward, what intentions can you set for cultivating reverence in your personal and professional life? What practices or commitments can support you in this intention?

References

1. Benedict, R. (1946). The Chrysanthemum and the Sword: Patterns of Japanese Culture. Houghton Mifflin, p. 191.

2. Buechner, F. (1993). Wishful Thinking: A Theological ABC. HarperOne, p. 119.

3. Confucius. (2003). Analects (E. Slingerland, Trans.). Hackett Publishing Company, 20.3.

4. Crawford, M. B. (2009). Shop Class as Soulcraft: An Inquiry into the Value of Work. Penguin Press, p. 81.

5. Einstein, A. (1931). Living Philosophies. Simon and Schuster, p. 5.

6. Harper, D. (2021). Reverence. In Online Etymology Dictionary.

7. Heschel, A. J. (1955). God in Search of Man: A Philosophy of Judaism. Farrar, Straus and Giroux, p. 88.

8. Merriam-Webster. (2021). Revere. In Merriam-Webster.com dictionary.

9. Plato. (1981). Five Dialogues: Euthyphro, Apology, Crito, Meno, Phaedo (G. M. A. Grube, Trans.). Hackett Publishing Company, 12e. (Original work published ca. 380 BCE)

10. Remen, R. N. (1996). Kitchen Table Wisdom: Stories That Heal. Riverhead Books, p. 141.

11. Woodruff, P. (2002). Reverence: Renewing a Forgotten Virtue. Oxford University Press, pp. 3-4, 185, 201

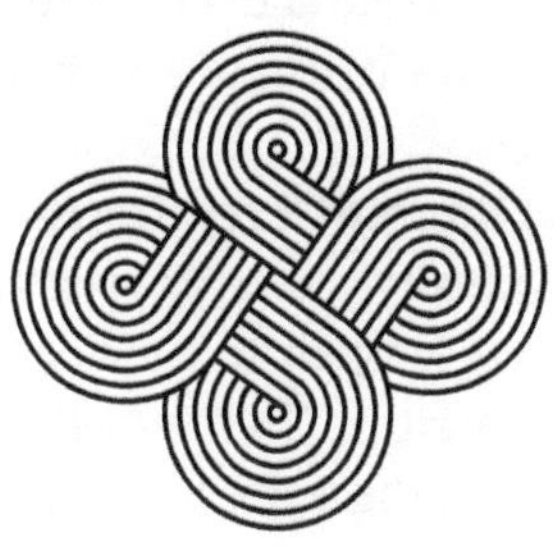

Chapter 10

Curious

"The important thing is not to stop questioning…
Never lose holy curiosity."
Albert Einstein

Curiosity is a vital trait for anyone in the healing profession. It drives the pursuit of knowledge, the desire to understand the root causes of disease, and the openness to explore new treatment approaches. This chapter delves into the nature of curiosity, its philosophical underpinnings, and its central role in the healing journey.

Etymology and Definitions of Curiosity
The word "curious" derives from the Latin "curiosus," meaning "careful, diligent, or inquisitive." It is related to the Latin noun "cura," meaning "care." In modern English, the term "curious" has several common definitions:

1. Eager to learn or know; inquisitive.
2. Prying; meddlesome.
3. Arousing interest because of novelty or strangeness.
4. Done, made, or designed to arouse curiosity.

It is important to distinguish healthy curiosity from mere distractibility or inattention. While curiosity involves a focused interest and desire to explore, distractibility and inattention represent a failure to prioritize our attention and actions. In Sanskrit, words related to curiosity include "jijñāsā" (desire to know) and "kutūhala" (eager desire, inquisitiveness).

Definition of Curiosity in Different Traditions

In the Buddhist tradition, curiosity is seen as a positive quality, a manifestation of the "beginner's mind" that is open to new experiences and insights. The Zen teacher Shunryu Suzuki writes, "In the beginner's mind, there are many possibilities, but in the expert's, there are few." [1]

In the Islamic tradition, curiosity is valued as a means of seeking knowledge, which is considered a religious duty. The Prophet Muhammad is reported to have said, "Seeking knowledge is a duty upon every Muslim." [2]

Western Philosophical Perspectives on Curiosity

Western philosophers have long grappled with the nature of curiosity, and there is a lack of consensus on its precise meaning and value. In his Metaphysics, Aristotle famously stated, "All men by nature desire to know. An indication of this is the delight we take in our senses; for even apart from their usefulness they are loved for themselves…not only with a view to action, but even when we are not going to do anything…." [3] Aristotle saw curiosity as a fundamental human drive, valuable in its own right apart from any practical utility.

However, other philosophers have taken a more ambivalent or hostile view of curiosity. Martin Heidegger, in his analysis of "curiosity" (Neugier) in Being and Time, described it as a superficial, fleeting interest in novelty that leads us away from authentic engagement with the world [4]. Similarly, Edmund Husserl critiqued "curiosity" (Neugier) as a naive, unreflective attitude that fails to grasp the deeper structures of conscious experience [5].

Eastern Perspectives on Curiosity

In Eastern philosophical traditions, curiosity is often seen as a positive quality, a means of overcoming ignorance and attachment. In the Confucian tradition, learning and self-cultivation are highly valued, and curiosity is necessary for growth. The Analects of Confucius state, "The Master said, 'To learn something and then put it into practice at the right time: is this not a joy?'" [6]

In the Taoist tradition, curiosity is associated with a childlike openness to the world, free from preconceptions and judgments. The Tao Te Ching advises, "In caring for others and serving heaven, there is nothing like using restraint. Restraint begins with giving up one's ideas." [7]

The Difference Between Curiosity and Distractibility

Despite differing philosophical perspectives, curiosity plays an essential role in the pursuit of knowledge and the process of healing. It is crucial, however, to distinguish between "knowing" and "knowledge." Knowing describes an experiential state of openness to what manifests in the present moment. It is a fertile ground for the emergence of new insights and understanding. Conversely, knowledge refers to a more fixed state shaped by pre-existing information and beliefs. While knowledge can provide a sense of certainty and confidence, it can also limit growth and the emergence of new possibilities if one becomes too rigidly attached to it.

Curiosity and the Distinction Between Knowing and Knowledge

Curiosity is the fuel that drives scientific discovery, propelling us to ask questions, test hypotheses, and expand the boundaries of what is known. The scientific method manifests curiosity, a systematic way of exploring the world through observation, experimentation, and analysis.

However, an overly narrow scientific materialism can paradoxically stifle curiosity by suggesting that current scientific methods limit reality to what can be measured and verified. The curiosity of revolutionary scientists like Galileo and Einstein, willing to question established dogmas, has opened up ever-widening horizons of understanding.

Galileo's curiosity led him to challenge the prevailing geocentric model of the universe, advocated by the Church and based on the authority of Aristotle and Ptolemy. Through his observations with the telescope, Galileo found evidence supporting the heliocentric model proposed by Copernicus. Despite facing persecution from the Inquisition, Galileo's curiosity drove him to defend the truth of his discoveries.

Similarly, Einstein's curiosity led him to question the absolute nature of space and time, which had been taken for granted in classical physics. His theory of relativity emerged from a deep curiosity about the fundamental nature of reality, and it revolutionized our understanding of the universe. Einstein himself once said, "I have no special talent. I am only passionately curious." [8]

Curiosity and the Limitations of Expertise

Curiosity provides a doorway beyond the restrictions imposed by experts and established knowledge. The figure of the dilettante, often derided as a superficial dabbler, can be seen more positively as someone whose curiosity refuses to be contained within a single field or discipline.

The polymath Leonardo da Vinci embodied this spirit of wide-ranging curiosity. His notebooks reveal a mind constantly inquiring into the nature of light, the structure of the human body, the flow of water, and countless other phenomena. Da Vinci's curiosity led him to make groundbreaking contributions in art, science, engineering, and beyond.

In the words of the philosopher Bertrand Russell, "In all affairs it's a healthy thing now and then to hang a question mark on the things you have long taken for granted." [9] Curiosity allows us to question the assumptions and dogmas that can limit our understanding and to approach the world with fresh eyes.

Curiosity as a Manifestation of the Universe's Telos
Curiosity can be seen as a manifestation of the universe's telos or inherent purpose. The Jesuit priest and philosopher Pierre Teilhard de Chardin observed, "Driven by the forces of love, the fragments of the world seek each other so that the world may come into being." [10] Curiosity is an expression of this evolutionary drive towards greater wholeness and integration.

Curiousness is an essential first ingredient in healing. It compels us to explore the depths of our being, understand the roots of disease and suffering, and discover new pathways to wholeness. The questions "Who am I? How did I arrive here? Where am I going?" reflect curiosity about the nature of disease, its etiology, and the way forward to healing.

Questions versus Answers
As we discussed in an earlier chapter of this text, an education of the heart is defined by the questions we ask and not the answers we generate. A healer's effectiveness is not determined by the answers they possess but by the questions they ask. Each medical technology and therapeutic modality offers a set of answers, but the scope of the technology itself limits these answers. A healer who relies solely on the answers provided by their particular medical toolkit risks becoming a technician rather than a true healer.

In contrast, a healer shaped by their questions remains open to new possibilities and perspectives. They recognize that each patient is unique and that the complexities of health and illness cannot be reduced to a simple formula or protocol. By asking deep, probing questions – about the patient's experience, beliefs, and values – the curious healer creates space for insight, discovery, and individualized care.

Sir William Osler observed, "The good physician treats the disease; the great physician treats the patient who has the disease." [11] Curious healers embrace this patient-centered approach, using their questions to guide the understanding of the whole person, not just the disease.

Curiosity, Optimism, and Spaciousness

Curiosity and optimism are closely intertwined. When we are curious, we are open to new possibilities and perspectives. There is always more to discover, learn, and explore. This sense of openness and possibility is the foundation of optimism.

In contrast, anxiety narrows our visual field and constrains our exploratory behavior. When we are anxious, we become focused on potential threats and dangers, and our experience of the world shrinks. We become less curious, less open, and less able to engage with the fullness of life.

Cultivating curiosity and optimism is essential for healers to maintain a sense of spaciousness and possibility in their work. By remaining open to new ideas and approaches, the curious healer avoids becoming stuck in rigid patterns of thought and behavior. They can approach each patient with fresh eyes, seeing beyond diagnoses and labels to the unique individual before them.

This spaciousness is crucial for healing because it creates room for creativity, imagination, and hope. When we are curious and optimistic, we are better able to envision new possibilities and find creative solutions to complex problems. Our openness and enthusiasm are contagious, so we can also better connect with others.

As the psychologist Rollo May wrote, "Creativity is a yearning for immortality. We human beings know that we must die. We have, strangely enough, a word for death. We know that our organism is going to die, but we believe in our heart of hearts that our creativity will live on." [12] By embracing curiosity and optimism, healers tap into this creative, life-affirming energy, even in the face of illness and mortality.

Each Patient is a Curiosity

For the curious healer, each patient is a unique and fascinating mystery. Rather than seeing patients as a collection of symptoms or diagnoses, the curious healer recognizes that every person's experience of illness is shaped by their history, beliefs, and circumstances.

This recognition demands a deep curiosity about each patient's story. The curious healer listens attentively, asking questions and seeking to understand the patient's perspective. They are interested not just in the "what" of the illness but also in the "how" and the "why."

By exploring each patient's unique experience, the curious healer is better able to tailor their approach to the individual's needs and goals. They can draw on a wide range of therapeutic modalities and resources, choosing the interventions that are most likely to support healing in each particular case.

This individualized approach contrasts the "one-size-fits-all" mentality that can emerge when healers see themselves primarily as experts rather than as curious explorers. As the saying goes, "When all you have is a hammer, everything looks like a nail." [13] Healers who are overly identified with their expertise may become rigid and inflexible, applying the same techniques and interventions to every patient regardless of their unique situation.

Curiosity and Vitality

Curiosity is a source of vitality and renewal for healers. When we are curious, we are engaged with the world and open to new experiences and perspectives. This engagement is energizing and life-affirming, helping us to stay present and connected even in the face of challenge and adversity.

In contrast, a lack of curiosity can lead to stagnation, burnout, and despair. When we lose our sense of wonder and possibility, we become disconnected from the vitality of the universe and our creative potential. As the poet Rainer Maria Rilke observed, "If we surrender to earth's intelligence, we could rise up rooted like trees. But if we continue to close ourselves off from the elemental life of our origins, it is all finished for him, he is just like an old man." [14]

For healers, maintaining a sense of curiosity is essential for avoiding burnout and maintaining a sense of purpose and meaning in their work. By remaining open to new ideas and experiences, the curious healer stays engaged with the ever-unfolding mystery of life. They can find joy and inspiration in their interactions with patients, even in the midst of suffering and loss.

This contagious sense of vitality and engagement inspires patients to become more curious and proactive in their healing journeys. Patients seeing their healers as interested and enthusiastic are more likely to feel hopeful and empowered. They may be more willing to explore new treatment options, make lifestyle changes, and engage in self-care practices that support their healing.

The Role of Curiosity in Healing

Curiosity plays a central role in the healing process, both for the healer and the one being healed. For the healer, curiosity drives the quest to understand the nature of health and disease, explore new treatment modalities, and tailor interventions to each individual's unique needs.

In her book "God's Hotel," the physician and author Victoria Sweet describes the importance of curiosity in her practice: "I was curious. I wanted to know what was going on with my patients, not just medically, but in their lives. [...] Curiosity, I found, was the key to empathy, and empathy was the key to healing." [15] The healer creates a space for deep understanding and connection by approaching each patient with genuine interest and care.

For the one being healed, curiosity is a powerful ally in the journey towards wholeness. By inquiring into the root causes of one's suffering, exploring the mind-body connection, and remaining open to new possibilities for growth and change, the individual becomes an active participant in their own healing process.

Author and spiritual teacher Eckhart Tolle writes, "The power for creating a better future is contained in the present moment: You create a good future by creating a good present." [16] Curiosity allows us to be fully present with what is rather than being trapped in regret about the past or anxiety about the future. By embracing curiosity, we open ourselves to the transformative potential of the present moment.

Cultivating Curiosity in Healing

How can we cultivate curiosity in the context of healing? One key is approaching each moment with a sense of wonder and openness, setting aside preconceptions and judgments. The Zen teacher Thich Nhat Hanh advises, "The mind can go in a thousand directions, but on this beautiful path, I walk in peace. With each step, the wind blows. With each step, a flower blooms." [17] By bringing a curious and attentive presence to each step, we can find beauty and meaning in the most ordinary aspects of life.

Another way to cultivate curiosity is through the practice of questioning. The philosopher and scientist David Bohm writes, "The ability to perceive or think differently is more important than the knowledge gained." [18] We keep our minds flexible and adaptable by asking questions that challenge our assumptions and invite new perspectives.

Engaging in creative pursuits, such as art, music, or writing, can also foster curiosity by allowing us to explore new modes of expression and perception. The artist Pablo Picasso once said, "I am always doing that which I cannot do, in order that I may learn how to do it." [19] By stepping outside our comfort zones and trying new things, we expand our capacity for curiosity and growth.

Finally, cultivating curiosity requires a willingness to embrace uncertainty and ambiguity. The poet John Keats described this quality as "negative capability," the ability to remain in "uncertainties, mysteries, doubts, without any irritable reaching after fact and reason." [20] By resting in the space of not knowing, we create room for new insights and possibilities to emerge.

The Relationship Between Curiosity and Creativity

Curiosity and creativity are intimately linked, with curiosity as the spark that ignites the creative process. When we are curious, we are driven to explore, to ask questions, and to seek out new ideas and possibilities. This openness and willingness to engage with the unknown is the foundation of all creative endeavors.

As the psychologist Carl Rogers observed, "The very essence of the creative is its novelty, and hence we have no standard by which to judge it." [21] Curiosity allows us to embrace this novelty, to venture into uncharted territory without being constrained by preconceived notions of what is possible or acceptable.

In healing, creativity is essential for developing individualized treatment plans, adapting to unique patient needs, and finding solutions to complex, multi-faceted health challenges. The curious healer is not content to rely solely on standard protocols or one-size-fits-all approaches but instead sees each patient as an opportunity for creative problem-solving.

The neurologist and author Oliver Sacks embodied this curious, creative approach to healing. In his book "The Man Who Mistook His Wife for a Hat," Sacks describes his encounters with patients suffering from a wide range of neurological conditions. Rather than seeing these patients as mere collections of symptoms, Sacks approached each case with deep curiosity and a desire to understand the individual's unique experience.

This curiosity led Sacks to develop creative, unconventional treatment approaches tailored to each patient's needs. For example, when working with a patient suffering from severe amnesia, Sacks discovered that the man had retained his ability to learn and remember new music. By incorporating singing and piano playing into their sessions, Sacks was able to help the patient establish new neural pathways and improve his overall functioning. [22]

Sacks' work demonstrates how curiosity and creativity can open up new possibilities for healing, even in the face of seemingly intractable challenges. By remaining open to the unknown and willing to explore uncharted territory, the curious, creative healer can help patients find paths to recovery and wholeness that might otherwise remain hidden.

The poet and philosopher Ralph Waldo Emerson described this creative power of curiosity when he wrote, "In the morning a man walks with his wholebody; in the evening, only with his legs. In the morning his eyes are open and his mind expands; in the evening he lets himself drift along like a log. This is the secret of the wise: live each day as if it were your last, and each morning as if it were your first." [23] By approaching each patient encounter with the fresh eyes of curiosity, the healer can tap into the creative potential of the present moment, unencumbered by the assumptions and habits of the past.

President John F. Kennedy also recognized the vital importance of curiosity and creativity in the face of complex challenges. In a 1962 speech at Rice University, he declared, "We choose to go to the moon in this decade and do the other things, not because they are easy, but because they are hard, because that goal will serve to organize and measure the best of our energies and skills, because that challenge is one that we are willing to accept, one we are unwilling to postpone, and one which we intend to win." [24]

Just as the Apollo missions required bold curiosity and creative problem-solving to overcome seemingly impossible obstacles, the curious, creative healer must be willing to embrace the hard work of exploring the unknown and finding innovative solutions to complex health and disease challenges.

Curiosity and creativity are essential for the healer who seeks to truly understand and address the root causes of their patient's suffering. As the physician and author Rachel Naomi Remen writes, "The most basic and powerful way to connect to another person is to listen. Just listen. Perhaps the most important thing we ever give each other is our attention." [25] By listening with curiosity and engaging with creativity, the healer can develop a deep understanding of each patient's unique experience and work collaboratively to find personalized pathways to healing.

Curiosity is The Antidote to Frustration and Boredom
Curiosity is a powerful antidote to the frustration and boredom that can sometimes arise during the healing journey. When faced with complex, chronic, or seemingly intractable health challenges, it can be easy for healers to become discouraged or disengaged, losing sight of the human being behind the diagnosis or the potential for growth and transformation.

In these moments, cultivating curiosity can help reignite the healer's sense of purpose and possibility. By approaching each patient encounter with fresh eyes and an open mind, the curious healer remains engaged and energized, even in the face of difficulty or uncertainty.

In his book "Flow: The Psychology of Optimal Experience," the psychologist Mihaly Csikszentmihalyi describes the importance of curiosity in maintaining a sense of engagement and meaning in one's work. He writes, "The best moments usually occur when a person's body or mind is stretched to its limits in a voluntary effort to accomplish something difficult and worthwhile. Optimal experience is thus something we make happen." [26] By embracing the challenges of the healing journey with curiosity and a willingness to stretch oneself, the healer can transform potential sources of frustration into opportunities for growth and discovery.

Curiosity also helps to counter the sense of stagnation or routine that can sometimes creep into the healer's work. When we approach each patient encounter as a unique opportunity for learning and connection, we maintain a sense of freshness and vitality in our practice.

Zen teacher Shunryu Suzuki speaks to this quality of beginner's mind when he writes, "In the beginner's mind there are many possibilities, but in the expert's there are few." [1] By cultivating curiosity and openness, the healer can avoid the trap of assuming that they already know all there is to know about a particular patient or condition.

This beginner's mind is essential for the healer who seeks to truly understand and address the root causes of their patient's suffering. As the physician and author Victoria Sweet writes, "Beginner's mind is the Zen attitude that allows docs to pay closer attention, untethered by what they know. [...] Beginner's mind lets doctors see beyond their specialties, beyond their expertise, even beyond their hospital, and into the actual life of the patient." [27]

By remaining curious and open to each individual's unique story and experience, the healer can develop a more holistic, compassionate, and practical approach to care. This curiosity helps to sustain the healer's commitment and engagement, even in the face of frustration, boredom, or burnout.

As the poet Rainer Maria Rilke writes in his "Letters to a Young Poet," "Have patience with everything that remains unsolved in your heart. Try to love the questions themselves, like locked rooms and like books written in a foreign language. Do not now look for the answers. They cannot now be given to you because you could not live them. It is a question of experiencing everything. At present, you need to live the question." [28]

By embracing the questions and uncertainties of the healing journey with patience, curiosity, and care, the healer can maintain a sense of vitality and purpose in their work, trusting that the answers will emerge in due time. This curious, open-hearted approach is the foundation of all true healing for the patient and the healer.

A Definition of the Curious Healer

The curious healer approaches their work with a sense of wonder, openness, and a desire to understand each patient's unique experience. They are driven by questions rather than answers, always seeking to explore the root causes of suffering and discover new pathways to wholeness. The curious healer is committed to ongoing growth and learning. They remain open to new ideas and experiences and continually expand their knowledge and skills. They approach their work with a beginner's mind, setting aside preconceptions and judgments to be fully present with what is unfolding in the moment.

Concluding Remarks

In conclusion, curiosity is not a luxury but a necessity for the healer seeking to catalyze genuine transformation. By approaching each patient with a sense of wonder, openness, and a desire to understand, the curious healer creates a space for deep connection, insight, and healing.

Curiosity is the antidote to the stagnation and burnout that can so easily arise in the face of the complex challenges of modern healthcare. By remaining engaged with the ever-unfolding mystery of life, the curious healer taps into a renewable source of vitality, creativity, and purpose.

As the theologian and mystic Howard Thurman wrote, "Don't ask what the world needs. Ask what makes you come alive, and go do it. Because what the world needs is people who have come alive." [29] May we all have the courage to embrace our curiosity, stay alive to the world's wonder and mystery, and bring this aliveness to all we do.

Self-Reflection Questions

1. How would you describe your current level of curiosity in your healing work? Do you feel more like a curious explorer or a knowledgeable expert?

2. Think of a patient or case that challenged or frustrated you recently. How might approaching that situation with a beginner's mind and curiosity have shifted your perspective or opened up new possibilities?

3. In what ways does your professional training and expertise help fuel your curiosity? In what ways might it sometimes limit your openness to new ideas?

4. Recall a time when you connected deeply with a patient's unique story and experiences. How did curiosity and a desire to understand their perspective enrich your work?

5. What practices or habits help you cultivate a sense of wonder, creativity and engagement in your day-to-day healing work? What tends to dull your curiosity?

6. How comfortable are you with ambiguity, uncertainty and 'not knowing' in your healing practice? How might embracing these qualities support your growth?

7. Think of a complex healing challenge you're facing with a patient right now. What new questions could you ask about the root causes and context of their illness to deepen your understanding?

8. In what ways does your clinical environment and health system support clinicians' open-ended curiosity? In what ways does it limit it in favor of efficiency, protocol, or expertise?

9. What untapped interests, talents, or experiences outside of medicine enliven your sense of curiosity and creativity? How might you bring those into your healing work?

10. What would it look like for you to approach each patient encounter with the fresh eyes and open mind of a curious beginner? What would be the benefits and challenges?

References

1. Suzuki, S. (1970). Zen mind, beginner's mind. Weatherhill.

2. Ibn Majah. (n.d.). Sunan Ibn Majah. (M. T. Ansari, Trans.). Hadith Collection. https://hadithcollection.com/ibnmajah.html

3. Aristotle. (1998). Metaphysics. (J. Lear, Trans.). In Aristotle: Selections. Hackett Publishing Company. (Original work published ca. 350 B.C.E.)

4. Heidegger, M. (1962). Being and time. (J. Macquarrie & E. Robinson, Trans.). Harper & Row. (Original work published 1927)

5. Husserl, E. (1983). Ideas pertaining to a pure phenomenology and to a phenomenological philosophy. (F. Kersten, Trans.). Martinus Nijhoff Publishers. (Original work published 1913)

6. Confucius. (1997). The Analects of Confucius. (S. Leys, Trans.). W.W. Norton & Company. (Original work published ca. 500 B.C.E.)

7. Lao Tzu. (1988). Tao Te Ching. (S. Mitchell, Trans.). Harper Perennial. (Original work published ca. 6th century B.C.E.)

8. Einstein, A. (n.d.). Albert Einstein quotes. BrainyQuote. https://www.brainyquote.com/quotes/albert_einstein_125368

9. Russell, B. (1925). What I believe. Kegan Paul, Trench, Trubner & Co.

10. Teilhard de Chardin, P. (1955). The phenomenon of man. (B. Wall, Trans.). Harper & Row.

11. Osler, W. (1904). Aequanimitas, with other addresses to medical students, nurses and practitioners of medicine. P. Blakiston's Son & Co.

12. May, R. (1975). The courage to create. W. W. Norton & Company.

13. Maslow, A. H. (1966). The psychology of science: A reconnaissance. Harper & Row.

14. Rilke, R. M. (1996). Rilke's book of hours: Love poems to God. (A. Barrows & J. Macy, Trans.). Riverhead Books.

15. Sweet, V. (2012). God's hotel: A doctor, a hospital, and a pilgrimage to the heart of medicine. Riverhead Books.

16. Tolle, E. (1999). The power of now: A guide to spiritual enlightenment. New World Library.

17. Nhat Hanh, T. (2005). Being peace. Parallax Press.

18. Bohm, D. (1996). On creativity. Routledge.

19. Picasso, P. (n.d.). Pablo Picasso quotes. BrainyQuote. https://www.brainyquote.com/quotes/pablo_picasso_103963

20. Keats, J. (1958). The letters of John Keats, 1814-1821. Harvard University Press.

21. Rogers, C. R. (1954). Toward a theory of creativity. ETC: A Review of General Semantics, 11(4), 249-260.

22. Sacks, O. (1998). The man who mistook his wife for a hat: And other clinical tales. Touchstone.

23. Emerson, R. W. (1995). Emerson's prose and poetry. (J. Porte & S. Morris, Eds.). W. W. Norton & Company.

24. Kennedy, J. F. (1962). Address at Rice University on the nation's space effort. John F. Kennedy Presidential Library and Museum. https://www.jfklibrary.org/learn/about-jfk/historic-speeches/address-at-rice-university-on-the-nations-space-effort

25. Remen, R. N. (1996). Kitchen table wisdom: Stories that heal. Riverhead Books.

26. Csikszentmihalyi, M. (1990). Flow: The psychology of optimal experience. Harper & Row.

27. Sweet, V. (2017). Slow medicine: The way to healing. Riverhead Books.

28. Rilke, R. M. (1934). Letters to a young poet. (M.D. Herter Norton, Trans.). W.W. Norton & Company.

29. Thurman, H. (1980). The creative encounter: An interpretation of religion and the social witness. Friends United Press.

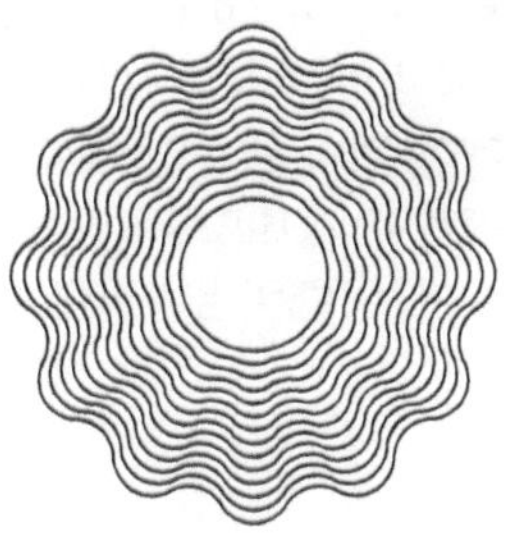

CHAPTER 11

Creative

"You can't use up creativity. The more you use, the more you have."
Maya Angelou

The word "creativity" has its roots in the Latin term "creare," meaning "to create, make" [1]. Over time, the concept of creativity has evolved to encompass the generation of novel and valuable ideas, solutions, or products across various domains [2]. In essence, creativity is the ability to transcend traditional ways of thinking or acting and to develop original, imaginative approaches to problems or situations [3].

Psychologist Mihaly Csikszentmihalyi, a prominent researcher in positive psychology, defines creativity as "any act, idea, or product that changes an existing domain or that transforms an existing domain into a new one" [4]. This definition highlights the transformative power of creativity and its potential to drive progress and innovation.

The Routinization of Healing

The practice of healing has undergone significant changes over the past century. As medical knowledge has expanded and evidence-based practices have gained prominence, treatment protocols, and algorithms have become increasingly standardized [5]. This routinization aims to ensure consistent, high-quality care and to minimize variations in treatment outcomes [6]. However, critics argue that an overreliance on protocols can stifle individualized care and creativity in the healing process [7].

Albert Einstein once remarked, "Imagination is more important than knowledge. For knowledge is limited, whereas imagination embraces the entire world, stimulating progress, giving birth to evolution" [8]. While standardized protocols are essential for ensuring a baseline of care, creative thinking remains crucial for addressing unique patient needs and driving innovation in healthcare.

The Psychology of Creativity

The psychology of creativity is a complex and multifaceted area of study that explores the mental processes, personality traits, and environmental factors that contribute to creative thinking and behavior [9]. Researchers have identified several key components of creativity, including divergent thinking (the ability to generate multiple unique ideas), cognitive flexibility (the capacity to switch between different perspectives or approaches), and openness to experience (a willingness to explore new and unconventional ideas) [10].

Psychologist J. P. Guilford, a pioneer in the study of creativity, proposed that creative thinking involves both convergent and divergent thinking processes [11]. Convergent thinking is the ability to find a single, correct solution to a problem, while divergent thinking involves generating multiple, diverse solutions. Guilford argued that both types of thinking are essential for creativity, as they allow individuals to explore a wide range of possibilities before converging on the most promising ideas.

Another important aspect of the psychology of creativity is the role of motivation and passion. Individuals who are intrinsically motivated, meaning they engage in creative activities for the inherent satisfaction and enjoyment they provide, tend to be more creative than those who are extrinsically motivated by external rewards or pressures [12]. As psychologist and author Scott Barry Kaufman notes, "Passion is one of the most important predictors of success in any field" [13].

The Neural Basis of Creativity

Recent advances in neuroscience have provided new insights into the neural basis of creativity. Studies using functional magnetic resonance imaging (fMRI) and other brain imaging techniques have identified several key brain regions and networks that are involved in creative thinking and problem-solving [14].

One of the most important brain networks for creativity is the default mode network (DMN), which is active when individuals are engaged in internally focused tasks such as daydreaming, mind-wandering, and self-reflection [15]. Research has also shown that the DMN is highly active during creative tasks, suggesting that the ability to generate novel ideas may be related to the brain's capacity for introspection and imaginative thinking [16].

Another key brain region for creativity is the prefrontal cortex, which involves higher-order cognitive functions such as planning, decision-making, and abstract reasoning [17]. Studies have found that the prefrontal cortex is particularly active during divergent thinking tasks and that individuals with greater prefrontal activity tend to generate more creative ideas [18].

The neurotransmitter dopamine has also been implicated in creative thinking and behavior. Dopamine is involved in reward-seeking behavior and plays a role in motivation, attention, and cognitive flexibility [19]. Research has shown that individuals with higher dopamine levels in the prefrontal cortex tend to perform better on creative tasks [20], suggesting that dopamine may facilitate creative thinking by enhancing cognitive flexibility and motivation.

The Impact of Artificial Intelligence on Creative Healthcare

Integrating artificial intelligence (AI) into healthcare is expected further to accelerate the trend towards routinization [21]. AI-driven systems can analyze vast amounts of patient data, identify patterns, and generate treatment recommendations based on established protocols [22]. This can potentially improve diagnostic accuracy, optimize treatment selection, and enhance overall efficiency in healthcare delivery [23].

However, as AI becomes more prevalent, it is essential to consider the role of human creativity in the healing process. While AI excels at data-driven decision-making, it lacks the intuition, empathy, and creative problem-solving abilities that are inherent to human healers [24]. As physician and author Rachel Naomi Remen notes, "Healing may not be so much about getting better, as about letting go of everything that isn't you – all of the expectations, all of the beliefs – and becoming who you are" [25]. This type of personalized, holistic approach to healing requires the creative insights and compassion that only human practitioners can provide.

Creativity in the Arts and Sciences

Creativity is a fundamental aspect of both the arts and the sciences, although the nature and expression of creativity may differ between these domains. In the arts, creativity often involves the generation of novel and original works that express the artist's unique perspective, emotions, and experiences [26]. Artistic creativity is often characterized by a high degree of subjectivity, intuition, and personal expression [27].

In contrast, scientific creativity typically involves the generation of new theories, hypotheses, and experiments that expand our understanding of the natural world [28]. Scientific creativity is often driven by a desire to solve problems, explain phenomena, and develop new technologies [29]. However, unlike artistic creativity, scientific creativity is constrained by the principles of scientific inquiry, such as empirical observation, logical reasoning, and experimental verification [30].

Despite these differences, artistic and scientific creativity share some common elements. Both require the ability to think beyond conventional boundaries, see problems from new perspectives, and generate original solutions [31]. As Albert Einstein, one of the most creative scientists in history, once said, "The greatest scientists are artists as well" [32].

Scientific Materialism and Creativity

Scientific materialism is the philosophical view that the natural world is all that exists and that all phenomena can be explained in terms of physical processes and interactions [33]. This perspective has been highly influential in shaping the scientific method, which emphasizes empirical observation, hypothesis testing, and experimental verification as the primary means of acquiring knowledge [34].

While the scientific method has been enormously successful in advancing our understanding of the natural world, some critics argue that an overemphasis on scientific materialism can stifle creativity and limit the scope of scientific inquiry [35]. As philosopher Thomas Nagel argues in his book "Mind and Cosmos," the reductionist approach of scientific materialism may be inadequate for explaining the subjective, first-person aspects of consciousness and experience [36].

Despite these limitations, the scientific method remains a powerful tool for creative problem-solving and discovery. By encouraging researchers to think critically, question assumptions, and explore alternative explanations, the scientific method can facilitate the generation of novel and valuable ideas [37]. As Carl Sagan, the renowned astronomer and science communicator, once said, "Science is a way of thinking much more than it is a body of knowledge" [38].

The Uniqueness of Creativity in Sentient Beings

Whether creativity is unique to sentient beings has been a topic of philosophical and scientific inquiry for centuries. While some argue that creativity is a purely human trait, others suggest that it may be present, to varying degrees, in other sentient beings [39].

Recent neuroscience research has shed light on how the human brain has evolved to enable creativity. Studies have shown that the prefrontal cortex, which is responsible for higher-order cognitive functions, plays a crucial role in creative thinking [40]. The human brain's ability to form complex neural networks and engage in abstract reasoning allows us to break free from sense-driven habit patterns and generate novel ideas [41].

As neuroscientist David Eagleman explains, "The human brain is a complex organ with the wonderful power of enabling man to find reasons for continuing to believe whatever it is that he wants to believe" [42]. This ability to transcend immediate sensory input and engage in imaginative thinking is a key factor in human creativity.

Creativity and Personal Development

Creativity is not only important for driving progress and innovation in the arts and sciences but also plays a crucial role in personal development and well-being. As humanistic psychologist Abraham Maslow argued in his theory of self-actualization, creativity is a fundamental human need and a key component of psychological health and fulfillment [43].

Engaging in creative activities can provide a sense of meaning and purpose, enhance self-esteem and self-efficacy, and promote personal growth and self-discovery [44]. As expressive arts therapist Cathy Malchiodi notes, "Creativity is a means of personal transformation, a way of remaking oneself and one's relationship to the world" [45].

Creativity can also be a powerful tool for coping with adversity and navigating life's challenges. By enabling individuals to find innovative solutions to problems, reframe negative experiences in a more positive light, and express difficult emotions in a healthy way, creativity can foster resilience and adaptability [46]. As author and poet Maya Angelou once said, "You can't use up creativity. The more you use, the more you have" [47].

Creativity and Health

The link between creativity and health is a growing area of research in psychology and medicine. Studies have shown that engaging in creative activities can have numerous physical and mental health benefits, including reduced stress and anxiety, improved mood and emotional well-being, and enhanced cognitive function [48].

In the context of healthcare, creativity can be a valuable tool for promoting healing and recovery. Expressive therapies, such as art therapy, music therapy, and dance/movement therapy, have been shown to be effective in treating a wide range of physical and mental health conditions [49]. These therapies provide patients with a means of self-expression, emotional release, and meaning-making, which can facilitate the healing process [50].

Creativity can also be important for healthcare providers in delivering compassionate and individualized care. As neurologist and author Oliver Sacks wrote in his book "The Man Who Mistook His Wife for a Hat," "In examining disease, we gain wisdom about anatomy and physiology and biology. In examining the person with disease, we gain wisdom about life" [51]. By approaching each patient as a unique individual with their own stories, experiences, and perspectives, healthcare providers can develop more effective and empathetic treatment plans.

Disease as a Breakdown in Creativity

From a holistic perspective, disease can be conceptualized as a breakdown in an individual's capacity to respond creatively to the shifting demands and challenges of their life circumstances [52]. When faced with stressors or changes in their environment, a healthy individual can adapt and find new ways of coping and thriving [53]. However, when this creative capacity is compromised, either by physical, psychological, or social factors, disease and dysfunction can result [54].

This perspective is reflected in the work of various thinkers and practitioners across different fields. Psychiatrist and psychoanalyst Carl Jung, for example, viewed neurosis as a result of individuals' inability to find creative solutions to their psychological conflicts and challenges [55]. As Jung wrote in his book "Modern Man in Search of a Soul," "The creative mind plays with the objects it loves" [56].

Similarly, traditional Chinese medicine, as interpreted by Taoist scholar Jeffrey Yuen, sees health as a dynamic balance between yin and yang, and disease as a result of stagnation and lack of flow [57]. From this perspective, cultivating creativity and flexibility is essential for maintaining health and preventing disease [58].

In the realm of poetry and philosophy, writer David Whyte has explored the idea of "conversational nature," or the ways in which individuals can engage in a creative dialogue with their inner and outer worlds [59]. As Whyte writes in his book "The Heart Aroused," "The antidote to exhaustion is not necessarily rest, it is wholeheartedness" [60]. By approaching life with curiosity, openness, and a willingness to embrace change and uncertainty, individuals can tap into their innate creativity and find new ways of flourishing.

The Importance of Creativity in Vitality and Healing

Creativity is not only essential for innovation and problem-solving but also plays a pivotal role in promoting vitality and well-being. Engaging in creative activities has been shown to reduce stress, improve mood, and enhance overall quality of life [61]. As psychologist Mihaly Csikszentmihalyi notes,

"Creativity is a central source of meaning in our lives ... most of the things that are interesting, important, and human are the results of creativity" [62].

Creativity is particularly crucial in the context of healing. Creative approaches to treatment, such as art therapy, music therapy, and narrative medicine, have been shown to promote emotional healing, foster resilience, and improve patient outcomes [63]. These creative interventions allow patients to express their experiences, find meaning in their struggles, and tap into their inner resources for healing.

Furthermore, creativity is essential for healthcare providers in delivering compassionate, individualized care. As physician and author Abraham Verghese states, "The good physician treats the disease; the great physician treats the patient who has the disease" [64]. Creative healers can see beyond the diagnosis and connect with the unique needs, values, and aspirations of each patient.

A Definition of a Creative Healer
The creative healer transcends conventional thinking, connects empathetically with patients, and develops innovative, individualized solutions to address their unique needs and promote holistic well-being. Creative healers recognize the importance of treating the whole person—mind, body, and spirit—and employ a flexible, adaptable approach to healing that goes beyond standardized protocols. They draw upon their imagination, intuition, and compassion to find new ways of facilitating healing and personal transformation in their patients.

Concluding Remarks
In conclusion, creativity is a vital and multifaceted aspect of human experience that plays a crucial role in the practice of healing, the advancement of knowledge, and the development of individuals and societies. By understanding the psychology and neuroscience of creativity, the ways in which creativity manifests in different domains, such as art and science, and the importance of creativity for personal growth and health, we can develop a more comprehensive and nuanced view of this essential human capacity.

As we navigate the complexities and challenges of the modern world, cultivating creativity and supporting the creative potential of individuals and communities will be increasingly important. By valuing and nurturing creativity in all its forms, we can foster a more vibrant, innovative, and fulfilling future for all. As philosopher and psychologist Erich Fromm once said, "Creativity requires the courage to let go of certainties" [65].

While the routinization of healthcare, driven by evidence-based protocols and AI, has the potential to improve efficiency and standardize care, it is essential to recognize the enduring importance of human creativity in healing. Creative healers possess the ability to transcend traditional ways of thinking, connect empathetically with patients, and develop innovative solutions to complex problems. By embracing creativity in healthcare, we can foster a more holistic, compassionate, and effective approach to healing that nurtures the mind, body, and spirit.

As Jungian analyst James Hollis writes in his book "The Middle Passage," "The goal of life is to make your heartbeat match the beat of the universe, to match your nature with Nature" [66]. By cultivating creativity and aligning ourselves with the transformative power of the creative process, we can tap into the innate healing potential within ourselves and the world around us.

Self-Reflection Questions
1. How do you define creativity in your own life and work? In what ways do you express your creativity?
2. Reflect on a time when you faced a challenging situation or problem. How did you use creative thinking to navigate or solve it? What did you learn about yourself and your creative capabilities in the process?
3. Consider the relationship between routinization and creativity in your personal or professional life. How do you balance the need for structure and consistency with the desire for innovation and originality? What strategies do you use to maintain a creative mindset within established routines?
4. The essay discusses the role of motivation and passion in driving creative pursuits. What intrinsically motivates you to engage in creative activities? How do you cultivate and sustain your passion for creativity?
5. Reflect on the idea that creativity is a fundamental human need and a key component of psychological well-being. In what ways does engaging in creative activities contribute to your sense of meaning, purpose, and fulfillment? How do you prioritize creativity in your self-care and personal development practices?
6. The essay explores the relationship between creativity and health, both in terms of individual well-being and healthcare practices. How has creativity played a role in your own health and healing journey? In what ways do you think healthcare systems could benefit from integrating more creative approaches to treatment and care?
7. Consider the concept of disease as a breakdown in an individual's capacity to respond creatively to life's challenges. Have you ever experienced a health issue or personal crisis that required you to tap into your creative resources to adapt and cope? What insights did you gain from this experience?
8. The essay highlights the importance of cultivating creativity in both the arts and sciences. How do you think creativity manifests differently in these

domains? What can artists and scientists learn from each other about the creative process?

9. Reflect on the role of the default mode network and the prefrontal cortex in creative cognition. Have you noticed any patterns or practices in your own life that seem to facilitate creative thinking and problem-solving? How can you create more opportunities for your brain to engage in creative processes?

10. The essay concludes by emphasizing the need to find a balance between the benefits of routinization and the transformative power of creativity in various aspects of life. What does this balance look like for you? How can you create space for creativity to flourish while still maintaining the necessary structures and routines that support your well-being and productivity?

11. Consider the quote by James Hollis: "The goal of life is to make your heartbeat match the beat of the universe, to match your nature with Nature." How do you interpret this statement in relation to creativity and personal growth? In what ways can aligning yourself with the creative rhythms of life contribute to your overall sense of meaning and purpose?

12. Reflect on your own creative journey and the people, experiences, or ideas that have influenced your creative development. Who are your creative role models or mentors? What lessons have you learned from them about the nature of creativity and its role in personal and professional growth?

References

1. Merriam-Webster. (n.d.). Creativity. In Merriam-Webster.com dictionary. Retrieved from https://www.merriam-webster.com/dictionary/creativity

2. Runco, M. A., & Jaeger, G. J. (2012). The standard definition of creativity. Creativity Research Journal, 24(1), 92-96.

3. Sternberg, R. J., & Lubart, T. I. (1999). The concept of creativity: Prospects and paradigms. In R. J. Sternberg (Ed.), Handbook of creativity (pp. 3-15). Cambridge University Press.

4. Csikszentmihalyi, M. (1996). Creativity: Flow and the psychology of discovery and invention. HarperCollins.

5. Timmermans, S., & Berg, M. (2003). The gold standard: The challenge of evidence-based medicine and standardization in health care. Temple University Press.

6. Woolf, S. H., Grol, R., Hutchinson, A., Eccles, M., & Grimshaw, J. (1999). Potential benefits, limitations, and harms of clinical guidelines. BMJ, 318(7182), 527-530.

7. Greenhalgh, T., Howick, J., & Maskrey, N. (2014). Evidence based medicine: a movement in crisis?. BMJ, 348, g3725.

8. Einstein, A. (n.d.). Albert Einstein quotes. BrainyQuote. Retrieved from https://www.brainyquote.com/quotes/albert_einstein_125368

9. Simonton, D. K. (2000). Creativity: Cognitive, personal, developmental, and social aspects. American psychologist, 55(1), 151-158.

10. Kaufman, J. C., & Sternberg, R. J. (2010). The Cambridge handbook of creativity. Cambridge University Press.

11. Guilford, J. P. (1967). The nature of human intelligence. McGraw-Hill.

12. Amabile, T. M. (1996). Creativity in context: Update to the social psychology of creativity. Westview Press.

13. Kaufman, S. B. (2013). Ungifted: Intelligence redefined. Basic Books.

14. Jung, R. E., & Vartanian, O. (Eds.). (2018). The Cambridge handbook of the neuroscience of creativity. Cambridge University Press.

15.15. Buckner, R. L., Andrews-Hanna, J. R., & Schacter, D. L. (2008). The brain's default network: Anatomy, function, and relevance to disease. Annals of the New York Academy of Sciences, 1124(1), 1-38.

16. Beaty, R. E., Benedek, M., Wilkins, R. W., Jauk, E., Fink, A., Silvia, P. J., ... & Neubauer, A. C. (2014). Creativity and the default network: A functional connectivity analysis of the creative brain at rest. Neuropsychologia, 64, 92-98.

17. Miller, E. K., & Cohen, J. D. (2001). An integrative theory of prefrontal cortex function. Annual review of neuroscience, 24(1), 167-202.

18. Benedek, M., Jauk, E., Sommer, M., Arendasy, M., & Neubauer, A. C. (2014). Intelligence, creativity, and cognitive control: The common and differential involvement of executive functions in intelligence and creativity. Intelligence, 46, 73-83.

19. Flaherty, A. W. (2005). Frontotemporal and dopaminergic control of idea generation and creative drive. Journal of Comparative Neurology, 493(1), 147-153.

20. Manzano, Ö. D., Cervenka, S., Karabanov, A., Farde, L., & Ullén, F. (2010). Thinking outside a less intact box: Thalamic dopamine D2 receptor densities are negatively related to psychometric creativity in healthy individuals. PLoS One, 5(5), e10670.

21. Topol, E. J. (2019). High-performance medicine: the convergence of human and artificial intelligence. Nature medicine, 25(1), 44-56.

22. Rajkomar, A., Dean, J., & Kohane, I. (2019). Machine learning in medicine. New England Journal of Medicine, 380(14), 1347-1358.

23. Yu, K. H., Beam, A. L., & Kohane, I. S. (2018). Artificial intelligence in healthcare. Nature biomedical engineering, 2(10), 719-731.

24. Obermeyer, Z., & Emanuel, E. J. (2016). Predicting the future—big data, machine learning, and clinical medicine. The New England journal of medicine, 375(13), 1216.

25. Remen, R. N. (2001). Recapturing the soul of medicine: Physicians need to reclaim meaning in their working lives. Western Journal of Medicine, 174(1), 4.

26. Kandel, E. R. (2016). Reductionism in art and brain science: Bridging the two cultures. Columbia University Press.

27. Zeki, S. (2001). Artistic creativity and the brain. Science, 293(5527), 51-52.

28. Simonton, D. K. (2004). Creativity in science: Chance, logic, genius, and zeitgeist. Cambridge University Press.

29. Sawyer, R. K. (2011). Explaining creativity: The science of human innovation. Oxford University Press.

30. Gaut, B. (2010). The philosophy of creativity. Philosophy Compass, 5(12), 1034-1046.

31. Root-Bernstein, R., & Root-Bernstein, M. (1999). Sparks of genius: The thirteen thinking tools of the world's most creative people. Houghton Mifflin Harcourt.

32. Einstein, A. (1923). Letter to Gestalt psychologist Max Wertheimer.

33. Lange, M. D. (2013). What is scientific materialism?. In M. D. Lange (Ed.), Philosophy of science: An anthology (pp. 204-210). John Wiley & Sons.

34. Godfrey-Smith, P. (2003). Theory and reality: An introduction to the philosophy of science. University of Chicago Press.

35. Sheldrake, R. (2012). The science delusion. Coronet Books.

36. Nagel, T. (2012). Mind and cosmos: Why the materialist neo-Darwinian conception of nature is almost certainly false. Oxford University Press.

37. Kuhn, T. S. (1962). The structure of scientific revolutions. University of Chicago Press.

38. Sagan, C. (1990). Guest comment: Why we need to understand science. Skeptical Inquirer, 14(3).

39. Kaufman, J. C., & Sternberg, R. J. (Eds.). (2006). The international handbook of creativity. Cambridge University Press.

40. Beaty, R. E., Benedek, M., Wilkins, R. W., Jauk, E., Fink, A., Silvia, P. J., ... & Neubauer, A. C. (2014). Creativity and the default network: A functional connectivity analysis of the creative brain at rest. Neuropsychologia, 64, 92-98.

41. Jung, R. E., & Haier, R. J. (2007). The Parieto-Frontal Integration Theory (P-FIT) of intelligence: converging neuroimaging evidence. Behavioral and Brain Sciences, 30(2), 135-154.

42. Eagleman, D. (2011). Incognito: The secret lives of the brain. Pantheon.

43. Maslow, A. H. (1968). Toward a psychology of being. Nostrand.

44. Runco, M. A. (2014). Creativity: Theories and themes: Research, development, and practice. Elsevier Science.

45. Malchiodi, C. A. (2007). The art therapy sourcebook. McGraw-Hill Education.

46. Pirson, M., & Langer, E. J. (2016). The mindful way in management. In M. G. Gonzalez-Morales & C. Scharmer (Eds.), Personal growth and transcendence in the workplace: Exploring wellbeing and performance (pp.

68-81). Routledge.

47. Angelou, M. (1983). Shaker, why don't you sing?. Random House.

48. Stuckey, H. L., & Nobel, J. (2010). The connection between art, healing, and public health: A review of current literature. American journal of public health, 100(2), 254-263.

49. Malchiodi, C. A. (2013). Expressive therapies. Guilford Publications.

50. Caddy, L., Crawford, F., & Page, A. C. (2012). 'Painting a path to wellness': Correlations between participating in a creative activity group and improved measured mental health outcome. Journal of Psychiatric and Mental Health Nursing, 19(4), 327-333.

51. Sacks, O. (1998). The man who mistook his wife for a hat and other clinical tales. Simon & Schuster.

52. Puchalski, C. M. (2001). The role of spirituality in health care. Proceedings (Baylor University. Medical Center), 14(4), 352-357.

53. Frankl, V. E. (1985). Man's search for meaning. Simon and Schuster.

54. Benson, H., & Stark, M. (1996). Timeless healing: The power and biology of belief. Simon and Schuster.

55. Jung, C. G. (1966). The practice of psychotherapy: Essays on the psychology of the transference and other subjects. Princeton University Press.

56. Jung, C. G. (1933). Modern man in search of a soul. Harcourt, Brace & World.

57. Yuen, J. (2010). Taoist healing gestures and postures. Jade Remedies.

58. Yuen, J. (2003). The ten classical formulas of traditional Chinese medicine. Jade Remedies.

59. Whyte, D. (2002). Crossing the unknown sea: Work as a pilgrimage of identity. Penguin.

60. Whyte, D. (1994). The heart aroused: Poetry and the preservation of the soul in corporate America. Crown Business.

61. Csikszentmihalyi, M. (2013). Creativity: The psychology of discovery and invention. Harper Perennial Modern Classics.

62. Csikszentmihalyi, M. (1990). Flow: The psychology of optimal experience. Harper & Row.

63. Caddy, L., Crawford, F., & Page, A. C. (2012). 'Painting a path to wellness': Correlations between participating in a creative activity group and improved measured mental health outcome. Journal of psychiatric and mental health nursing, 19(4), 327-333.

64. Verghese, A. (2010). Cutting for stone. Vintage.

65. Fromm, E. (1959). The creative attitude. In H. H. Anderson (Ed.), Creativity and its cultivation (pp. 44-54). Harper & Row.

66. Hollis, J. (1996). Swamplands of the soul: New life in dismal places. Inner City Books.

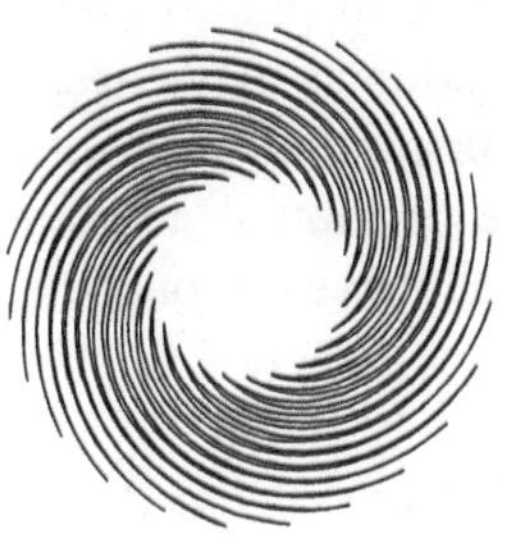

CHAPTER 12

Inspiring

"Inspiration is God making contact with itself."
Ram Dass

*I*nspiration is a vital yet often overlooked quality that can transform the healer-patient relationship. More than a momentary flash of motivation, true inspiration is a deep and sustained connection to the very breath of life. It is a force that enlivens, expands, and awakens us to possibilities beyond our perceived limitations.

Cultivating the capacity to inspire is an essential part of the healing art. By embodying presence, compassion, and an unwavering faith in human potential, the inspiring healer becomes a catalyst for their patients' innate healing capacities. They serve as a mirror, reflecting back the wholeness and radiance that may have been obscured by suffering. Yet, inspiration is not a one-way street. Patients are often profound sources of inspiration for their healers, demonstrating remarkable courage, resilience, and wisdom in the face of adversity. By attuning to these inspiring qualities, healers not only support their patients' healing journeys—they also nourish their own ability to serve with renewed passion and dedication. This chapter explores the nature and role of inspiration in the healing relationship. We will trace the roots of the word "inspire," uncover its core characteristics, and examine its transformative impact across various healing traditions. We will also investigate the shadow side of inspiration, recognizing that it is a morally neutral force that must be consciously channeled with clear intention and compassion.

Crucially, the mutuality of inspiration between healer and patient can both offer and receive inspiration as they engage in a sacred dance of shared awakening. By embodying inspiration, we can transform the healer-patient relationship into a crucible of mutual awakening, kindling the flames of wholeness and resilience in all those we touch.

Etymology of "Inspire"
The English word "inspire" derives from the Latin verb *inspirare*, which means "to breathe or blow into" [1]. This Latin root itself comes from the prefix *in-*, meaning "into," combined with *spirare*, meaning "to breathe" [2]. So, at its core, to inspire means to impart life or vitality as if by breathing. The concept of "spire" also has intriguing parallels across different cultural and spiritual traditions:

In Christianity, the Holy Spirit (from Latin Spiritus Sanctus*) is the third person of the Trinity who imparts divine grace and inspiration to believers [3].

In Hinduism, prana is the vital life force or breath that permeates the universe. Yogic breathing practices aim to cultivate and harmonize this inner wind [4].

In traditional Chinese medicine, *qi* is the essential life energy that flows through meridians in the body. Proper circulation of *qi* is seen as fundamental to health and vitality [5].

In many shamanic traditions, the breath is a conduit between ordinary and non-ordinary states of consciousness. Shamanic practices often use breathing techniques to access inspiration and guidance [6].

Across these diverse traditions, "spire" points to an animating essence, a vitalizing force transmitted through the breath. To inspire, then, is to enliven and uplift by connecting to this core of aliveness.

Definition of "Inspire"
Leading dictionaries define "inspire" as [7][8]:

1. To spur on, motivate, or encourage
2. To exert a stimulating or beneficial effect upon
3. To breathe life into, animate
4. To infuse or suggest ideas or impulses
5. To guide or prompt by divine influence
6. To inhale air into the lungs

While the first definitions relate to influence and motivation, the latter touch on the more existential meanings—enlivening, connecting to deeper ideas, and drawing in the breath of life. Fully understood, inspiration goes beyond surface-level encouragement to awaken untapped possibilities.

Core Characteristics of Inspiration

At its essence, inspiration involves a sense of expanded potential and heightened receptivity. When inspired, we feel elevated beyond our usual limitations, yet paradoxically more attuned to our depths. Inspiration dissolves stagnation and fills us with the impulse to express, create, and actualize. A key characteristic of inspiration is that it is non-hierarchical. While motivation often involves a power differential between the motivator and the motivated, inspiration arises through resonance. The inspirer and inspired mutually ignite each other's latent potential. As the poet Rainer Maria Rilke wrote, "The only journey is the one within" [9]. Encountering an inspiring presence catalyzes our inward unfolding.

Compared to motivation, inspiration draws more from intrinsic rather than extrinsic factors [10]. Motivation relies on goals, incentives, and willpower, while inspiration stems from a deeper source. Motivation compels us to act through reasons and explanations, while inspiration moves us before the thinking mind even grasps the why. When motivated, we push ourselves forward; when inspired, we are pulled into possibilities that already resonate within us. Put another way, motivation is linear and quantitative while inspiration is nonlinear and qualitative.

Ultimately, inspiration springs from a place of abundance rather than lack. It arises not to compensate for a deficit, but to express our own innate wholeness. In this sense, it is more about allowing than striving. As Michelangelo eloquently stated, "I saw the angel in the marble and carved until I set him free" [11]. The inspiring healer helps awaken us to the radiant potential already shimmering within.

Impact of Inspiration

When we feel inspired, our sense of limitation and separation softens. We tap into an expansive energy that enlivens us from within. Time recedes, self-consciousness dims, and we become absorbed in our present-moment experience.

Ralph Waldo Emerson described inspiration as the "influx of spirit," an enlivening force that dissolves our sense of limitation: "We lie in the lap of immense intelligence, which makes us receivers of its truth and organs of its activity" [15].

Perhaps no tradition has expressed the inspiring power of presence more eloquently than the Sufi poets. For them, inspiration is triggered through resonance with the beloved, the human manifestation of divine beauty.

In one of his short discourses, Rumi writes:

"When lover and beloved unite,
their ego dissolves in love's embrace.
Two bodies become one soul—
how could this be called two?" [16]

Rumi beautifully conveys how inspiration dissolves the boundaries of the limited self, immersing us in a larger field of love and abundance. Importantly, his transformation as a poet only occurred after encountering his mysterious teacher Shams-e Tabrizi. Before meeting Shams, Rumi was a sober Islamic scholar. But after just a few encounters with this wild mystic, a tectonic shift occurred in Rumi's consciousness. Rumi became intoxicated with the living presence of the divine beloved, a transfiguration he expressed in thousands of ecstatic poems.

As Rumi's journey attests, the external inspirer is ultimately a mirror for our luminous depths. In one famous poem, he proclaims: "You are not a drop in the ocean. You are the entire ocean in a drop" [17]. True inspiration helps us recognize the ocean of aliveness already surging within us.

Inspiration in the Healing Relationship

In the context of healing, inspiration plays a vital role. Beyond addressing ailments, the inspiring healer transmits a quality of presence that calls forth our intrinsic wholeness. Drawing on the root meaning of "inspire," the healer serves as a conduit for the breath of life. By connecting to a rejuvenating energy beyond the ordinary self, the healer invites that same energy to flow through the patient. As theologian Albert Schweitzer expressed, "In everyone's life, at some time, our inner fire goes out. It is then burst into flame by an encounter with another human being. We should all be thankful for those people who rekindle the inner spirit" [18].

This transfer of vital, healing energy has been recognized across therapeutic traditions:

- In Reiki, practitioners serve as channels for universal life force energy (*ki*), facilitating the recipient's self-healing capacities [19].
- In Therapeutic Touch, nurses are attuned to the patient's energy field, working to balance and harmonize it. Practitioners often report feeling a sense of energy flowing through them during sessions [20].
- Psychologist Carl Rogers emphasized the healing power of unconditional

positive regard. By meeting patients with a nonjudgmental, accepting presence, therapists create an optimal climate for growth and change [21].

Fundamentally, the inspiring healer transmits a felt sense of possibility. By embodying an expanded state, the healer becomes a mirror for the patient's potential. The Tibetan Buddhist teacher Chögyam Trungpa expresses this poignantly: "The only thing that could inspire you is a glimpse of your enlightened nature ... The healer is the external appearance of your inherent strength of mind" [22].

Again, the Sufi poets capture this mirroring dynamic beautifully. Hafiz writes:

"I wish I could show you,
When you are lonely or in darkness,
The Astonishing Light
Of your own Being!" [23]

The inspiring healer provides this reflective glimpse, rekindling the light of our radiance. They serve not as the source of that light but as a catalyst for its recognition.

Core Characteristics of the Inspiring Healer

Drawing on the themes explored, we can distill several core characteristics of the inspiring healer:

1. *Presence*: The inspiring healer embodies an unwavering quality of presence. Anchored in the here and now, they become a conduit for healing energy.
2. *Unconditional positive regard*: Meeting patients with spacious acceptance, the inspiring healer reflects each person's intrinsic value and potential. Judgment and pathologizing are replaced with nonjudgmental compassion.
3. *Resonance*: More than applying techniques, the inspiring healer works through resonance. By touching their own depths, they become a tuning fork that awakens the patient's innate healing capacities.
4. *Beginner's mind*: The inspiring healer approaches each encounter with fresh eyes. Preconceptions are surrendered to meet the living mystery of this unique person and moment.
5. *Authenticity*: Incongruence or role-playing can hamper inspiration. The inspiring healer commits to genuine expression, allowing their humanity to serve as an invitation for authentic relating.

6. *Humility*: Recognizing that healing emerges from within the patient, the inspiring healer assumes a humble posture of service. They get out of the way, creating space for each person's unfolding process.
7. *Faith*: The inspiring healer carries an unwavering faith in human potential. Even in suffering, they trust each person's capacity for resilience and transcendence.

Ultimately, the inspiring healer's way of being is itself the healing catalyst. As Gandhi memorably put it: "Be the change you wish to see in the world" [24]. By embodying inspiration, the healer awakens that same potential in those they serve.

Inspiration Can Be a Two-Edged Sword

While inspiration can catalyze profound healing and growth, it's crucial to recognize that it is a neutral force. The resonance between people can energize both constructive and destructive potentials, depending on the intentions and clarity of those involved.

History abounds with examples of inspiration's double-edged impact:

Mahatma Gandhi inspired millions to engage in nonviolent resistance, helping India achieve independence and providing a model for civil rights movements worldwide [25]. Yet his assassin, Nathuram Godse, was inspired by a vision of Hindu nationalism that saw Gandhi as a threat [26].

Martin Luther King Jr.'s inspiration galvanized the American civil rights movement, leading to landmark legislation and societal transformation [27]. However, FBI director J. Edgar Hoover was so threatened by King's influence that he sought to undermine him through surveillance and blackmail [28].

The environmental activist Wangari Maathai inspired a grassroots movement that planted over 50 million trees in Kenya, advanced women's rights, and opposed political corruption [29]. Yet, Kenya's government repeatedly suppressed her efforts, sometimes brutally.

In each case, the same inspiring presence evoked radically different responses based on the perceiver's mental state. Those attuned to love and justice resonated with the higher potentials, while those identified with fear and control felt threatened by the very same message.

This duality is perhaps most starkly embodied by Adolf Hitler. Hitler's fiery oration and vision of a restored Germany inspired millions to support his destructive ambitions. By tapping into the collective shadow—the unhealed wounds and prejudices of the populace—Hitler channeled inspiration towards horrific ends. As psychologist Carl Jung observed, "The phenomenon we have witnessed in Germany was nothing less than the first outbreak of epidemic insanity, an irruption of the unconscious into what seemed to be a tolerably well-ordered world" [30].

Hitler's example is a sobering reminder that inspiration itself is amoral. When an inspiring figure lacks a clear ethical grounding, their charisma can unleash the unchecked shadow. The greater the wounds and repressions in the collective psyche, the more susceptible it is to false prophets offering catharsis through violence or domination. Recognizing this duality highlights the importance of individual responsibility. Both the inspiring figure and those inspired must vigilantly attune to their underlying intentions. Is the inspiration rooted in love and the impulse to heal? Or is it feeding the ego's desire for power and control? The inspiring healer bears a special responsibility in this regard. By virtue of their role, they are entrusted with the vulnerable depths of those they serve. It is incumbent on the healer to continually refine their motivations, anchoring inspiration in a compassion that embraces both light and shadow. When the healer's presence is rooted in clear, loving intention, it is less prone to unconscious distortion.

Ultimately, we cannot control how our inspiration will be metabolized by others. We can only commit to refining our own intentions, radiating a compassion that excludes nothing and no one. In the words of Etty Hillesum, who perished in Auschwitz yet whose diaries reveal an astonishing love for life" "We have just one moral duty: to reclaim large areas of peace in ourselves, more and more peace, and to reflect it towards others. And the more peace there is in us, the more peace there will also be in our troubled world.' [31]

The inspiring healer is called to be a beacon of this inner peace. By marrying inspiration to all-embracing compassion, the healer becomes a joyful warrior, bearing witness to the highest in self and others.

Our Inspiring Patients

While healers rightly focus on inspiring their patients, it's vital to recognize that inspiration flows in both directions. Our patients are often our greatest teachers, embodying remarkable courage, resilience, and wisdom in the face of profound challenges. By attuning to their inspiring qualities, we not only support their healing—we also nourish our own capacity to serve.

Witnessing remarkable courage: Our patients constantly inspire us through their courage in meeting suffering head-on. Whether facing a life-threatening illness, grappling with trauma, or managing chronic pain, they demonstrate a willingness to confront adversity that is humbling to behold. As Brené Brown writes, "Courage is contagious. Every time we choose courage, we make everyone around us a little better and the world a little braver" [32]. Recognizing this courage is a profound gift to our patients. It affirms their intrinsic dignity and inner strength, especially when they feel most vulnerable or broken. By mirroring back their bravery, we help kindle the flame of inspiration within them.

Sustaining our work: The demanding nature of caring professions can lead to burnout, empathy fatigue, and cynicism if we're not mindful. Regularly connecting to inspiration is crucial for sustaining our work with passion and presence. As Mother Teresa wisely noted, "To keep a lamp burning, we have to keep putting oil in it" [33]. Experiencing our patients' inspiring qualities is a powerful form of this replenishing "oil." Their determination, heart, and tenacity renew our faith in the human spirit. Drinking from this well of inspiration allows us to return again and again to serving, with a sense of grounded vitality.

Embracing humility and vulnerability: Acknowledging our patients as inspiring requires a willingness to step down from the pedestal of the all-knowing expert. It invites us to embrace humility—to recognize that we are all pilgrims on the path of life, each with gifts to offer and lessons to learn. As the Zen saying goes, "In the beginner's mind there are many possibilities, in the expert's mind there are few" [34].

Claiming the beginner's mind takes vulnerability. It means softening our professional armor and reconnecting to our shared humanity. In this undefended space, we can receive our patients' teachings with an open heart. This vulnerability is not weakness; rather, it is the ground of authentic connection and mutual healing. As psychologist Carl Rogers understood, "What is most personal is most universal" [35].

Ultimately, when we open to our patients' inspiring qualities, we engage in a dance of mutual awakening. We become mirrors for each other's wholeness, reflecting back and forth the light of our essential nature. In this sacred dance, the boundaries between healer and healed dissolve, revealing the healing power of interconnection.

As the physician Rachel Naomi Remen writes: "Befriending life is less about powerful interventions than about*Befriending life is less about powerful interventions than about learning to bring forth the strength, wisdom, and healing power that is latent within everyone. The healer's task is to strengthen the life within ... and to remember that the life within the patient is the same as the life within the healer." [36]

By embracing our patients as inspiring, we honor the life we share. We affirm that, even in the midst of suffering, seeds of luminosity are always ready to blossom.

A Definition of an Inspiring Healer

The inspiring healer is a healthcare professional who embodies presence, unconditional positive regard, and an unwavering faith in human potential.

They serve as a catalyst for their patients' innate healing capacities by creating a resonant field of compassion and acceptance.

Concluding Remarks

This chapter has explored the profound potential of inspiration in the healing arts. By tracing the etymology and cross-cultural expressions of "inspire," we discovered a common theme—transmitting essential, enlivening energy through the breath of presence.

Examining the core characteristics of inspiration revealed its non-hierarchical, expansive nature. In contrast to motivation's linearity, inspiration dissolves the boundaries between self and other, awakening a sense of limitless potential. The Sufi poets, epitomized by Rumi, beautifully expressed how the encounter with an inspiring presence can shatter our illusory limitations.

In the healing relationship, inspiration serves as a catalyst for recognizing our intrinsic wholeness. By embodying presence, unconditional regard, and faith in human potential, the inspiring healer reflects each person's latent capacity for self-healing. More than any technique, the healer's way of being is itself the transformative elixir.

Yet inspiration is a morally neutral force. The healer must root their presence in clear intention, remaining vigilant not to unconsciously energize destructive potentials. By marrying inspiration to all-embracing compassion, the healer becomes a joyful warrior, humbly bearing witness to the highest in each person.

Crucially, we explored how patients themselves are often our greatest sources of inspiration. By honoring their courage, resilience, and wisdom, we nourish our capacity to serve with passion and presence. In this way, healer and healed engage in a sacred dance of mutual awakening.

Ultimately, inspiration is an invitation to radical aliveness. In a world that often settles for conformity, the inspiring healer shows the courage to inhabit each moment fully. This bravery is itself a healing gift, encouraging us to drop our masks and embrace the vulnerable radiance of our shared being.

Self-Reflection Questions

1. Recall a time when you felt deeply inspired. What qualities were present in that experience? How can you cultivate more of those qualities in your daily life?

2. Who have been sources of inspiration in your own life? What was it about their presence that ignited something within you?

3. In your own role, how can you serve as a mirror for others' potential? What shifts in perspective would allow you to see through the lens of inspiration more often?

4. Where do you find yourself getting stuck in hierarchical or motivational approaches? How can you move towards inspiration and resonance in those situations?

5. Reflect on the core characteristics of the inspiring healer. Which ones feel most resonant for you? Which feel most challenging or aspirational? What steps can you take to embody those qualities more fully?

References

1. "Inspire." Etymology Online Dictionary.
https://www.etymonline.com/word/inspire
2. Ibid.
3. "Holy Spirit." Britannica. https://www.britannica.com/topic/Holy-Spirit
4. "Prana." Yogapedia. https://www.yogapedia.com/definition/4994/prana
5. "What is Qi?" TCM World. https://www.tcmworld.org/what-is-tcm/qi/
6. Walsh, R. (2007). The World of Shamanism. Woodbury, MN: Llewellyn Publications.
7. "Inspire." Merriam-Webster Dictionary.
https://www.merriam-webster.com/dictionary/inspire
8. "Inspire." Oxford Advanced Learner's Dictionary.
https://www.oxfordlearnersdictionaries.com/definition/english/inspire
9. Rilke, R.M. (1932). Letters to a Young Poet. New York: W.W. Norton & Company.
10. Thrash, T.M. & Elliot, A.J. (2003). Inspiration as a psychological construct. Journal of Personality and Social Psychology, 84(4), 871-889.
11. Attributed to Michelangelo, though the source is disputed.
12. Plato. (1997). Complete Works (J.M. Cooper & D.S. Hutchinson, Eds.). Indianapolis: Hackett.
13. Shantideva. (2006). The Way of the Bodhisattva (Padmakara Translation Group, Trans.). Boston: Shambhala.
14. Witherspoon, G. (1977). Language and Art in the Navajo Universe. Ann Arbor: University of Michigan Press.
15. Emerson, R.W. (1841). The Over-Soul. In Essays: First Series. Boston: James Munroe & Co.
16. Rumi, J.D. (2004). Discourses of Rumi (A.J. Arberry, Trans.). London: RoutledgeCurzon.
17. Barks, C. (Trans.). (1995). The Essential Rumi. New York: HarperCollins.
18. Schweitzer, A. (1955). Memories of Childhood and Youth (C.T. Campion, Trans.). London: George Allen & Unwin.
19. "What is Reiki?" International Association of Reiki Professionals. https://iarp.org/what-is-reiki/
20. Krieger, D. (1979). Foundations for Holistic Health Nursing Practices: The

Renaissance Nurse. Philadelphia: J.B. Lippincott.

21. Rogers, C.R. (1961). On Becoming a Person. Boston: Houghton Mifflin.

22. Trungpa, C. (2010). The Sanity We Are Born With: A Buddhist Approach to Psychology. Boston: Shambhala.

23. Ladinsky, D. (Trans.). (1999). The Gift: Poems by Hafiz. New York: Penguin.

24. Attributed to Mahatma Gandhi, though the source is disputed.

25. Fischer, L. (2010). The Life of Mahatma Gandhi. New York: Harper.

26. Jayakar, P. (1998). Nathuram Godse and the Gandhi Murder. Mumbai: Rupa.

27. Carson, C. (2001). The Autobiography of Martin Luther King, Jr. New York: Grand Central Publishing.

28. Gage, B. (2014). The Day the Music Died: The Last Tour of Buddy Holly, the "Big Bopper," and Ritchie Valens. Chicago: Chicago Review Press.

29. Maathai, W. (2006). Unbowed: A Memoir. New York: Anchor.

30. Jung, C.G., & Jaffé, A. (1965). Memories, Dreams, Reflections. New York: Vintage.

31. Hillesum, E. (2001). Etty: The Letters and Diaries of Etty Hillesum 1941-1943. Grand Rapids, MI: Eerdmans.

32. Brown, B. (2015). Rising Strong. New York: Random House.

33. Mother Teresa. (2010). Where There Is Love, There Is God: A Path to Closer Union with God and Greater Love for Others. New York: Doubleday.

34. Suzuki, S. (1970). Zen Mind, Beginner's Mind. Boston: Shambhala.

35. Rogers, C.R. (1980). A Way of Being. Boston: Houghton Mifflin.

36. Remen, R.N. (1996). Kitchen Table Wisdom: Stories That Heal. New York: Riverhead.

37. Attributed to Hippocrates, though the source is disputed.

Section Two
The Yoga of Medicine

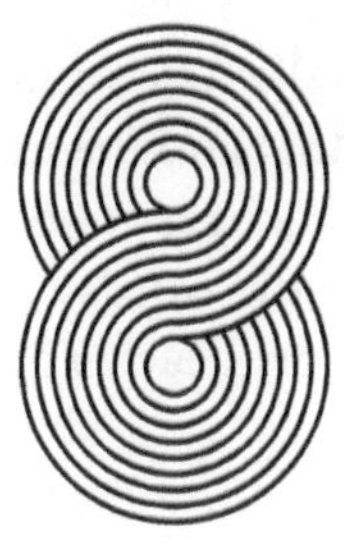

CHAPTER 13

The Yoga of Medicine

*"Yoga is the art of conscious self-finding through work,
through knowledge, through devotion or through
psychological self-analysis and self-control."*
Sri Aurobindo

Having explored the theoretical foundations of integral healthcare in Volume One, we now focus on the practical application of these principles in the clinical setting. This section, "The Yoga of Medicine," is dedicated to the *praxis* of integral healthcare—the embodiment of theory in action.

Understanding Yoga: Beyond Hatha Yoga in the West

The term "yoga" is central to this section, serving as a bridge that binds seemingly disparate elements together. The word "yoga" is derived from the Sanskrit root *yuj*, which means "to yoke, harness, or bind together" [1]. This binding together is not merely a superficial connection but a deep integration. As Christopher Wallis elaborates, "Yoga is the practice of accessing and integrating all facets of our true nature—body, mind, and spirit—in the pursuit of inner harmony" [2].

However, in the West, the term "yoga" has often been misunderstood and narrowly associated with the physical practice of Hatha yoga. While

171

Hatha yoga is one aspect of the broader yoga tradition, it is not the entirety. As Sadhguru explains, "Yoga is not just a practice. It is a way of being. It is not about twisting your body or holding your breath. It is about learning to live in ultimate harmony with existence" [3].

The true essence of yoga lies in its ability to facilitate a profound connection between the individual and the universal, the microcosm and the macrocosm. It is a path of self-discovery and self-realization, leading to unity and oneness with all creation. In the words of Swami Satchidananda, "Yoga is the uniting of consciousness in the heart. Yoga is the union of the individual with the whole of creation" [4].

This more profound understanding of yoga is essential for healthcare providers seeking to integrate contemplative practices into their clinical work. By recognizing yoga as a holistic approach to well-being that encompasses body, mind, and spirit, we can begin to appreciate its potential for facilitating healing on multiple levels.

Healing as Sadhana - Healing as a Spiritual Practice
"When we say sadhana, we are not talking about any particular aspect. We are talking about using every aspect of life - both internal and external - so that it is a continuous nurturing for your life. Because the very nature of a human being is such, unless there is some dynamism, some movement in his life towards betterment within and outside himself, he will feel frustrated. He has to keep moving to a newer and newer possibility. Sadhana is that which facilitates that." Swami Sadhguru [23]

The Yoga of Medicine aims to describe a sadhana of healing that will transform our experience as healers and enliven ourselves and our work. The term "sadhana" comes from the Sanskrit root "sadh," which means "to go straight to the goal, to attain" [5]. In spiritual practice, sadhana refers to the disciplined and dedicated effort towards personal growth and self-realization.

Traditionally, sadhana has been associated with meditation, prayer, and yoga, often conducted in temples or religious gatherings. However, the principles of sadhana need not be restricted to these contexts. As Sri Aurobindo states, "All life is a Yoga of Nature seeking to manifest God within itself. Yoga marks the stage at which this effort becomes capable of self-awareness and, therefore, of the right completion in the individual. It is a gathering up and concentration of the movements dispersed and loosely combined in the lower evolution" [6].

In this light, sadhana can be understood as a conscious, concentrated effort to align one's life with a higher purpose. It is a means of infusing every action and role with a sense of the sacred. A sadhana practice, therefore, does not need to be restricted to temples or religious gatherings. It can be integrated into all aspects of life, including our professional work.

In many ways, a sadhana is akin to a ritual. Both involve intentional, repeated actions that focus the mind, evoke certain qualities, and connect us to something greater than ourselves. As the anthropologist Bobby Alexander writes, "Ritual is a planned or improvised performance that effects a transition from everyday life to an alternative context within which the everyday is transformed" [7].

For those in the healing professions, our work offers a uniquely potent opportunity for sadhana, ritualized action that transforms the everyday routine into the sacred. Every interaction with a patient, every procedure or prescription, can become an act of worship, an offering of our skills and compassion in healing.

As healers, we are profoundly fortunate to have this opportunity to help others. In the words of Mother Teresa, "It is not how much we do, but how much love we put in the doing. It is not how much we give, but how much love we put in the giving" [8]. When we approach our work with this spirit of love and dedication, it becomes the highest form of sadhana, a means of uniting with the Divine through selfless service.

In spiritual practice, sadhana refers to the disciplined and dedicated effort towards personal growth and self-realization. For those in the healing professions, work can be a particularly potent form of sadhana, offering a precious opportunity to practice Karma Yoga, the yoga of selfless action. By integrating the four pillars of sadhana - Seva (selfless service), Swadhyaya (self-study), Santosh (contentment), and Satsang (association with truth) - along with the principles of Karma Yoga into our healing work, we can transform our daily responsibilities into a spiritual practice, a "Yoga of Medicine," that nourishes both ourselves and those we serve.

The First Pillar of Sadhana: Seva (Selfless Service)
The first pillar of sadhana, Seva, and the related practice of Karma Yoga offers a powerful antidote to the growing problems of burnout and compassion fatigue in healthcare. Burnout, characterized by emotional exhaustion, depersonalization, and reduced personal accomplishment, affects a significant proportion of healthcare professionals [9]. Compassion fatigue, a related concept, describes the cumulative emotional toll of caring for others in distress [10].

By shifting our focus from personal gain to selfless service, Seva and Karma Yoga help us find renewed meaning and purpose in our work. As the Bhagavad Gita reminds us, "Work done with selfish motives is inferior by far to the selfless service or Karma-Yoga. Therefore be a Karma-Yogi,

O Arjuna. Those who seek [to secure] the welfare of the world should not abandon their duties" [11].

When we approach our healing work as a form of worship, as an offering to the Divine, we tap into a source of energy and resilience beyond our limited personal reserves. This shift in perspective allows us to serve with greater joy, compassion, and equanimity, even in the face of challenges.

The Second Pillar of Sadhana: Swadhyaya (Self-Study)

The second pillar, Swadhyaya, addresses the need for continuous learning and self-awareness in healthcare. In an era of rapid technological and scientific advances, healers must engage in lifelong learning to maintain and improve their skills. Moreover, the complex interpersonal and emotional demands of healing require high self-awareness and emotional intelligence.

Swadhyaya, the practice of self-study and self-reflection, supports both goals. We grow as healers and human beings by regularly reflecting on our work, seeking feedback, and pursuing ongoing education. As Mahatma Gandhi noted, "The best way to find yourself is to lose yourself in the service of others" [12]. Through Seva and swadhyaya, we discover our strengths, limitations, and areas for growth.

Furthermore, self-awareness is essential for providing compassionate, patient-centered care. As physician and author Rachel Naomi Remen writes, "The most basic and powerful way to connect to another person is to listen. Just listen. Perhaps the most important thing we ever give each other is our attention" [13]. By cultivating self-awareness through swadhyaya, we enhance our ability to be fully present and attuned to the needs of those we serve.

The Third Pillar of Sadhana: Santosh (Contentment)

The third pillar, Santosh, is particularly relevant to the challenges of moral distress and the need for resilience in healthcare. Moral distress occurs when healthcare professionals know the ethically appropriate action but are constrained from taking it due to institutional barriers or conflicting obligations [14]. Over time, unresolved moral distress can lead to burnout, compassion fatigue, and even leaving the profession.

Santosh, finding contentment in the face of life's challenges can help us navigate these difficult situations with greater stability. By focusing on the intrinsic value of our service rather than attachment to specific outcomes, we can maintain a sense of purpose and perspective even when faced with systemic obstacles.

Moreover, cultivating Santosh supports the development of resilience, the ability to adapt and recover in the face of adversity. As the Bhagavad Gita counsels, "Perform your obligatory duty, because action is indeed better than inaction" [15]. By embracing our responsibilities with a spirit of acceptance and detachment, we find the strength to persevere through challenges.

The Fourth Pillar of Sadhana: Satsang (Associating with a Supportive Community)
The fourth pillar, Satsang, speaks to the importance of community and shared purpose in healthcare. In the face of increasing specialization and fragmentation of care, interprofessional collaboration is essential for providing high-quality, patient-centered care [16]. However, effective collaboration requires more than just structural arrangements; it demands a sense of shared purpose and mutual respect among all healthcare team members.

Satsang, the practice of associating with truth and surrounding ourselves with those who support our growth, can help foster this sense of community and shared purpose. Creating spaces for genuine dialogue, mutual support, and shared reflection among colleagues strengthens the bonds of trust and understanding essential for true collaboration.

Moreover, by coming together in the spirit of Satsang, we remind ourselves that we are part of a larger community of healers united by a shared commitment to service. Mother Teresa said, "None of us, including me, ever do great things. But we can all do small things, with great love, and together we can do something wonderful" [17]. Through satsang, we draw strength and inspiration from our shared dedication to the healing arts.

The Yoga of Medicine: Transforming Healing Work into Spiritual Practice
Integrating the four pillars of sadhana and the principles of Karma Yoga into our healing work transforms it into a comprehensive spiritual practice, a "Yoga of Medicine." This approach recognizes that our daily responsibilities as healers, from mundane tasks to profound interactions, are all opportunities for spiritual growth and selfless service.

As the Indian sage Swami Sivananda stated, "The practice of medicine is Yoga - a method of uniting the individual soul with the Supreme Soul. True service is worship" [18]. By approaching our healing work as a form of worship, as a path of Yoga, we imbue it with a deeper meaning and purpose.

This Yoga of Medicine is not a separate practice from our daily work but rather a way of approaching and experiencing our responsibilities. It involves bringing a quality of presence, compassion, and dedication to every aspect of our healing work, from listening to patients to collaborating with colleagues.

The principles of ritual design and behavioral change discussed later in this section find a powerful application in the concept of "The Yoga of Medicine." This approach describes a series of contemplative skills that can be seamlessly integrated into clinical work, transforming mundane tasks into a spiritual practice that enlivens and empowers both the healer and the patient. As the Bhagavad Gita states, "Yoga is a skill in action" [19]. It is a means of bringing mindful presence and intentionality to every aspect of our work.

Just as an asana in Hatha yoga describes the mechanics of a posture and the inner experience of being in that posture, the Yoga of Medicine is concerned with the quality of our presence and awareness amid our clinical duties. It invites us to ask, "Who are we being as we engage in this work? What is the state of our mind, heart, and spirit?"

By cultivating skills such as presence, acceptance, affirmation, intention, beneficence, mindfulness, and equanimity, we transform our experience of ourselves, our work, and our relationship to the transcendent. We move beyond the surface level of symptom management and enter into a space of deep healing and connection.

As a spiritual teacher and former physician, Ram Dass writes, "Healing does not mean going back to the way things were before, but rather allowing what is now to move us closer to God" [20]. The Yoga of Medicine is a path of healing - not just for our patients but also for ourselves.

By embracing this contemplative approach, we tap into a source of resilience and renewal in the face of the stresses and challenges of modern healthcare. As Thich Nhat Hanh, a Zen master and peace activist, notes, "The practice of mindfulness is a kind of ritual that allows us to heal ourselves and to live more deeply and more fully" [21].

In a time when burnout and disconnection are all too common in healthcare, the Yoga of Medicine offers a powerful antidote. By integrating the wisdom of ritual, the insights of behavioral science, and the practices of contemplative tradition, we can create a new paradigm of healing that honors the sacred in each moment and awakens the healer within us all.

Concluding Remarks

For those in the healing professions, our work offers a precious opportunity to practice sadhana and Karma Yoga. By integrating the four pillars of Seva, Swadhyaya, Santosh, and Satsang into our daily responsibilities, we transform our healing work into a comprehensive spiritual practice, a "Yoga of Medicine."

This approach allows us to find deeper meaning and purpose in our work, to grow personally and spiritually through our service, and to offer our skills as a selfless dedication to the Divine. As we navigate the challenges and joys of healing work, sadhana and Karma Yoga principles guide us towards a path of compassion, wisdom, and selfless loving-kindness. In the words of Swami Vivekananda, "The ideal person is one who, in the midst of the greatest silence and solitude, finds the most intense activity, and in the midst of the most intense activity, finds the silence and solitude of the desert. One has learned the secret of restraint; one has controlled oneself" [22]. By approaching our healing work as a spiritual practice, we learn this secret of restraint, this inner balance and poise, allowing us to serve with total dedication while maintaining a center of peace and stability.

Ultimately, the Yoga of Medicine is a path of transformation, not only for ourselves but for all those we serve. As we bring a quality of presence, compassion, and selfless service to our work, we create ripples of healing that extend far beyond the clinic or hospital walls. We become instruments of love and grace, contributing to the healing and elevation of consciousness on this planet.

Self-Reflection Questions
1. How can I integrate the principles of sadhana and Karma Yoga into my daily work as a healer? What specific practices or rituals might support this integration?
2. In what ways has my healing work served as a mirror for self-discovery and personal growth? What strengths, limitations, and areas for development has it revealed?
3. How can I cultivate a sense of contentment (Santosh) and equanimity in the face of the challenges and stresses of my work? What practices help me maintain a sense of perspective and purpose?
4. How can I foster a sense of community and shared purpose (Satsang) among my colleagues and within my healthcare organization? How might this support our collective ability to serve and heal?
5. How can I approach my interactions with patients and colleagues as opportunities for mindful presence, compassionate listening, and selfless service (Seva)?
6. How can I navigate situations of moral distress in my work, drawing on the principles of sadhana and Karma Yoga? What resources or supports might I turn to for guidance and resilience?
7. In what ways has my healing work served as a path of personal and spiritual growth? How has it challenged me to confront my limitations and develop my capacities?
8. How can I balance the demands of selfless service (Seva) with the need for self-care and personal renewal? What practices might help me maintain this balance?
9. What does it mean for me to approach my healing work as a form of worship, as a path of Yoga? How might this perspective transform my experience of my daily responsibilities and interactions?

References

1. Grimes, J. (1996). A Concise Dictionary of Indian Philosophy: Sanskrit Terms Defined in English. State University of New York Press.

2. Wallis, C. (2019). The Mattamayūra Tantra: And the Path to Deification. Mattamayura Press.

3. Hanh, T. N. (1998). The Heart of the Buddha's Teaching: Transforming Suffering Into Peace, Joy & Liberation: the Four Noble Truths, the Noble Eightfold Path, and Other Basic Buddhist Teachings. Harmony.

4. Watson, B. (2009). The Lotus Sutra and Its Opening and Closing Sutras. Columbia University Press.

5. Buswell, R. E., & Lopez, D. S. (2013). The Princeton Dictionary of Buddhism. Princeton University Press.

6. Aurobindo, Sri. (1997). The Synthesis of Yoga. Sri Aurobindo Ashram Publication Department.

7. Alexander, B. C. (1997). Ritual and current studies of ritual: Overview. Anthropological Studies of Religion: An Introductory Text, 139-160.

8. Teresa, Mother. (2001). No Greater Love. New World Library.

9. Shanafelt, T. D., & Noseworthy, J. H. (2017). Executive leadership and physician well-being: nine organizational strategies to promote engagement and reduce burnout. Mayo Clinic Proceedings, 92(1), 129-146.

10. Sinclair, S., Raffin-Bouchal, S., Venturato, L.,Mijovic-Kondejewski, J., & Smith-MacDonald, L. (2017). Compassion fatigue: A meta-narrative review of the healthcare literature. International Journal of Nursing Studies, 69, 9-24.

11. Prasad, R. (2007). Bhagavad Gita: The Song of God. Sura Books.

12. Gandhi, M., & Desai, M. H. (1927). An Autobiography or The story of my experiments with truth. Navajivan Publishing House.

13. Remen, R. N. (1996). Kitchen table wisdom. Riverhead Books.

14. Hamric, A. B., Borchers, C. T., & Epstein, E. G. (2012). Development and testing of an instrument to measure moral distress in healthcare professionals. AJOB Primary Research, 3(2), 1-9.

15. Easwaran, E. (2007). The Bhagavad Gita (Vol. 1). The Blue Mountain Center of Meditation.

16. World Health Organization. (2010). Framework for action on interprofessional education & collaborative practice.

17. Kolodiejchuk, B. (2007). Mother Teresa: Come be my light: The private writings of the Saint of Calcutta. Crown Publishing Group.

18. Sivananda, S. (1958). Practice of Karma Yoga. Divine Life Society Publication.

19. Easwaran, E. (2007). The Bhagavad Gita (Vol. 1). The Blue Mountain Center of Meditation.

20. Dass, R. (1976). The Only Dance There Is. Anchor Books.

21. Hanh, T. N. (2009). You Are Here: Discovering the Magic of the Present Moment. Shambhala Publications.
22. Vivekananda, S. (1991). Karma Yoga. Advaita Ashrama Publication.
23. Sadhguru. (2016). Inner Engineering: A Yogi's Guide to Joy. Spiegel & Grau.

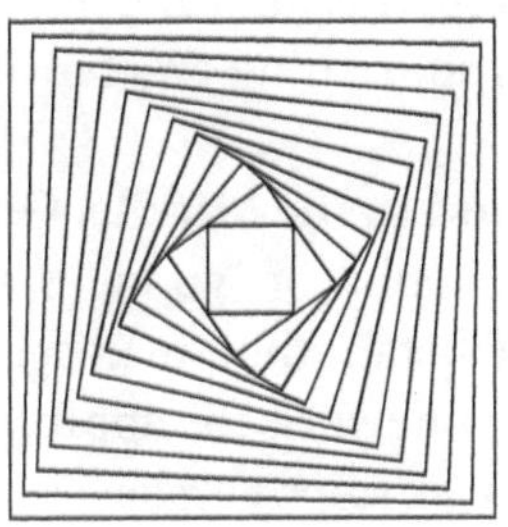

CHAPTER 14

The Importance of Ritual in Healing

"One purpose of creative ritual was to experience the connection to "the other" as well as a deeper connection to oneself. That's why ancient people would say: that ritual made me more aware of how I'm connected to life, to the earth, to the spirits, to the song of creation, and made me more aware of who I am inside, at the level of my own being. What we've lost is partly the sense that we are each connected to the whole thing, that each human soul is secretly connected to the living soul of the world."
Michael Meade

During my travels and work with healers from many ancient medical traditions, it became clear that rituals are essential to each tradition. As someone who was raised a Catholic altar boy and constantly in fear that I would make a mistake at some point in the religious ceremony, I was very averse to the idea that rituals are a vital aspect of healing practice. However, experience has led me to acknowledge the role of ritual in healing.

The Yoga of Medicine describes seven contemplative clinical skills intended to become a stable ritual of our clinical practice. At first blush, adding a ritual to our clinical practice may sound dehumanizing. Rituals have been integral to healing practices across cultures and throughout

181

history. They provide meaning, structure, and a sense of connection in the face of the challenges and uncertainties of the healing process. As Malidoma Somé, a West African elder and author, explains, "Ritual is the way in which the community can come together and move as one body, with one voice, acknowledging that there is something greater than themselves" [8].

Good in the Beginning, Good in the Middle, Good in the End

The Tibetan Buddhist philosophy of "good in the beginning, good in the middle, good in the end" (Tibetan: thog mar dge ba, bar du dge ba, tha mar dge ba) offers a profound framework for approaching any task, particularly in the realm of healing. This concept emphasizes maintaining a positive and mindful approach throughout an activity [5].

In the context of healing, this framework is particularly relevant and beneficial:

Good in the Beginning

This refers to setting the right intention and preparing correctly for the healing process. For a healer, it might involve centering oneself, reviewing the patient's history, and approaching the interaction with compassion and presence. For the patient, it could mean coming to the healing session with an open mind and a willingness to engage in the process.

Good in the Middle

This emphasizes maintaining focus, compassion, and skill throughout the healing process. It reminds both healer and patient to stay present and engaged, even when facing challenges or discomfort.

Good in the End

This aspect highlights the importance of concluding the healing session thoughtfully, ensuring that both healer and patient are clear about the next steps, and taking time to reflect on and integrate the experience.

The importance of this framework in healing cannot be overstated. It encourages a holistic approach that values every aspect of the healing interaction, from preparation to conclusion. This comprehensive mindset can lead to better outcomes, as it ensures nothing is overlooked and that both healer and patient remain fully engaged throughout the process. Moreover, it cultivates a sense of reverence and mindfulness that can transform routine medical interactions into more meaningful, healing experiences.

Etymology and Definitions of Ritual

The word "ritual" comes from the Latin "ritualis," meaning "relating to (religious) rites," which itself derives from "ritus," meaning "rite, ceremony" [6]. Over time, the term has evolved to encompass a broader range of formalized, symbolic actions, both religious and secular.

Various definitions of ritual highlight its multifaceted nature:

1. Merriam-Webster defines ritual as "a formal ceremony or series of acts that are always performed in the same way" [7].
2. Anthropologist Victor Turner describes rituals as "prescribed formal behavior for occasions not given over to technological routine, having reference to beliefs in mystical beings or powers" [8].
3. Sociologist Émile Durkheim viewed rituals as "rules of conduct which prescribe how a man should comport himself in the presence of sacred objects" [9].
4. The Oxford Dictionary of Archaeology offers a more critical perspective: "A favorite but deplorable term commonly used by archaeologists looking to explain unfamiliar patterns in material culture that seem to have no functional explanation" [10].
5. William Ayot provides a more poetic and psychological definition: "A ritual is a symbolic action through which we can give our soul, or psyche, an important message" [11].

These varied definitions reflect the complexity and diversity of rituals across cultures and disciplines. They highlight rituals' formal, symbolic nature, connection to beliefs and values, and potential to convey meaning beyond mere functional utility.

The Universality of Rituals in Healing Traditions

Rituals have been integral to healing practices across cultures and throughout history. Their universality speaks to a fundamental human need to imbue the act of healing with meaning and significance beyond its mere physical aspects.

Examples of healing rituals around the globe and across time include:

1. Native American Sweat Lodge ceremonies, used for physical and spiritual purification [12].
2. Ayurvedic panchakarma rituals for detoxification and rejuvenation [13].
3. Ancient Greek healing temples dedicated to Asclepius, where patients would sleep to receive healing dreams [14].
4. Traditional Chinese Medicine's acupuncture rituals involve specific needle placements to balance qi [15].

5.   Shamanic soul retrieval rituals in various indigenous cultures [16].

Even in modern scientific medicine, we have created many rituals, often under the guise of protocols or procedures. Examples include:

1.   The ritualized "scrubbing in" process before surgery.
2.   The structured format of patient interviews and physical examinations.
3.   The ceremonial aspects of medical school graduations and white coat ceremonies.

Interestingly, modern medicine increasingly encourages rituals to prevent errors and improve patient care. In his book "The Checklist Manifesto," surgeon Atul Gawande advocates for using checklists in medical settings, which can be seen as ritual. He writes:

"We have the means to make some of the most complex and dangerous work we do—in surgery, emergency care, and I.C.U. Medicine—more effective than we ever thought possible. But the prospect pushes against the traditional culture of medicine, with its central belief that in high risk and complexity, what you want is a kind of expert audacity—the right stuff, again" [17].

While primarily functional, these checklists also serve a ritual purpose by focusing attention, ensuring completeness, and marking the gravity of the medical procedure about to be undertaken.

What is Not a Ritual

To fully understand the concept of ritual, it's essential to distinguish it from related but distinct phenomena:

1.   *A Habit*: While rituals can become habitual, not all habits are rituals. Habits are often unconscious and may lack the symbolic significance of rituals.

      Mahatma Gandhi recognized the power of habits in the personal and political realms. He famously said, "I have three enemies. The first is the British colonialists. The second is the Indian people. The third is my own habits" [18]. This quote highlights how our habits can become obstacles to our goals and values just as much as external forces.

      In contrast, rituals are intentional practices that aim to align our actions with our deeper intentions. They are chosen and imbued with meaning rather than being unconscious patterns.

2.   *A Compulsion*: Compulsions are repetitive behaviors driven by anxiety or other psychological distress. Unlike rituals, they are not freely chosen and do not typically carry more profound meaning.

3. *An Obsession*: Obsessions are persistent, intrusive thoughts or urges. While rituals may be associated with particular thought patterns, they are actions rather than thoughts.
4. *Muscle Memory*: This refers to the automatic performance of a physical task through repetition. While rituals may involve physical actions, their significance goes beyond motor skills.
5. *Fear-Based Action*: While some rituals may originate from fears (e.g., superstitions), actual rituals are not primarily motivated by fear but by a desire for meaning, connection, or transformation.

Rituals are intentional, meaningful actions that often carry symbolic significance. They are chosen and performed with awareness, even if that awareness has become implicit through long practice. Unlike habits or compulsions, rituals serve a purpose beyond the action itself, often connecting the individual to a larger context, community, or set of values. Understanding these distinctions can help practitioners and patients recognize the value of rituals in healing. It can guide the development of meaningful practices that enhance the healing process rather than fall into rote behaviors or anxiety-driven compulsions.

The Functions of Ritual

Rituals serve several essential functions in our lives:

1. Provide a doorway out of our habitual patterns: By interrupting our automatic behaviors and thoughts, rituals create a space for new possibilities and perspectives.
2. Connect us with something beyond ourselves: Whether it's a higher power, a community, or a set of values, rituals help us transcend and connect with something more significant.
3. Shape our relationship to time and space: Rituals can "stop time" by creating a sense of timelessness and presence. They can also transform ordinary spaces into sacred or significant places.
4. Disengage us from technology: In a world increasingly dominated by screens and devices, rituals provide a way to unplug and reconnect with ourselves and others.
5. Generate a positive and transformative experience: Well-designed rituals can evoke powerful emotions, insights, and changes in perspective that carry over into our daily lives.

The Structure of Ritual

Rituals typically involve three key elements: intention, attention, and repetition.

1. *Intention*: This is the purpose or meaning behind the ritual. It's what we aim to invoke or embody through ritual actions. Intention setting is often an explicit part of the ritual, such as stating one's goal or dedication at the beginning.
2. *Attention*: Rituals require presence and focus. Unlike habits, which can be performed mindlessly, rituals invite us to bring our full awareness to the action. This attention allows the ritual to "stop time" and create a sense of timelessness or presence.
3. *Repetition*: Rituals often involve repeated actions, words, or gestures. This repetition can deepen the experience, ingraining both the action and its significance into our being. However, it's essential that this repetition doesn't become rote or empty. Patanjali, the author of the Yoga Sutras, warns, "Losing awareness of self is the trap of Karma. The hunter becomes the hunted, the architect becomes the bonded laborer, the creator becomes the creation. A spider trapped in a web of its own making is a tragedy" [19]. Maintaining presence and awareness is crucial in preventing ritual from devolving into mere habit.

When these elements are combined, ritual can become what the Bhagavad Gita calls "impeccable action"—righteous, skillful, and performed without attachment to outcome [20]. The Gita teaches that such action is a path to freedom and enlightenment, as it aligns us with our deepest nature and divine will.

Individual and Collective Rituals in Healing

Rituals can be performed individually or collectively; both types play essential roles in healing practices.

One engages in individual rituals alone, often for personal healing, growth, or transformation. Examples of healing might include:

1. A daily meditation practice to reduce stress and promote mental well-being.
2. A personal prayer or intention-setting before a medical procedure.
3. A self-care routine that includes mindful activities like journaling or yoga.

The power of individual ritual lies in its ability to foster a deep connection with oneself and one's healing process. It provides a space for introspection, self-discovery, and personal transformation.

On the other hand, collective rituals are performed by groups of people and connect individuals to a larger community or shared purpose. In healing, collective rituals can:

1. Create a sense of support and solidarity among people facing similar health challenges.
2. Tap into the power of collective intention and prayer for healing.
3. Provide a space for shared catharsis, grief, or celebration in the face of illness or recovery.

Examples of collective healing rituals might include:

1. A support group for cancer patients that begins each meeting with a shared affirmation or moment of silence.
2. A community prayer circle for someone undergoing a health crisis.
3. A celebratory ritual to mark the end of a course of treatment or a milestone in recovery.

Collective rituals remind us that we are not alone in our healing journeys. They can provide a profound sense of connection, support, and shared meaning in the face of even the most private and personal health struggles.

Both individual and collective rituals have their place in healing. Individual practices allow personal transformation and self-discovery, while collective rituals foster connection, support, and shared meaning-making. The interplay between the two often creates the most potent and comprehensive healing experiences.

For example, a person undergoing a major surgery might engage in personal rituals like meditation and intention-setting to prepare emotionally and spiritually for the procedure. At the same time, they might be supported by collective rituals like prayers from their faith community or a pre-surgery ritual with their medical team. Combining individual and collective practices can provide a multi-layered, holistic approach to healing.

In the end, whether a ritual is performed alone or with others, its power lies in its ability to connect us more deeply to ourselves, each other, and something greater than ourselves. In the face of the challenges and uncertainties of the healing process, rituals can provide a grounding, meaning, and transformation that supports us on every level of our being.

Creating Supportive Rituals in Your Healing Practice

1. Start with "Why" and the Power of Purpose
Simon Sinek, author of "Start With Why," argues that the most successful and inspiring individuals and organizations start by clarifying their core purpose or belief - their "Why" [21]. This principle is particularly relevant when creating rituals in a healing context.

The fundamental "why" in healthcare is compassion—the desire to alleviate suffering and promote well-being. When designing a supportive ritual, it's essential to keep this core purpose at the forefront. Ask yourself: How does this ritual express and embody compassion? How does it align with the more profound mission of healing?

This focus on the "Why" is a crucial difference between a ritual and a mere habit. As Sobonfu Somé, a teacher and author on African spirituality, notes, "Ritual is a container for the sacred. It is a way of making visible the invisible" [9]. By starting with the "Why" of compassion, we ensure that our rituals are not just empty routines but profound expressions of our commitment to healing.

2. Build Rituals with Habits
Once we have clarified our "Why," we can start to build our rituals using James Clear's "Atomic Habits" model [22]. This model suggests that habits (and, by extension, rituals) are formed through a three-step process:

1. Cue: The trigger that initiates the behavior.
2. Routine: The behavior itself.
3. Reward: The benefit gained from the behavior.

To create a supportive ritual, we can design each of these steps with the intention:

1. Cue: Choose a clear, consistent trigger for your ritual. This might be a specific time of day, a particular location, or a preceding action. For example, you may begin each patient interaction with a moment of centering and intention-setting.
2. Routine: Design the ritual actions to be meaningful, focused, and aligned with your "Why." This could involve deep breathing, silent reflection, or a verbal affirmation. The key is to choose actions that feel authentic and supportive to you.
3. Reward: Identify your ritual's intrinsic rewards. These might be a sense of grounding, connection, or renewed purpose. By focusing on these

internal benefits rather than external incentives, you reinforce the ritual's inherent value. By intentionally crafting each stage of the habit loop, we can create meaningful, sustainable, and integrated rituals into our daily healing practices.

3. Leverage Behavioral Design

Adopting a new ritual can be challenging even with a clear "Why" and a well-designed routine. This is where behavioral design comes in - the science of creating environments and systems that shape behavior. B.J. Fogg, a pioneer in this field, has developed a model for behavior change that can be applied to ritual adoption [23].

Fogg's model suggests that three elements must converge for a behavior to occur: motivation, ability, and a prompt. In other words, we must want to do the behavior, be able to do it, and be reminded to do it. This model has been used extensively in designing cell phone apps and social media platforms to create compelling user behaviors.

We can apply these same principles to creating supportive healing rituals:

1. Motivation: Connect your ritual to your deeper "Why" of compassion and healing. This intrinsic motivation will fuel your desire to engage in the practice.
2. Ability: Design your ritual to be simple, accessible, and easy to integrate into your existing routine. Start with small, manageable steps and build up over time. Fogg refers to these as "tiny habits" - small, easily achievable behaviors that can be built upon over time.
3. Prompt: Use clear, consistent cues to remind yourself to engage in your ritual. This could be a visual reminder (like a note on your desk), a time-based cue (like an alarm), or an action-based prompt (like taking a deep breath before entering a patient's room.

By aligning these three factors - motivation, ability, and prompts - we create an environment that supports the adoption and maintenance of meaningful healing rituals.

Malidoma Somé emphasizes the importance of consistency and repetition in ritual: "Ritual is a way of remembering, and it is in the remembering that the power of ritual lies. [...] It is through repetition that we are able to access the deeper layers of ourselves" [8]. We create the conditions for sustained, transformative ritual practice by aligning motivation, ability, and prompts.

Concluding Remarks

As we navigate the challenges and opportunities of modern healthcare, integrating rituals provides a path to reconnect with the deeper essence of healing. By creating spaces for meaning, connection, and transcendence within our medical practices, we improve outcomes and honor the fundamental human dimensions of the healing relationship.

The invitation is to bring a spirit of curiosity, creativity, and reverence to developing rituals in our personal and professional healing practices. In doing so, we tap into a timeless wisdom that can transform our individual experiences and the larger landscape of healthcare. As we embrace the sacred art of ritual, we reconnect with the heart of healing and rediscover the profound transformation potential within each clinical encounter.

Self-Reflection Questions

1. What role have rituals played in your healing journey as a patient or healer?
2. How might the Tibetan Buddhist concept of "good in the beginning, good in the middle, good in the end" be applied to your current healing practices?
3. Reflect on a habit or routine in your life. How might you transform it into a meaningful ritual by infusing it with intention, attention, and wise repetition?
4. Consider a challenging aspect of your healing work. How might the principles of ritual design (starting with "Why," building atomic habits, leveraging behavioral design) help you create a supportive practice to navigate this challenge?
5. Imagine integrating the principles of the Yoga of Medicine into your healing practice. What would bringing mindful presence and intentionality to every aspect of your work look like? What impact might this have on your well-being and your patients?

References

[1] Bhagavad Gita, Chapter 3, Verse 19.
[2] Bhagavad Gita, Chapter 2, Verse 51.
[3] Swami Sivananda, "The Practice of Medicine as Yoga," from the book "Bliss Divine."
[4] Swami Vivekananda, "Karma Yoga," Chapter 5.
[5] Patrul Rinpoche. (1994). The Words of My Perfect Teacher. HarperOne.
[6] Online Etymology Dictionary. (n.d.). Ritual. Retrieved from https://www.etymonline.com/word/ritual
[7] Merriam-Webster. (n.d.). Ritual. In Merriam-Webster.com dictionary.
[8] Somé, M. (1999). The Healing Wisdom of Africa: Finding Life Purpose Through Nature, Ritual, and Community. TarcherPerigee.
[9] Somé, S. (2002). Falling Out of Grace: Meditations on Loss, Healing, and

Wisdom. North Bay Books.

[10] Darvill, T. (2008). Oxford Concise Dictionary of Archaeology. Oxford University Press.

[11] Ayot, W. (2015). Re-enchanting the Forest: Meaningful Ritual in a Secular World. Vala Publishing Cooperative Ltd.

[12] Bucko, R. A. (1998). The Lakota Ritual of the Sweat Lodge. University of Nebraska Press.

[13] Svoboda, R. E. (1992). Ayurveda: Life, Health and Longevity. Penguin Books India.

[14] Askitopoulou, H., Konsolaki, E., Ramoutsaki, I., & Anastassaki, E. (2002). Surgical cures by sleep induction as the Asclepieion of Epidaurus. The history of anesthesia: proceedings of the Fifth International Symposium, by José Carlos Diz, Avelino Franco, Douglas R. Bacon, J. Rupreht, Julián Alvarez. Elsevier Science B.V., International Congress Series 1242, pp. 11-17.

[15] Kaptchuk, T. J. (2000). The Web That Has No Weaver: Understanding Chinese Medicine. Contemporary Books.

[16] Ingerman, S. (1991). Soul Retrieval: Mending the Fragmented Self. HarperOne.

[17] Gawande, A. (2009). The Checklist Manifesto: How to Get Things Right. Metropolitan Books.

[18] Gandhi, M. K. (1927). An Autobiography or The Story of My Experiments with Truth. Navajivan Publishing House. p. 295.

[19] Patanjali. (2009). The Yoga Sutras of Patanjali. Integral Yoga Publications. p. 156.

[20] Easwaran, E. (2007). The Bhagavad Gita. Nilgiri Press. pp. 61-63.

[21] Sinek, S. (2009). Start with Why: How Great Leaders Inspire Everyone to Take Action. Portfolio/Penguin.

[22] Clear, J. (2018). Atomic Habits: An Easy & Proven Way to Build Good Habits & Break Bad Ones. Avery.

[23] Fogg, B. J. (2020). Tiny Habits: The Small Changes That Change Everything. Houghton Mifflin Harcourt.

[24] Dass, R. (1976). Be Here Now. Lama Foundation. p. 87.

[25] Hanh, T. N. (2015). How to Walk. Parallax Press. p. 42.

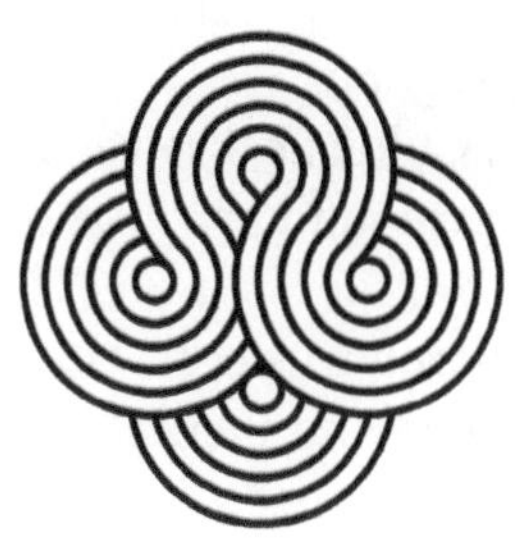

CHAPTER 15

Contemplative Clinical Skills

"The best definition I know for contemplation is as follows:
Contemplation is a long, loving look at what really is..."
Richard Rohr

"The Yoga of Medicine" describes seven essential contemplative skills that can be integrated into the clinical encounter. These contemplative clinical skills embody the critical elements of contemplative practice and are vehicles for the contemplative experience within a clinical setting. These skills are not meant to replace conventional medical training but to complement and enhance it. By developing these capacities, healthcare professionals can foster deeper connections with their patients, gain insight into the root causes of illness, and ultimately facilitate more profound healing.

The seven contemplative skills that make up the Yoga of Medicine are:

1. Create Intention: Set a clear and purposeful direction for the clinical encounter.
2. Create a Safe Space: Establish an environment of trust, respect, and non-judgment.
3. Become Present: Cultivate a state of being fully present in the moment.
4. Make Connection: Build rapport and foster a deep understanding and

connection with the patient.

5. Be Courageous: Having the courage to sit with difficult emotions and experiences, both one's own and the patient's.
6. Close and Dedicate: Close the clinical encounter and dedicate the fruits of one's efforts to the highest good.
7. Be Joyful and Celebrate: Cultivate a sense of joy and celebration in one's work and recognize the profound privilege of serving others.

These skills will be explored in depth later in this text, with practical guidance on cultivating and applying them in the clinical setting. The rituals described by the yoga of medicine:

1. Align our intention with our behaviors
2. Create a space that provides fertile ground for healing and transformation.
3. Connect the healer and their patient with their greatest potential for flourishing.
4. Foster the self-cultivation of the healer.
5. Energize the healer and the patient.
6. Support the development of the healer's craft.

As Sadhguru reminds us, "Yoga is the science of activating your inner energies in such a way that your body, mind, and emotions function at their highest peak" [1]. By embracing the principles and practices outlined in this section, healthcare providers can tap into their inner resources and create a space for genuine healing.

One realistic concern raised by clinicians is that the seven "asanas" of the yoga of medicine will require even more time in an already tight clinical schedule. However, no additional time is necessary, and each asana may enhance the clinician's efficiency and efficacy.

Contemplative experience inhabits a space outside the purview of language and concepts. Any attempt to use language to define or describe contemplation will inevitably be inadequate or even misleading. However, visual imagery and imagination can be more helpful in capturing the ineffable quality of contemplative experience. Imagine you're a physician rushing through a busy day in the hospital. Visualize and hear the clang of beeping monitors and urgent pages. Visualize yourself as you experience the sympathetic arousal and fear you must inhabit to maintain your constant reactivity state designed to respond to both real and imagined emergencies. This is the "survival mode" that describes the daily experience of most modern healers.

Now, take a long, slow, deep breath and open a space of safety, clarity, kindness, and joy. Inhabit this space of spacious abundance and confidence in ourselves and the universe. This is where contemplative practice and contemplative experience come in. Contemplation is not just an impractical ancient practice for monks and philosophers; it's a tool that could transform your medical practice and your life. Contemplative practice is the key to accessing vitality and avoiding the "burnout" that has become the hallmark of modern healers' experience.

Common Themes Across Contemplative Practices: Finding the Thread

There is currently no consensus definition of the term contemplation, and a long list of various descriptors has been used to describe the characteristics of contemplation. However, like the thread of a rosary or mala beads, these commonalities lend coherence and a guideline for understanding the organizing principles of the world's contemplative practices. It does appear that the world's contemplative traditions have a consensus on the following characteristics of contemplation:

1. Focused attention
2. Inner Exploration
3. Transformation
4. Insight
5. Expanded awareness
6. Present-moment focus
7. Connection
8. Non-judgmental observation
9. Cultivation of positive mental states
10. Integration

The Five Key Elements of Contemplation

Different traditions all describe the five key elements of contemplative practice as: attention, presence, concentration, alertness, and discernment. I will now describe each of these in more detail.

Attention

Attention is the ability to focus on a chosen object or experience. As William James wrote, "Attention is the taking possession by the mind, in clear and vivid form, of one out of what seem several simultaneously possible objects or trains of thought" [2]. Attention can be focused externally on sensory stimuli or internally on thoughts, emotions, or sensations. The practice of sustained, voluntary attention is a core element of many contemplative practices.

Attention as an element of contemplation involves several interrelated capacities:

1.   Selective attention
2.   Sustained attention
3.   Shifting attention
4.   Divided attention

Optimizing and balancing these attentional capacities is crucial for effectively navigating both our inner lives and the external world. In a healthcare context, clinicians must be able to attend to relevant clinical data selectively, sustain attention through long shifts and complex procedures, shift attention between multiple patients and changing priorities, and divide attention between a patient's words, non-verbal cues, and clinical reasoning.

The growing prevalence of attentional disorders like ADHD highlights the importance of attention. As psychologist Daniel Brown argues in his book on ADHD, "Attention serves as the foundation for our ability to organize thoughts, perceptions, and behaviors into coordinated, systematic effort. Attention is like the conductor of our mental orchestra...It helps to direct a complex set of attentional skills so that our minds work well" [3].

Cultivating attentional skills is thus essential for clinicians and human flourishing more broadly. Brown describes a model of attentional development called "The Elephant Path," which integrates insights from Western psychological science and Buddhist contemplative practices to outline a systematic path for optimizing attention [3].

Such integrative approaches offer great promise for addressing the attentional challenges of our time. As clinician-educators, we have a responsibility to cultivate our attentional capacities and find skillful ways to share these practices with our students, colleagues, and patients.

Presence

In a contemplative context, presence implies bringing one's full awareness to the here and now without being lost in thoughts of the past or future. Philosopher Bertrand Russell described contemplation as "that receptive attitude of mind which, in the words of Jacob Boehme, 'listens only to God, and to nothing else'" [4]. In Buddhist practice, presence is cultivated through mindfulness or paying careful attention to one's present-moment experience. The topic of presence and its particular importance in the healing encounter is explored in more depth elsewhere in this book.

Concentration

Concentration refers to the depth, stability, and continuity of attentional focus. B. Alan Wallace distinguishes concentration from attention, noting that "attention is the faculty of focusing on a particular object, whereas

concentration is the ability to sustain that attentional focus over time"
[5]. Buddhist texts like the Visuddhimagga map the progressive stages of
meditative concentration in detail.

In a clinical context, concentration allows the healthcare provider to
remain focused and grounded amidst the many distractions and stressors of
the medical environment. It supports clinical precision, clear communication,
and a stable therapeutic presence. Practitioners who can concentrate deeply
are better equipped to listen attentively to patients, pick up on subtle diagnostic
cues, and perform delicate procedures with care and skill.

Alertness

Alertness, in the context of contemplative practice, is a kind of meta-
awareness that monitors the quality of attention and notices when the mind
has wandered. Scholar John Dunne describes alertness as "the factor of the
mind that observes or witnesses the primary focus of attention" [6]. In the
Buddhist tradition, alertness (sampajanna) is paired with mindfulness (sati)
as two essential qualities of the mind.

In healthcare, alertness allows clinicians to monitor their mental states
and catch potential errors or oversights. It is a critical component of reflective
practice and supports ongoing learning and improvement. Alertness also
helps clinicians stay attuned to their patients' shifting needs and conditions
and respond flexibly as situations change.

Discernment

Discernment refers to the ability to clearly perceive and understand the
nature of one's contemplative experience. Buddhist scholar Joseph Goldstein
describes discernment as "seeing the truth of our experience, not being lost in
reactivity or judgments" [7]. Discernment is the fruit of deep contemplative
insight, which sees beyond surface appearances into the underlying nature
of reality.

In a clinical setting, discernment allows healthcare providers to see beyond
surface symptoms to discern the root causes of illness and suffering. It supports
accurate diagnosis, individualized treatment, and a holistic understanding of
the patient's lived experience. Discernment helps clinicians navigate complex
ethical dilemmas by clarifying core values and moral principles.

The 84,000 Medicines

In Buddhist tradition, it is said that the Buddha taught 84,000 different
practices or dharma doors. This vast number is not meant to be taken literally
but symbolically represents the innumerable ways the Buddha adapted his
teachings to suit sentient beings' diverse needs, capacities, and inclinations [8].

As the Buddha explained in the Lotus Sutra:

"I look upon all beings equally,
Without any distinction among them,
But in order to save them,
I employ various means." [9]

The 84,000 practices are like medicines prescribed by a skilled doctor. Just as a doctor diagnoses a patient's illness and prescribes the appropriate remedy, the Buddha recognizes each individual's unique "diseases" or afflictions and offers the specific antidote as a tailored spiritual practice [10].

Thich Nhat Hanh elaborates on this metaphor: "When a skilled doctor treats a patient, he has to find the cause of the illness before he can prescribe the proper medicine. If the cause is heat, he has to use a cooling medicine; if cold, then a warming medicine. The Buddha is like a skilled physician. He taught 84,000 Dharma doors because sentient beings have 84,000 afflictions." [11]

This underscores the pragmatic and compassionate nature of the Buddha's teachings. Rather than insisting on a one-size-fits-all approach, he acknowledged the diversity of human experiences and provided a wide range of entry points into the path of awakening.

In this light, meditation and contemplation can be seen as two broad categories within the 84,000 practices. Meditation encompasses the more structured, technique-driven approaches, while contemplation allows a more open-ended exploration of consciousness. Both serve as potent medicines for the mind, helping alleviate suffering and cultivating wisdom and compassion.

As the renowned Tibetan Dzogchen practitioner Tulku Urgyen Rinpoche notes: "There are numerous methods for training in meditation, but the key point of all of them is to realize the inseparability of samsara and nirvana, of the ordinary confused state of mind and the fully awakened state." [12]

Ultimately, whether through the focused lens of meditation or the expansive field of contemplation, the 84,000 practices all aim to guide us back to our inherent nature. This boundless, luminous awareness is our true home.

An Integral Definition of Contemplation

Contemplative practices are inevitably shaped and respond to the cultural conditions in which they are practiced. Based on these common themes, I suggest a definition of contemplation that might be particularly relevant for us in healthcare:

Contemplation is a practice of sustained, focused attention that involves inner exploration and present-moment awareness. It cultivates expanded consciousness, fostering insight, personal transformation, and a sense of connection beyond the individual self. Through non-judgmental observation, contemplation integrates various aspects of human experience, leading to enhanced understanding, positive mental states, and, potentially, spiritual realization.

What are Contemplative Clinical Skills?

Contemplative clinical skills represent a fusion of traditional contemplative practices with modern healthcare techniques. These skills enable healthcare professionals to bring heightened awareness, presence, and compassion to their clinical practice. By integrating contemplative approaches into healthcare, practitioners can enhance their ability to connect with patients, make more accurate diagnoses, and provide more holistic care.

Key aspects of contemplative clinical skills include:

1. Mindful Presence: The ability to be fully present with patients, listening deeply and attentively without judgment or distraction. This skill allows clinicians to pick up on subtle cues and create a safe, compassionate space for healing.
2. Emotional Regulation: involves using contemplative techniques to manage one's emotions and stress levels in challenging clinical situations. This skill helps prevent burnout and allows for more precise decision-making.
3. Empathic Attunement: Developing a more profound sense of empathy and connection with patients through practices that cultivate compassion and understanding.
4. Clinical Intuition: Honing the ability to tap into intuitive insights that complement analytical diagnosis and treatment planning thinking.
5. Ethical Discernment: Using contemplative practices to clarify values and navigate complex ethical dilemmas in healthcare.
6. Self-Reflection: Regularly self-examining to identify biases, improve clinical skills, and foster personal growth.
7. Holistic Perception: Developing the ability to see patients as whole persons, understanding the interconnections between physical, emotional, and spiritual aspects of health.
8. Therapeutic Presence: Cultivating a healing presence that can positively influence patient outcomes beyond specific interventions.
9. Resilience and Self-Care: Using contemplative practices to build resilience and maintain personal well-being in the face of healthcare challenges.

10. Inter-professional Awareness: Enhancing collaboration and communication with other healthcare professionals through increased self-awareness and presence.

Implementing contemplative clinical skills involves integrating practices such as mindfulness meditation, reflective writing, body awareness exercises, and contemplative dialogue into clinical training and daily practice. These skills can be developed through:

- Formal training programs in mindfulness-based interventions
- Regular personal contemplative practice
- Reflective practice groups or supervision
- Incorporating moments of mindfulness into daily clinical routines
- Using contemplative approaches in team meetings and case discussions

By developing these skills, healthcare professionals can enhance not only their clinical effectiveness but also their personal well-being and job satisfaction. Patients benefit from more attentive, compassionate care, potentially leading to improved health outcomes and increased satisfaction with their healthcare experience.

As healthcare continues to evolve, contemplative clinical skills offer a promising approach to addressing many challenges modern healthcare systems face, including burnout, fragmented care, and the need for more patient-centered approaches. By bridging ancient wisdom with contemporary medical practice, these skills can transform the experience of both healthcare providers and patients, fostering a more holistic, humane, and healing-oriented approach to care.

What Are The Benefits of Contemplative Clinical Skills?

The integration of contemplative clinical skills into healthcare practice can lead to several important benefits:

1. Improved Patient Outcomes: Contemplative clinical skills can lead to more effective treatments and better health outcomes by fostering deeper connections and more accurate perceptions of patients' needs.
2. Enhanced Patient Satisfaction: Patients often feel more heard, understood, and cared for when their healthcare providers demonstrate strong contemplative clinical skills.
3. Reduced Medical Errors: The increased awareness and presence associated with these skills can help clinicians catch potential errors and make more informed decisions.

4. Better Team Dynamics: When healthcare teams cultivate contemplative skills collectively, it can lead to improved communication, reduced conflict, and more effective collaboration.
5. Increased Job Satisfaction: Healthcare providers who develop these skills often report a greater sense of meaning and fulfillment in their work, which can help combat burnout and turnover.
6. Cultural Competence: Contemplative practices can enhance clinicians' ability to understand and respect diverse cultural perspectives, leading to more inclusive and equitable healthcare.
7. Improved Self-Care: The self-awareness and emotional regulation skills developed through contemplative practices can help healthcare providers better manage their stress and maintain their well-being.

Challenges in Implementing Contemplative Clinical Skills

While the benefits of contemplative clinical skills are significant, there are challenges to their widespread adoption in healthcare settings:

1. Time Constraints: The fast-paced nature of many healthcare environments can make it challenging to incorporate contemplative practices.
2. Skepticism: Some healthcare professionals may be skeptical of contemplative approaches' scientific validity or practical applicability.
3. Lack of Training: Many medical and nursing education programs do not yet include comprehensive training in contemplative skills.
4. Cultural Barriers: In some healthcare cultures, there may be resistance to practices perceived as "soft" or non-technical.
5. Measurement Difficulties: The benefits of contemplative skills can be challenging to quantify, making it difficult to demonstrate their value in evidence-based healthcare systems.

Overcoming these challenges requires a multi-faceted approach:

1. Education and Training: Integrating contemplative skills into medical and nursing curricula and offering continuing education opportunities for practicing clinicians.
2. Research: Conducting rigorous studies to demonstrate the efficacy of contemplative approaches in healthcare settings.
3. Organizational Support: Developing policies and structures that support the integration of contemplative practices in healthcare workplaces.
4. Leadership: Encouraging healthcare leaders to model and promote contemplative skills.
5. Technology Integration: Developing digital tools and apps that can

support the practice of contemplative skills in clinical settings.

Future Directions for Contemplative Clinical Skills

As healthcare evolves, contemplative clinical skills will likely play an increasingly important role. Some potential future developments include:

1. Personalized Contemplative Approaches: Tailoring contemplative practices to individual clinicians' and patients' needs and preferences.
2. Integration with Artificial Intelligence: Using AI to support the development and application of contemplative skills in clinical decision-making.
3. Virtual Reality Applications: Leveraging VR technology to create immersive environments for practicing contemplative skills.
4. Global Health Applications: Exploring how contemplative clinical skills can be adapted and applied in diverse global health contexts.
5. Interdisciplinary Collaboration: Fostering collaboration between healthcare professionals, contemplative scholars, and researchers from neuroscience and psychology to further develop and refine contemplative clinical skills.

Concluding Remarks

Contemplative clinical skills represent a powerful approach to enhancing healthcare delivery and outcomes. By bridging ancient wisdom with modern medical practice, these skills offer a path to more compassionate, effective, and sustainable healthcare. As we continue to face complex challenges in healthcare, cultivating contemplative clinical skills is essential to creating a healthcare system that truly serves the needs of patients and providers.

The journey of developing contemplative clinical skills is ongoing for individual practitioners and the healthcare system as a whole. It invites us to continually deepen our understanding, refine our practices, and expand our capacity for healing presence. As we move forward, let us embrace the potential of these skills to transform our clinical practice and our understanding of what it means to be truly present in the art and science of healing.

"There are a hundred ways to kneel and kiss the ground." - Rumi.

This quote from the 13th-century Persian poet Rumi reminds us that there are many paths to cultivating presence, compassion, and healing [13]. Contemplative clinical skills offer healthcare professionals a rich array of approaches to deepen their practice and enhance their ability to serve. As we continue to explore and develop these skills, we open new possibilities for healing, growth, and transformation in healthcare.

Self-Reflection Questions

1. How do I currently incorporate contemplative practices into my clinical work, and what opportunities do I see for deepening my engagement with these approaches?

2. Which of the five key elements of contemplation (attention, presence, concentration, alertness, discernment) do I feel most proficient in, and which do I need to cultivate further?

3. In what ways have I experienced the benefits of contemplative clinical skills in my practice, such as improved patient outcomes, enhanced job satisfaction, or better self-care?

4. What challenges or barriers do I face in integrating contemplative practices into my clinical work, and how might I address these obstacles?

5. How can I contribute to the growing field of contemplative clinical skills, whether through personal practice, research, teaching, or advocacy?

6. How do my cultural background and belief system shape my understanding and experience of contemplative practices, and how can I remain open to diverse perspectives?

7. As I reflect on the journey of developing contemplative clinical skills, what insights or aspirations arise regarding my growth as a healthcare provider and person?

References

[1] Sadhguru. (2016). Inner Engineering: A Yogi's Guide to Joy. Spiegel & Grau.

[2] James, W. (1902). The Varieties of Religious Experience. Longmans, Green & Co.

[3] Brown, D.P., & Engler, J. (1980). The stages of mindfulness meditation: A validation study. Journal of Transpersonal Psychology, 12(2), 143-192.

[4] Pascal, B. (trans. 1995). Pensées. Penguin Classics.

[5] Wallace, B.A. (2006). The Attention Revolution: Unlocking the Power of the Focused Mind. Wisdom Publications.

[6] Brown, D.P., & Engler, J. (1980). The stages of mindfulness meditation: A validation study. Journal of Transpersonal Psychology, 12(2), 143-192.

[7] Kabat-Zinn, J. (1994). Wherever You Go, There You Are: Mindfulness Meditation in Everyday Life. Hyperion.

[8] Buswell, R. E., & Lopez, D. S. (2013). The Princeton Dictionary of Buddhism. Princeton University Press.

[9] Watson, B. (2009). The Lotus Sutra and Its Opening and Closing Sutras. Columbia University Press.

[10] Thich, N. H. (1998). The Heart of the Buddha's Teaching: Transforming Suffering Into Peace, Joy & Liberation: the Four Noble Truths, the Noble

Eightfold Path, and Other Basic Buddhist Teachings. Harmony.
[11] Hanh, T. N. (2009). The Heart Of Understanding: Commentaries on the Prajñaparamita Heart Sutra. Parallax Press.
[12] Rinpoche, T. U. (1999). As It Is. Rangjung Yeshe Publications.
[13] Rumi, J. (trans. 2004). The Essential Rumi. HarperOne.

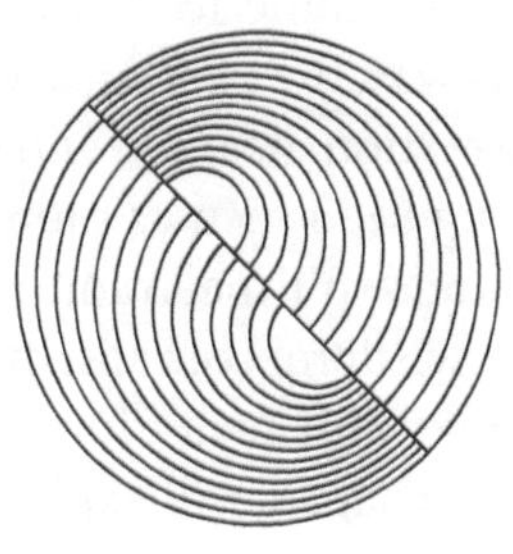

Chapter 16

Asana One: Have Clear Intention

Instruction: "Be mindful of your intention"

*"Waking up this morning, I smile. Twenty-four brand new
hours are before me. I vow to live fully in each moment
and to look at all beings with eyes of compassion."*
Thich Nhat Hahn

*O*ne intention is the central axis around which we align and assess our actions. Intention setting is a practice with deep psychological roots and transformative potential. By focusing attention, priming the mind, harnessing self-fulfilling prophecy and confirmation bias, enhancing self-awareness and self-regulation, tapping into neuroplasticity and mental rehearsal, and engaging social psychology and accountability, intention setting creates fertile ground for personal and collective change.

Too often, we behave in ways that leave us disappointed in ourselves. This can be particularly true in modern healthcare settings where healers react negatively to the constant barrage of challenges that describe their work. Having a clear intention for ourselves and our work helps to remind us of the north star that directs our path as healers. Intention is like the compass that guides us home. It is never more important than when we are in the storm of our life. Whether setting an intention for a particular conversation, a day's priorities, or a lifelong vision, the principles are the same. With clarity, commitment, and consistent practice, we can use the power of intention to shape our lived reality and contribute to a world that reflects our deepest values and aspirations. In this way, the psychology of intention setting offers a pathway to personal transformation, healing, and evolution.

The human heart has long been seen as more than a physical organ that pumps blood. Across cultures and spiritual traditions, the heart is viewed as the seat of emotion, authenticity, wisdom, courage, and intention. The "intention of the heart" refers to one's innermost aspirations and the principles that guide one's choices and actions. This chapter will explore the meaning of intention, its role in human psychology and behavior, and its spiritual significance, particularly in the Mahayana Buddhist tradition.

Etymology and Definitions of Intention

The English word "intention" derives from the Latin intentio, which means "a stretching out, straining, exertion, or effort; attention" [1]. It implies directing the mind toward some purpose or goal. Dictionary definitions of intention include:

1. A thing intended; an aim or plan.
2. The action or fact of intending [2].
3. A determination to act in a certain way [3].
4. Conceptions formed by directing the mind towards an object [4].

These definitions highlight that intentions arise from a purposeful focus of the mind. They exist as mental determinations or commitments that precede and guide our actions. Intentions give direction and coherence to behavior by organizing it around consciously chosen aims.

The Psychology of Intention

In psychology, intention has been studied as a critical factor in motivation, self-regulation, and goal-directed behavior. According to the Theory of Planned Behavior, intentions are the immediate antecedents and best predictors of voluntary actions [5, p. 179]. Intentions are shaped by one's attitudes (overall evaluations of the behavior), subjective norms (beliefs about how others view the behavior), and perceived behavioral control (the extent to which one believes they can perform the behavior) [6, p. 665].

Psychologists distinguish between goal intentions, which specify desired end states to be achieved, and implementation intentions, which are "if-then" plans that link anticipated situations to goal-directed responses [7, p. 493].

For example, one might form the goal intention to be more compassionate and then create an implementation intention such as "If I see someone suffering, then I will offer them comfort and support." Research has shown that forming implementation intentions significantly increases the likelihood of accomplishing one's goals by enabling people to initiate planned responses when specified situations arise automatically [8, p. 69; 9, p. 295].

The concept of intentions has also been central to understanding moral behavior. Rest's Four Component Model proposes that moral behavior arises from four inner psychological processes: 1) moral sensitivity, 2) moral judgment, 3) moral motivation, and 4) moral character [10]. Moral motivation refers to forming intentions to act morally and prioritizing moral values above other values and needs [11, p. 101]. This highlights how our intentions reflect what we ultimately care about and are committed to.

The Intention of the Heart and the Work

Michael Meade, a renowned storyteller, author, and mythology scholar, has written extensively about the power of living with intentionality and authenticity. For Meade, the "intention of the heart" represents our deepest calling and the unique gifts we will bring to the world. He writes:

"Each person comes into the world as a package deal; we each come with a seeded project, an inborn dream, and a way intended by the soul. We each have an inherent reason for being and a mythic identity trying to grow from the inside out. Following the clues to find a way to that inner treasure involves an initiatory adventure. When the heart becomes the initiating factor, intention becomes the key to real meaning and purpose" [24, p. 42].

Meade suggests that connecting with the heart's intention is an ongoing process of self-discovery and self-creation. It involves listening to the deep promptings of the soul and having the courage to follow where they lead, even when that path departs from social norms or expectations.

"When you know the intention of your heart, you can withstand all the pressure to conform and all the people who want to use you for their own purposes. The intention of the heart becomes an invisible protector, an inner light in a time of outer darkness" [26, p. 89].

Following the heart's intention may require going against social expectations or resisting external pressures. But it allows us to stay connected to our core sense of self and purpose. When we act with intention, we are less likely to get pulled off course by competing demands or distractions.

Intention in Buddhist Psychology

In Buddhism, the role of intention is paramount. The Buddha declared, "Intention, I tell you, is kamma. Intending, one does kamma through body, speech, & intellect" [12]. Karma (Sanskrit: karma) refers to voluntary or intentional action - the idea that our actions have moral weight and create consequences. The Buddha taught that our intentions are the ultimate source of our actions and shape our character and future experiences. He said, "All experiences are preceded by mind, led by mind, created by mind" [13].

The Buddha often used the metaphor of seeds to describe how intentions produce results: "Karma is like a field, our intentions are like seeds. Positive intentions bring positive results; negative intentions bring negative results" [14, p. 204]. Every intentional thought, word, and deed plants 'seeds' in the mind that will come to fruition when the proper conditions arise. Unwholesome intentions rooted in greed, hatred, and delusion lead to suffering, while wholesome intentions based on generosity, love, and wisdom lead to happiness and freedom.

Intention of the Heart and Bodhicitta
In Mahayana Buddhism, bodhicitta represents the pinnacle of positive intention. Bodhicitta is often translated as "awakening mind" or "the mind of enlightenment." It is the heartfelt aspiration to attain enlightenment for the benefit of all sentient beings [15, p. 11]. Bodhicitta is an altruistic intention that places the welfare of others above one's own and seeks to relieve the suffering of all.

The 8th-century Indian Buddhist master Shantideva wrote extensive praises of bodhicitta and the way of the bodhisattva (one who cultivates bodhicitta). He describes bodhicitta as a potent inner force:

> "Just as a flash of lightning on a dark, cloudy night
> For an instant brightly illuminates all,
> Likewise in this world, through the might of Buddha,
> A wholesome thought rarely and briefly appears.
> Hence virtue is perpetually feeble,
> The great strength of negativity being extremely intense,
> And except for a Fully Awakening Mind
> By what other virtue will it be overcome?" [16, Ch. 1, v. 5-7]

For Shantideva, bodhicitta is the ultimate "intention of the heart" - a radically compassionate resolve that can overcome all mental afflictions and lead to the perfect enlightened state of a Buddha. Cultivating bodhicitta transforms all of one's actions into causes for enlightenment.

In describing meditation on bodhicitta, Shantideva writes:

"Upon making such an aspiration,
A moment later, a miserable person
Becomes known as a child of the Sugatas [Buddhas].
Even by gods and humans, he is revered" [17, Ch. 3, v. 18-19].

Generating bodhicitta marks a fundamental shift in one's motivations and self-identity. One's intentions are no longer primarily self-oriented but are expanded to encompass the welfare of all beings. With bodhicitta, one's individual aims to align with the greater purpose of liberating all beings from suffering and leading them to enlightenment.

Sankalpa: Aligning Intention with Action in the Hindu Tradition
In addition to the Buddhist concept of bodhicitta, the Hindu tradition offers valuable insights into the role of intention through the practice of Sankalpa. Sankalpa can be translated as "will, purpose, or determination." It is the subtle power of intention and faith that enables us to harness our will to achieve our highest aspirations [34].

Hindu scholar Pandit Rajmani Tigunait describes the nature of Sankalpa:

"Sankalpa is the compound of san, which refers to a connection with the highest truth, and Kalpa, which means vow or commitment. Thus, sankalpa means a commitment we make to support our highest truth. It is a declaration of who we are, what we believe in, and what we stand for" [35, p. 59].

Sankalpa is not just a fleeting wish or desire but a deeper resolve that aligns our thoughts, words, and actions with our innermost values and beliefs. When we set a Sankalpa, we affirm our intentions and mobilize our willpower to manifest those intentions.

Sankalpa is traditionally part of yoga nidra, a meditative practice in a relaxed state of consciousness. In this receptive state, the sankalpa is "planted" deep in the subconscious mind, like a seed. With repetition, the sankalpa gathers strength, unfolds, and begins to bear fruit [36]. The regular practice of affirming one's sankalpa is a means of reprogramming the subconscious mind and changing deep-rooted behavior patterns.

The practice of sankalpa rests on the understanding that our thoughts and intentions can shape our reality. As Swami Sivananda explains:

"Thought is the greatest force on earth. Thought is the most powerful weapon in the armor of a Yogi. Constructive thought transforms, renews and builds. Negative thought destroys. Thought has much building and destroying power" [37, p. 76].

By consciously choosing and affirming a positive intention, we harness the creative power of thought. We replace self-limiting beliefs and habits with a more expansive sense of possibility.

There are three essential steps for cultivating sankalpa: sravana, manana, and nididhyasana [12]. Sravana is hearing or receiving the sankalpa. This involves listening to our deepest aspirations and allowing a clear intention to arise. Manana is reflecting upon the sankalpa, contemplating its meaning and significance. This step enables the Sankalpa to take root in our minds and hearts. Nididhyasana is applying the Sankalpa and embodying it in our actions. The fundamental transformation occurs in this final step, as our intentions shape our moment-to-moment choices.

For those on the healer's path, the practice of sankalpa can be a powerful tool for strengthening the intention of compassion. By repeatedly affirming the intention to relieve suffering, we weave that intention into the fabric of our being. Sankalpa practice can help us remember our deepest aspirations amid challenging circumstances. It empowers us to align our actions with our values, bridging the gap between what we believe and how we live.

Compassion as an Intention of the Heart

Compassion is a prime example of an "intention of the heart" and is the foundation for bodhicitta. It can be understood as the sympathetic wish for others to be free from suffering, coupled with a readiness to help relieve that suffering [18, p. 351]. Genuine compassion is more than a fleeting emotion—it is a stable intention that organizes one's priorities and actions around the aim of benefiting others.

The Dalai Lama, the spiritual leader of Tibetan Buddhism, has said, "For those who wish to follow the Bodhisattva path, compassion is the very basis and starting point" [19, p. 101]. Compassion propels bodhisattvas to make incredible sacrifices to help others, life after life until all beings are liberated. The Dalai Lama teaches that when compassion permeates every aspect of one's being, all of one's actions naturally work for the good of others: "When you have purity of motivation and purity of conduct, then even if you don't do much meditation practice, all your actions become Dharma [positive actions]. Because the motivation is pure and the way you lead your life is pure, every action becomes constructive and beneficial to others" [20].

Like a seed that grows to influence the shape of a tree, compassionate intention can grow to shape the entire course of one's life. When compassion becomes one's primary motivation, it lends a profound sense of meaning and direction. All of one's diverse activities become unified and consistent when they stem from the single intention to relieve suffering. In medicine, intention and compassion are essential in promoting healing and well-being. As several prominent medical and spiritual figures have emphasized, cultivating a genuine intention to alleviate suffering can transform healthcare.

The Hippocratic Oath, which includes the principle of "do no harm," is a step in the right direction but falls short of fully capturing the essence of intention in medicine. While refraining from causing harm is crucial, it does not actively promote the positive intention to do good. The Golden Rule, "Do unto others as you would have them do unto you," goes beyond the "silver rule" of simply avoiding harm and calls us to extend compassion and care [3] proactively.

Modern allopathic medicine, with its emphasis on scientific methods and evidence-based protocols, risks losing sight of the fundamental role of intention in healing. When the focus shifts primarily to techniques and technologies, the human element of compassion can become overshadowed. This leaves many medical practitioners feeling disconnected from the deeper purpose of their work [4]. Dr. Barry Kerzin, a Buddhist monk and medical doctor, emphasizes the importance of uniting compassion with medical knowledge. He teaches that when compassion and wisdom work together, patients feel genuinely cared for, and doctors find greater meaning in their work. Integrating compassion training into medical education could help prevent burnout and reignite the passion for healing [5].

Tibetan doctor Jampa Yonten echoes this sentiment, stating, "In my medical practice, I've found that holding the intention to relieve suffering is just as important as the treatments I provide" [6]. By setting a compassionate intention, healers create an environment that fosters trust and supports the body's innate healing capacities. Dr. David Shlim, an American doctor who spent decades practicing medicine in Nepal, writes about the power of compassion in his book Medicine and Compassion. He states, "Compassion is not just empathy or altruism. In medicine, compassion means the heartfelt motivation to relieve the suffering of others" [7]. Shlim argues that cultivating genuine compassion can help physicians provide better care and establish deeper patient connections.

Buddhist teacher Chokyi Nyima Rinpoche also stresses the importance of compassion, stating, "The essence of compassion is a desire to alleviate the suffering of others and to promote their well-being" [8]. In medicine, this translates to providing care with the sincere intention of helping patients heal physically, mentally, and emotionally.

The Intention of the Heart and the Path of the Healer
The path of the healer aligns closely with the intention of compassion. At its core, healing work arises from the aspiration to alleviate the pain and suffering of others. For those in helping professions, fostering a compassionate intention of the heart can enhance the efficacy of their work and protect against burnout.

Sun Simiao, a renowned 7th-century Chinese physician, wrote about the importance of compassionate intention in medical practice. In his "On the Absolute Sincerity of Great Physicians," he states:

"If you truly wish to be a great physician, you must first of all have a great heart of compassion, desiring to benefit all beings and wishing to heal all diseases. Those who lack this mind and aspiration, even if they know all the prescriptions, will only be mediocre physicians" [27, p. 52].

For Sun Simiao, compassionate intention is the very foundation of medical mastery. Technical knowledge alone is insufficient; great physicians must be motivated by a sincere wish to help others and relieve suffering.

Vasant Lad, a prominent teacher of Ayurveda, echoes this perspective. He emphasizes that healing is both a technical process and a sacred act rooted in compassion: "Healing is a sacred path, a spiritual journey. It is an act of love, compassion, unity, harmony, truth, and wisdom. The healer's task is not just to cure a disease but to assist in the spiritual unfoldment of the patient" [28, p. 11]. Lad suggests that the healer's intention shapes the quality and impact of their work. Healing is more profound when infused with compassion and a desire to support the patient's well-being.

Our Oath and Our Intention

In many healing traditions, practitioners take oaths articulating their core intentions and ethical commitments. The Hippocratic Oath, originating in ancient Greece, is one of the most well-known examples. It includes the promise to "prescribe regimens for the good of my patients according to my ability and my judgment and never do harm to anyone" [29].

This oath establishes beneficence (doing good) and non-maleficence (avoiding harm) as guiding intentions for medical practice. It calls upon healers to use their skills and judgment in service of the patient's well-being. The oath helps to shape a collective intention within the medical community and provides an ethical touchstone for individual practitioners.

Other healing traditions have their oaths that support compassionate intention. The Ayurvedic physician's oath includes the pledge, "I shall always promote the happiness of all creatures" [30, p. 2]. The traditional Chinese medicine practitioner's oath states, "I will serve all equally, the poor, the rich, and the noble, and make no distinction between their status and position" [31, p. 8].

These oaths reinforce the idea that healing should be rooted in a heartfelt desire to benefit others. They help align the healer's intentions with the greater purpose of their profession. By taking an oath, healers make a public commitment to living up to certain ideals and letting these ideals guide their work.

Identity and Intention in Healing

The identity from which we approach healing also plays a significant role in shaping our intentions. When we view healing as a job, we may feel like victims trapped in a cycle of fear. We risk becoming heroes trapped in an ego pattern when we see it as a career. However, when we recognize healing as a calling, we become vessels or pilgrims, conduits of a higher power. Ultimately, when we embody healing as our true nature, we become manifestations of boundless vitality [10].

Intention serves as our North Star, guiding us through the challenges and complexities of medical practice. As Dr. David Shlim writes in Medicine and Compassion, "Compassion is not just empathy or altruism. In medicine, compassion means the heartfelt motivation to relieve the suffering of others" [7]. When we anchor ourselves in this intention, we can navigate even the most difficult circumstances with greater clarity and resilience.

Cultivating Genuine Intention

Cultivating a genuine intention involves three essential steps. The first step, Sravana, is the willingness to hear the message and open ourselves to the call of compassion. Manana's second step is welcoming the message, embracing the intention to alleviate suffering. The third step, Nididhyasana, is actioning the message, embodying compassion in our thoughts, words, and deeds [12].

While compassion alone is insufficient for addressing serious health conditions, it becomes a powerful catalyst for healing when combined with medical expertise. As these experts suggest, uplifting compassion and intention as guiding principles in medicine can improve patient outcomes and bring more meaning to healthcare. Modern medical training would do well to place compassion on par with clinical knowledge and technical skills. Ultimately, healthcare is fundamentally about human beings caring for one another, a truth we forget at our peril.

We may not always have compassionate intentions. We must be honest with ourselves if we intend to make money, gain personal or academic accolades, or pursue another ego-based goal. When we are authentically aligned with our conscious intention, we avoid the cognitive and emotional dissonance that eventually produces increasing personal distress for ourselves and those around us.

Shared and Collective Intentions

While individuals have their intentions, we are also influenced by the shared intentions of the groups and systems we belong to. These collective intentions do not always align with our aims, which can create tension and challenges.

In healthcare systems, the intentions of individual practitioners may conflict with those of the larger organization. A healer may be motivated by a sincere desire to provide compassionate care, while the system may prioritize efficiency, cost-cutting, or profit. This misalignment can significantly contribute to moral distress and burnout among healthcare workers.

Rachel Naomi Remen writes about the toll of working in a system that does not share one's deepest values:

"Many of us have been trained to believe that we can serve our patients without being affected by their suffering. This myth of invulnerability denies our humanity and fosters attitudes and behaviors that separate us from our patients. It enables us to ignore and violate our own needs with impunity. Many of us leave our training imbued with a deep sense of unworthiness and loss of meaning... We have no idea how to keep ourselves from drowning in the ocean of suffering that washes endlessly through the medical system. Burned out, we become cynical, numb, and detached and learn to protect ourselves from further pain. Yet behind the mask of professionalism, we continue to ache." [33]

When the healer's intention to be present and caring clashes with a system that does not support this intention, it can lead to a profound sense of disconnection and exhaustion. Healers may feel unable to live out their values or bring their whole selves to their work.

To address this challenge, healthcare organizations must examine their collective intentions and strive to create cultures that align with the deeper purposes of healing. This may involve rethinking incentive structures, prioritizing patient-centered care, and providing more support for patients' and staff's emotional and spiritual needs.

Remen suggests that for healers to sustain their work, they need to be part of a community that shares their intentions: "A profession that demands so much needs the shelter of a committed community that shares the same purpose and serves the same values. So many of us feel isolated in our work, unsupported by our profession. We see each other as competitors rather than kindred spirits. We learn to live in our separateness, not in our belonging. But meaning lies in belonging, our connections to one another and the life around us." [33]

By coming together around shared intentions of service and compassion, healers can find renewed strength and inspiration. They can support each other in living out their deepest values, even in the face of systemic challenges.

Concluding Remarks

It is time to place compassion and intention at the heart of medical training and practice, recognizing that they are just as essential as clinical skills and scientific knowledge. By aligning our intentions with the profound aspiration to relieve suffering, we can tap into the immense potential for healing within each act of genuine care and kindness. As we awaken to the power of intention in medicine, we can transform healthcare into a sacred art that harnesses the genius of medical science with the wisdom of our compassionate intention.

The Buddha once said, "The whole world lives on the tip of intention" [1]. This profound statement indicates our intentions' immense power in shaping our reality. In medicine, purpose and compassion are essential in promoting healing and well-being. By placing the intention of the heart at the center of our work as healers, we can create a healthcare system that truly serves the needs of all beings. May we have the courage to let our deepest intentions guide us, and may we never lose sight of the sacred nature of our calling.

Self-Reflection Questions

1. What is my deepest intention as a healer? How does this intention shape my thoughts, words, and actions in my work?

2. In what ways do I currently cultivate compassion in my healing practice? What opportunities do I see to deepen my commitment to alleviating suffering?

3. How aligned do I feel with the collective intentions of the healthcare system I work in? What tensions or challenges arise when my intentions differ from organizational priorities?

4. When have I experienced the power of intention in my life, personally or professionally? What did I learn from those experiences?

5. Which of the three steps of cultivating genuine intention (sravana - hearing, manana - reflecting, nididhyasana - applying) do I feel most competent in, and which could I strengthen?

6. How do I navigate situations where my intention to provide compassionate care conflicts with time pressures, resource limitations, or other systemic constraints?

7. How does my sense of identity as a healer (e.g., seeing my work as a job, career, calling, or true nature) influence my intentions and approach to patient care?

8. How can I create more space in my daily routine to reconnect with my deepest intentions and reaffirm my commitment to compassion?

9. What support systems or practices help me to stay grounded in my intention to alleviate suffering, even in challenging circumstances? How can I strengthen those supports?

10. What would it look like to place intention and compassion at the heart of my healing work? What shifts, internal and external, would be required to embody this vision fully?

References
[1] Thich Nhat Hanh, The Heart of the Buddha's Teaching, p. 57
[2] "intention, n." OED Online. Oxford University Press, March 2022.
[3] Jeff Sebo, "The Silver Rule: Do No Harm," Psychology Today, 2018
[4] David Shlim, Medicine and Compassion, p. 22
[5] Barry Kerzin, "The Art of Compassion in Healthcare," TEDxDharmshala, 2018
[6] Jampa Yonten, personal communication, 2022
[7] David Shlim, Medicine and Compassion, p. 18
[8] Chokyi Nyima Rinpoche, Medicine and Compassion, p. xi
[9] Bhikkhu Bodhi, "Cetana: The Will to Do Good," Access to Insight, 2013
[10] Rachel Naomi Remen, "Recapturing the Soul of Medicine," Noetic Sciences Review, No. 45, p. 19
[11] Rest, J. R., Narvaez, D., Thoma, S. J., & Bebeau, M. J. (1999). Postconventional Moral Thinking: A Neo- Kohlbergian Approach. Mahwah, NJ: Lawrence Erlbaum Associates.
[12] Swami Sivananda, Vedanta for Beginners, p. 92
[13] "Dhammapada: The Path of Dhamma," Access to Insight, 2012
[14] Traleg Kyabgon, The Essence of Buddhism, p. 204
[15] Khunu Rinpoche Tenzin Gyaltsen, Vast as the Heavens, Deep as the Sea: Verses in Praise of Bodhicitta, p. 11
[16] Shantideva, Guide to the Bodhisattva's Way of Life, Ch. 1, v. 5-7
[17] Shantideva, Guide to the Bodhisattva's Way of Life, Ch. 3, v. 18-19
[18] Tania Singer & Olga M. Klimecki, "Empathy and compassion," Current Biology, Vol. 24, Issue 18, p. 351
[19] The Dalai Lama, An Open Heart: Practicing Compassion in Everyday Life, p. 101
[20] The Dalai Lama, A Policy of Kindness: An Anthology of Writings By and About the Dalai Lama
[24] Michael Meade, The Genius Myth, p. 42
[25] Michael Meade, Awakening the Soul, p. 31
[26] Michael Meade, The Genius Myth, p. 89
[27] Sun Simiao, On the Absolute Sincerity of Great Physicians, p. 52
[28] Vasant Lad, Ayurveda: The Science of Self-Healing, p. 11
[29] "Hippocratic Oath", Encyclopedia Britannica
[30] Charaka Samhita, Sutrasthana 8.13, p. 2
[31] Unschuld, Paul U., Medical Ethics in Imperial China, p. 8
[33] Rachel Naomi Remen, Kitchen Table Wisdom: Stories That Heal, p. 53
[32] Viktor Frankl, Man's Search for Meaning, p. 66
[5] Icek Ajzen, "The theory of planned behavior", Organizational Behavior and Human Decision Processes, Vol. 50, Issue 2, p. 179

[6] Martin Fishbein & Icek Ajzen, Predicting and Changing Behavior: The Reasoned Action Approach, p. 665

[7] Peter M. Gollwitzer & Paschal Sheeran, "Implementation Intentions and Goal Achievement: A Meta-analysis of Effects and Processes", Advances in Experimental Social Psychology, Vol. 38, p. 493

[8] Thomas L. Webb & Paschal Sheeran, "Does Changing Behavioral Intentions Engender Behavior Change? A Meta-Analysis of the Experimental Evidence", Psychological Bulletin, Vol. 132, Issue 2, p. 69

[9] Peter M. Gollwitzer, "Implementation intentions: Strong effects of simple plans", American Psychologist, Vol. 54, Issue 7, p. 295

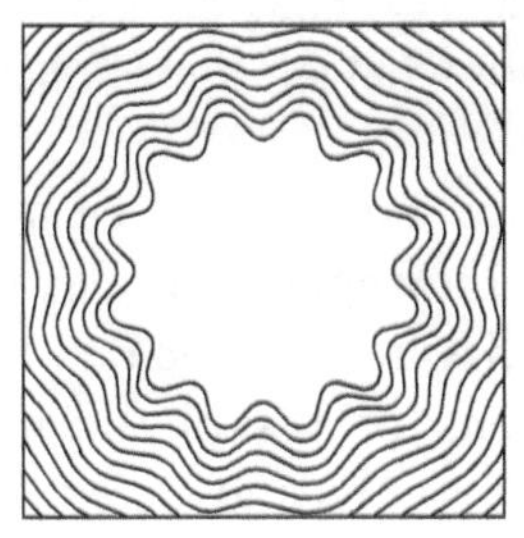

CHAPTER 17

Asana Two: Create Safe Space

Instruction: "Take a long, slow, and deep breath"

"What has to be taught first, is the breath".
Confucius

$\mathcal{R}$emarkable physician and inspirational teacher Rachel Remen described her experience with a young patient who was referred to her after he had been diagnosed with insulin-dependent diabetes but would not accept his condition. The 17-year-old boy refused to administer his insulin and refused to follow his diet, which he pursued recklessly. This resulted in him being admitted to the hospital on numerous occasions with keto acidosis and death experiences. Rachel was asked to see him in the hope that she would be able to convince him somehow to accept his diagnosis and follow the life-preserving prescription of his physicians. Rachel describes meeting the young man regularly in her office. On each occasion, he would be rude, irritable, and insulting. He repeatedly stated that he had no intention of accepting his diagnosis and would continue to leave his life the way he chose. As a result, he did not improve over the next few months and continued to experience recurrent medical crises.

One day, while in her office, Rachel recognized this young man's name on her schedule for the day. She decided it would be appropriate to discontinue her work with him as he was not making any outward progress, and it was costing his parents significant expense for her to continue seeing him. She, therefore, prepared herself for what she knew might be a difficult conversation with the young man.

Upon entering her office, Rachel noticed a pronounced change in her young patient's demeanor. They appeared relaxed and even in good spirits. He immediately told her that he had decided to accept his diagnosis and follow the recommendations of his physicians. He apologized for his rudeness over the previous months and stated that he was very grateful for the work that they had done together. Rachel expressed her confusion about his rapid change and asked whether he could explain how he had decided on this change, of course.

The young man stated that he recognized that everything had changed for him after he had a compelling dream a week earlier. He said that in the dream, he saw himself entering Dr. Remen's office, which he had done on many occasions. However, upon sitting down, a man brandishing a huge knife came running into Dr. Remen's office. The young man said that he was startled in his dream and fearful that the man was about to stab him. However, the man ran past the young boy and moved towards Dr. Remen. In his dream, the young man became terrified and angry that the man was apparently about to stab Dr. Remen in the chest. However, he did not. He ran past Dr. Remen and thrust the knife into the chest of a tiny Buddha statue sitting on the shelf behind Dr. Remen. He recounted that as he sat there, the Buddha became larger until it filled up the entire bookshelf. The butter continued growing until it filled the room, building, and town. At this point, he could no longer see the knife because the Buddha had become so large. And the Buddha continued to grow larger and larger. At this point, the Buddha noticed that not only could he no longer see the knife, but as he looked at the Buddha's face, he saw the Buddha smiling. At that point, he knew that everything would be all right.

The story speaks to me about the importance of space and healing. Once this young man recognized that space was always available to him, he realized that he never needed to feel trapped by a diagnosis or his suffering. He recognized that the more space he could create, the broader and wiser his perspective on the options open to him would be. He realized that while pain was inevitable, his suffering could be malleable to the extent of his perspective.

Becoming Aware of Space
Most of us move through our days snared in time's arrow as we pursue some real or imagined goal. This is particularly true of the modern healer, who

often lives a life measured in fifteen-minute increments and has productivity metrics that consistently demand more. We seldom notice our environment unless it stands in the way of our efficiency. We inhabit a world of straight lines and sharp corners that support our linear thinking and fence in our imaginations. As healers, we inhabit a world saturated with fear and negative emotions. Healers courageously and consciously enter the raging fires burning within the lives of their suffering patients. As the Tibetan Buddhist teacher Chögyam Trungpa said, "Enlightened people are not afraid to enter the fire—the fire of confusion, the fire of anger, the fire of passion. They just plunge into the fire, knowing it cannot harm them" (Trungpa 2013, 13).

Pema Chödrön writes, "When the ground is shaky, the impulse is to grab hold of something. Especially when things are challenging, the instructions tell us to do the opposite—to let go. Instead of tightening our grip, it's a chance to soften" (Chödrön 2010, 75). Creating and inhabiting this softening and holding environment is vital if healing is to occur.

Modern Western concepts of space traditionally emphasize functionality, individuality, and maximizing use. This is evident in architectural and urban planning practices where space is often organized to serve specific purposes, optimize efficiency, and accommodate the fast pace of modern life. For instance, in many Western homes, rooms are designated for particular functions — a kitchen for cooking, a bedroom for sleeping, a living room for socializing — and are often permanently separated by walls.

In Eastern cultures, space is not merely physical but deeply intertwined with spiritual, psychological, and cosmic significance. Feng Shui, a traditional Chinese practice, embodies this principle by emphasizing the harmonious alignment of space with the natural world. It is based on the belief that the arrangement of space can influence the flow of chi (energy) and, consequently, affect the health, wealth, and happiness of the people inhabiting that space. Feng Shui principles, such as using the five elements (wood, fire, earth, metal, and water) and the concept of yin and yang, are often incorporated into the design of healing spaces to create atmospheres that support the recovery of patients.

The Japanese concept of Ma, which translates to "gap," "space," "pause," or "the space between two structural parts," offers another perspective on space as a relational and experiential entity. Ma emphasizes the importance of negative space — the empty, the void — to highlight or enhance the positive, filled spaces. In the context of health and healing, Ma underscores the significance of the spaces within and between our bodies, believed to be channels through which energy flows. The mindful management of these spaces, through practices such as meditation and mindfulness, can aid in preventing and healing illness and promoting physical and mental well-being.

Western Concepts of Space Western concepts of space traditionally emphasize functionality, individuality, and the maximization of use. This is evident in architectural and urban planning practices where space is often organized to serve specific purposes, optimize efficiency, and accommodate the fast pace of modern life. In healthcare settings, this approach to space is reflected in the clinical and often sterile design of hospitals and clinics, prioritizing cleanliness, order, and the efficient delivery of medical care.

However, there is a growing recognition in Western healthcare of the importance of creating healing environments that go beyond the purely functional. Evidence-based design principles, which draw on research linking the built environment to patient outcomes, are increasingly being applied to transform hospitals and clinics into spaces that promote comfort, reduce stress, and support holistic recovery. This shift reflects a broader understanding of the role of space in shaping our physical, mental, and emotional well-being.

Indigenous Perspectives: The Aboriginal Songlines Indigenous cultures offer profound insights into space's sacred and interconnected nature. For example, the Aboriginal concept of songlines encapsulates the complex relationships between the land, its people, and its rich spiritual and cultural heritage. Songlines are intricate maps of the landscape, stories of creation, and laws by which to live, all woven into a comprehensive oral tradition that guides the Aboriginal people in their interactions with the land and each other.

The songlines reflect an Aboriginal understanding of space that is profoundly relational and animated. The land is alive and storied, and each element is interconnected through the ancestral journeys. This perspective fosters a sense of stewardship and respect for the environment, with the songlines providing a spiritual and practical guide for living in harmony with the land. In the context of healing, the songlines offer a holistic approach that recognizes the interconnectedness of physical, emotional, spiritual, and environmental dimensions of well-being.

Integrating Space Awareness into Modern Healthcare
Integrating Eastern, Western, and Indigenous spatial concepts into modern healthcare environments holds transformative potential for creating spaces that genuinely support healing and well-being. Applying Feng Shui principles, for example, can guide the design of patient rooms, waiting areas, and gardens to create atmospheres that promote relaxation, harmony, and positive energy flow. The incorporation of Ma can inspire the creation of spaces that respect the value of emptiness, silence, and pause, allowing for moments of reflection and inner peace amidst the often hectic hospital environment.

Western evidence-based design principles, such as the use of natural light, views of nature, and the incorporation of art and music, can complement these Eastern concepts to create healthcare spaces that are both functional and nurturing. Furthermore, the Indigenous understanding of space as sacred and interconnected can inform the development of healing environments that honor the spiritual dimensions of well-being and foster a sense of connection to the natural world.

Every Moment is a Doorway into a New Space
In the context of the healer-patient relationship, it is essential to approach each interaction with a fresh perspective, unencumbered by the experiences of previous encounters. Every patient deserves the full, undivided attention of the healer, and this can only be achieved by consciously letting go of any lingering thoughts, emotions, or judgments from prior interactions. As the Buddhist monk Thích Nhất Hạnh teaches, "Every morning we are born again. What we do today is what matters most" (Nhất Hạnh 2012, 7).

Seeing each patient with fresh eyes is crucial to maintaining a wise mind that perceives things as they are, free from the distortions of past conditioning. The Buddhist concept of "beginner's mind" (shoshin) encourages us to approach each moment with openness, curiosity, and nonjudgment as if encountering it for the first time (Suzuki 2011, 21). By embracing this beginner's mind, the healer can be fully present with each patient, listening deeply and responding with compassion and skill.

The Buddhist concept of the "bardos" beautifully captures the idea that every moment is a doorway into a new space. While the term is often associated with the "bardo of dying," as described in the Tibetan Book of the Dead, the bardos encompass much more. Chögyam Trungpa Rinpoche, a renowned Tibetan Buddhist teacher, explains that the bardos refer to any transitional state or "gap" between one moment and the next (Trungpa 2013, 3).

Trungpa Rinpoche teaches that every moment of our lives is a bardo, an opportunity to awaken to the present and let go of the past. He states, "The past is past, the future has not yet come, and there is only the present moment. That is the bardo" (Trungpa 2002, 20). By recognizing each moment as a bardo, a space between the dissolution of the old and the emergence of the new, we can cultivate the ability to meet each experience freshly without the baggage of the past.

Just as it is essential to consciously enter each patient interaction with a clear and open mind, it is equally crucial to mindfully "close the space" at the end of each encounter. This involves taking a moment to acknowledge the shared experience, express gratitude, and consciously release any energy or emotions that may have arisen during the interaction. As the Buddhist teacher Jack Kornfield reminds us, "The practice of letting go is essential for our freedom and well-being. We can learn to let go gracefully, with ease and kindness" (Kornfield 2010, 67).

By consciously closing the space after each patient interaction, the healer can prevent residual energy from carrying over into subsequent encounters. This energetic hygiene practice helps maintain a clear and balanced state of mind, allowing the healer to be fully present and available for the next patient. As the Dalai Lama advises, "We must learn to let go, to give up, to make room for the things we have prayed for and desired" (Dalai Lama XIV 2012, 43).

Recognizing every moment as a doorway into a new space is a powerful way for healers to approach each patient interaction with freshness, presence, and compassion. By embracing the Buddhist concept of the bardos and cultivating a beginner's mind, healers can let go of past experiences and meet each patient anew. Consciously closing the space after each encounter further supports this practice, promoting energetic clarity and resilience. As healers, it is through this ongoing practice of opening and closing, of letting go and beginning again, that we can truly be of service to those in our care.

We are never alone. Healing is often frightening. Standing on the sharp edge of transformation requires us to step out of our assumptions' false security. This is typically a lonely place. Unfortunately, the modern healer has to walk this sharp ledge alone and has learned that such feelings are a sign of weakness that should be suppressed. Other healing traditions have recognized that loneliness does not need to be the healer's path. Their recognition and reverence for their lineage hold them in a community where they never " fly solo."

THE 4 STEPS TO SAFE SPACE

Step One: Prepare the Space - Create a Supportive Environment

Consciously observe your working environment. Become aware of how you feel in this space. Do you feel enlivened and creative, or do you feel dull and uninspired? Observe your sensory experience. Sight, sound, touch, smell. Explore how these sensory experiences support or inhibit your work as a healer.

Using this information, seek out simple ways to revitalize your workspace. Simple but evocative images of nature? Perhaps a small plant? Softening the lighting? Aromatherapy? Natural materials? If you cannot do these things, bring into your mind a vision of how you would like your healing space to manifest in the room. A place in nature where you experienced safety and joy, a gathering of supportive souls?

Western Concepts of Space Western concepts of space traditionally emphasize functionality, individuality, and the maximization of use. This is evident in architectural and urban planning practices where space is often organized to serve specific purposes, optimize efficiency, and accommodate the fast pace of modern life. In healthcare settings, this approach to space is reflected in the clinical and often sterile design of hospitals and clinics, prioritizing cleanliness, order, and the efficient delivery of medical care.

However, there is a growing recognition in Western healthcare of the importance of creating healing environments that go beyond the purely functional. Evidence-based design principles, which draw on research linking the built environment to patient outcomes, are increasingly being applied to transform hospitals and clinics into spaces that promote comfort, reduce stress, and support holistic recovery. This shift reflects a broader understanding of the role of space in shaping our physical, mental, and emotional well-being.

Eastern Concepts of Space: Feng Shui and Ma In Eastern cultures, space is not merely physical but deeply intertwined with spiritual, psychological, and cosmic significance. Feng Shui, a traditional Chinese practice, embodies this principle by emphasizing the harmonious alignment of space with the natural world. It is based on the belief that the arrangement of space can influence the flow of chi (energy) and, consequently, affect the health, wealth, and happiness of the people inhabiting that space. Feng Shui principles, such as using the five elements (wood, fire, earth, metal, and water) and the concept of yin and yang, are often incorporated into the design of healing spaces to create atmospheres that support the recovery of patients.

The Japanese concept of Ma, which translates to "gap," "space," "pause," or "the space between two structural parts," offers another perspective on space as a relational and experiential entity. Ma emphasizes the importance of negative space — the empty, the void — to highlight or enhance the positive, filled spaces. In the context of health and healing, Ma underscores the significance of the spaces within and between our bodies, believed to be channels through which energy flows. The mindful management of these spaces, through practices such as meditation and mindfulness, can aid in preventing and healing illness and promoting physical and mental well-being.

Indigenous Perspectives: The Aboriginal Songlines Indigenous cultures offer profound insights into space's sacred and interconnected nature. For example, the Aboriginal concept of songlines encapsulates the complex relationships between the land, its people, and its rich spiritual and cultural heritage. Songlines are intricate maps of the landscape, stories of creation, and laws by which to live, all woven into a comprehensive oral tradition that guides the Aboriginal people in their interactions with the land and each other.

The songlines reflect an Aboriginal understanding of space that is profoundly relational and animated. The land is alive and storied, and each element is interconnected through the ancestral journeys. This perspective fosters a sense of stewardship and respect for the environment, with the songlines providing a spiritual and practical guide for living in harmony with the land. In the context of healing, the songlines offer a holistic approach that recognizes the interconnectedness of physical, emotional, spiritual, and environmental dimensions of well-being.

Integrating Spatial Concepts in Modern Healthcare Integrating Eastern, Western, and Indigenous spatial concepts into modern healthcare environments holds transformative potential for creating spaces that genuinely support healing and well-being. Applying Feng Shui principles, for example, can guide the design of patient rooms, waiting areas, and gardens to create atmospheres that promote relaxation, harmony, and positive energy flow. The incorporation of Ma can inspire the creation of spaces that respect the value of emptiness, silence, and pause, allowing for moments of reflection and inner peace amidst the often hectic hospital environment.

Practical Suggestions for Enlivening the Modern Healthcare Work Environment

Western evidence-based design principles, such as the use of natural light, views of nature, and the incorporation of art and music, can complement these Eastern concepts to create healthcare spaces that are both functional and nurturing. Furthermore, the Indigenous understanding of space as sacred and interconnected can inform the development of healing environments that honor the spiritual dimensions of well-being and foster a sense of connection to the natural world.

Unless they work in a private practice environment, the modern healer will unlikely have much control over their physical working environment. Given this reality, there are simple things that we can explore:

Meaningful Images and Artwork

Visual stimuli play a significant role in shaping our emotional and mental states. By incorporating meaningful images and artwork into their work environment, healthcare professionals can create a more uplifting and supportive atmosphere. Research has shown that viewing nature scenes can reduce stress, lower blood pressure, and improve overall mood (Ulrich et al., 1991, p. 224). As such, choosing artwork depicting natural landscapes, such as mountains, forests, or beaches, can provide a calming and restorative influence amidst the chaos of a busy healthcare setting.

Moreover, displaying images that hold personal significance, such as photos of loved ones, inspiring quotes, or artwork that reflects one's values and aspirations, can be a source of motivation and encouragement. As Dr. Rachel Naomi Remen notes in her book "Kitchen Table Wisdom," "The most important tool a healthcare professional has is not what is in their bag, but what is in their heart" (Remen, 1996, p. 52). By surrounding oneself with visual reminders of what matters most, healthcare professionals can tap into a more profound sense of purpose and compassion.

Optimizing Lighting

The quality and quantity of light in one's work environment can significantly impact mood, energy levels, and cognitive function. Poor lighting can lead to eye strain, headaches, and fatigue, while exposure to natural light has been linked to improved mood, reduced stress, and better sleep quality (Boyce, 2014, p. 213). Whenever possible, healthcare professionals should strive to work in spaces with ample natural light, such as near windows or skylights. If natural light is limited, using full-spectrum light bulbs that mimic the quality of sunlight can be a helpful alternative.

In addition to optimizing the quality of light, healthcare professionals can also use light to create a more soothing and nurturing environment. For example, incorporating soft, warm lighting in break rooms or staff lounges can promote relaxation and restoration during rest. As Florence Nightingale, the founder of modern nursing, observed, "Little as we know about the way in which we are affected by form, by color, and light, we do know this, that they have an actual physical effect" (Nightingale, 1860, p. 34). By being mindful of the impact of lighting on their well-being, healthcare professionals can create work environments that are more conducive to healing and resilience.

Aromatherapy

Engaging the sense of smell through aromatherapy can be a powerful way to promote relaxation, reduce stress, and enhance cognitive function in the healthcare work environment. Certain essential oils, such as lavender, chamomile, and bergamot, have been shown to have calming and anxiety-reducing effects (Sayorwan et al., 2012, p. 667). By using diffusers or personal inhalers to disperse these scents in their immediate surroundings, healthcare professionals can create a more soothing and supportive atmosphere.

Certain scents can promote relaxation and boost energy and mental clarity. For example, the smell of peppermint has been found to enhance memory, attention, and alertness (Moss et al., 2008, p. 1091). By incorporating energizing scents into their work environment, healthcare professionals can help counteract the fatigue and mental fog accompanying long shifts and demanding workloads.

The Power of Non-verbal Cues in Creating Sacred Space

Beyond the physical elements of one's work environment, non-verbal cues can play a crucial role in supporting the experience of sacred space and promoting a sense of connection, compassion, and healing. Non-verbal cues, such as facial expressions, gestures, and tone of voice, are essential components of human communication and can convey various emotions and intentions (Mehrabian, 1972, p. 44).

For healthcare professionals, cultivating awareness of their non-verbal communication can create a more nurturing and supportive environment for patients and colleagues. Simple acts, such as maintaining eye contact, offering a warm smile, or using a gentle touch, can convey a sense of presence, empathy, and care beyond words. As Dr. Jodi Halpern notes in her book "From Detached Concern to Empathy," "Non-verbal attunement is the foundation of empathy in the clinical encounter" (Halpern, 2001, p. 67).

Moreover, non-verbal cues can create a sense of sacred space in healthcare. By adopting a calm and centered demeanor, speaking in a soft and soothing tone, and using gestures that convey openness and compassion, healthcare professionals can transform even the most sterile and impersonal environments into spaces of healing and connection. As chaplain and author Debbie Augenthaler observes, "Sacred space is not just a physical location; it is a state of being, a way of showing up in the world with reverence and intention" (Augenthaler, 2018, p. 92).

When implemented with intention and care, these simple strategies can profoundly impact the quality of care provided to patients and the overall well-being of healthcare professionals. Dr. Rachel Naomi Remen reminds us, "The secret of the care of the patient is in caring for the patient" (Remen, 1996, p. 144). By creating work environments that nurture the human spirit, healthcare professionals can more fully embody this ethos of compassionate care.

Never forget the Power of Your Presence.

We discussed in the next chapter the power of presence in creating sacred and safe spaces cannot be overstated. By bringing our full attention and care to the present moment, we open up the possibility for genuine connection, empathy, and transformation. Through mindfulness, deep listening, and loving-kindness, we can cultivate a presence that naturally fosters a sense of sacredness and safety in our interactions and environments. As we move through the world with this quality of presence, we become agents of healing and connection, helping to create a more compassionate and sacred world, one moment at a time.

Step Two: Recall Your Intention

Before you encounter your next patient, very consciously recall your intention statement and silently repeat this to yourself three times.

As discussed in the previous chapter, establishing clarity on our intention is the first asana of the yoga of medicine. Our intention offers a vision for our journey and a north star to guide us through challenging seas. It anchors us to a higher purpose beyond the perceived constraints of the current moment. As Thích Nhất Hạnh said, "The most precious gift we can offer anyone is our attention. When mindfulness embraces those we love, they will bloom like flowers" (Nhất Hạnh 2014, 62). Regularly recalling our intention to be fully present and of service reconnects us to the heart of healing work. Rumi wrote, "Let yourself be silently drawn by the strange pull of what you really love. It will not lead you astray" (Rumi 2004, 45).

It is helpful to have simple reminders—your intention. For example, you can include your intention statement on your screensaver or place a sticky note on your computer or mirror.

Step Three: Open the Doorway to the Next Space by Taking a Breath

Before you engage with your next patient, stop, remain, and consciously take a breath. Observe your breath as you breathe through your nose, take two or three in-breaths, and then relax into the out-breath for at least 7 seconds and without effort. At the end of the out-breath, remain until your body lets you know it is time to take the next in-breath. Repeat this three times.

The Breath is the Doorway into Equanimity

We have discussed the concept of equanimity earlier in this text. However, it is worth repeating. Equanimity is the foundation for our ability to respond and not simply react. "In the space between the in-breath and the out-breath... Quote Viktor Frankl. This space is the doorway into spacious repose where we are not caught in the cycle of being and becoming. A spaciousness where time itself seems to dissolve into a boundless horizon that is no longer defined by our restless mind and the stories we tell ourselves.

In Buddhism, equanimity (upekkhā) is one of the four brahmaviharas or "divine abodes," along with compassion (karunā), lovingkindness (mettā), and empathetic joy (muditā). Buddhists acknowledge the inescapable reality of change and suffering in life. Equanimity provides the steady, nonreactive mind to meet that suffering with wisdom. In Islam, everything that occurs is seen as God's will. Trusting this allows the believer to let go of worry and rest in the peace of acceptance. The Arabic root of "Islam" (aslama) refers to the peace of surrendering to the divine. Equanimity is also valued in Jewish spiritual life, known as menuhat ha-nefesh ("calmness of mind") or yishuv ha-da'at ("settled mindfulness"). Rabbis consider it essential for spiritual development. Stoic philosophy made equanimity its central focus, advocating responding rather than unthinkingly reacting to life's uncontrollable events. Finally, Many yogic paths cultivate equanimity (upekṣā) through daily meditation and āsana practice. The Upeksha school of yoga holds it as the primary aim of practice.

The great physician Sir William Osler said: "Equanimity is the grace of life...In the first place, there is in it a strong sense of the true values in life and the insignificance of the trivial things that disturb our peace..." (Osler 2013, 64). Buddhist teacher Ethan Nichtern adds, "Equanimity is not about pretending things don't affect you. Equanimity is actually about fully acknowledging our experience while understanding how reactivity and storylines can undermine our ability to respond skillfully and with care" (Nichtern 2017, 127)

In Pema Chödrön's words: "Equanimity gives us a wider perspective. It balances the other qualities of unconditional friendship, compassion, and joy, giving them stability and strength. Without equanimity, compassion can become over-sentimentality; lovingkindness can become attachment, and joy can lead to craving when it fades. Equanimity supplies the ground for the other three to grow in a healthy way" (Chödrön 2001, 64).

The healer encounters numerous challenges during their typical day. Commenting on the stabilizing role of equanimity under these challenging circumstances, Sadhguru says, "Learning to maintain your balance is what will get you through life" (Sadhguru 2016, 117).

Repeatedly observe and regulate your breath during the day.
Breathing is a fundamental physiological process that sustains life, but how we breathe can significantly impact our overall health and well-being. In recent years, the science of nasal breathing has gained increasing attention for its role in promoting parasympathetic tone, rest, and digestion. The ancient wisdom traditions have long recognized the vital role of breath in health and healing. In Ayurveda, the traditional medical system of India, breath is seen as the bridge between the body and mind. Vasant Lad, an Ayurvedic physician and author, explains, "Prana, the life force, is the breath. It is the physical and subtle

connection, the bridge between body and mind. By regulating the breath, we can influence our physical and mental states" (Lad 1999, 63).

Similarly, in Traditional Chinese Medicine, the concept of qi, vital energy, is intimately linked to breath. The NeiJing, an ancient Chinese medical text, states: "Life is breath, and breath is life. When the breath is gone, life is gone" (Neal 2015, 17). David Frawley, a Vedic scholar and Ayurvedic practitioner, elaborates on this idea: "The quality of our breath reflects the quality of our qi. When our breath is smooth, deep, and relaxed, our qi flows freely, nourishing the body and mind" (Frawley 2018, 109).

For the modern healer, who often faces high-stress environments and demanding workloads, maintaining a balanced breath pattern is crucial for both personal well-being and the ability to provide effective care. Many healers go through their lives with rapid, shallow breaths, which can heighten their subjective distress and lead to burnout. Tenzin Wangyal, a Tibetan Bön teacher, notes, "When we are not aware of our breath, we are not aware of ourselves. By learning to breathe consciously and deeply, we can transform our relationship with stress and cultivate inner peace" (Wangyal 2011, 57). It is important to remember that our breathing pattern is essentially a deeply entrenched habit shaped by breathing more than twenty thousand times a day. As we move through life, every unresolved (undigested) emotional trauma is trapped in our energy system and impacts the natural flow of our breath cycle. Unfortunately, many of us are unaware of our unhealthy breathing patterns that are generating and entrenching our physical, emotional, and even spiritual dysregulation.

Nasal breathing, as opposed to mouth breathing, has been shown to have numerous benefits for the body and mind. When we breathe through the nose, the air is filtered, humidified, and warmed before it enters the lungs (McKeown 2015, 28). This process helps protect the delicate tissues of the respiratory system and enhances oxygen absorption. Additionally, nasal breathing stimulates the production of nitric oxide, a vasodilator that improves blood flow and oxygenation throughout the body (Lundberg et al. 1999, 7121).

Breathing is closely tied to our autonomic nervous system, which consists of the sympathetic (fight-or-flight) and parasympathetic (rest-and-digest) branches. Slow, deep nasal breathing activates the parasympathetic nervous system, promoting relaxation, calmness, and restoration (Russo et al. 2017, 5). In contrast, rapid, shallow breathing, often through the mouth, is associated with the sympathetic nervous system and a heightened stress response.

As Patrick McKeown, a leading expert on the Buteyko breathing method, explains, "The way we breathe is a reflection of our mental and emotional state. When stressed, our breathing becomes faster and shallower, and we tend to breathe more through the mouth. This type of breathing perpetuates the stress response, creating a vicious cycle" (McKeown 2019, 42).

In stressful situations, we unconsciously hold the in-breath, leading to rapid, shallow breathing. This breath pattern can contribute to feelings of anxiety, tension, and exhaustion. Lama Yondong, a Tibetan Buddhist teacher, emphasizes the importance of awareness and relaxation in breathing: "When we are under stress, we tend to hold our breath or breathe in a shallow, irregular way. By bringing mindfulness to our breathing and consciously relaxing, we can shift our state of being" (Yondong and Wangyal 2012, 86).

Cultivating a practice of slow, deep nasal breathing can profoundly affect parasympathetic tone, rest, and digestion. By consciously engaging in diaphragmatic nasal breathing, we stimulate the vagus nerve, a vital component of the parasympathetic nervous system. This activation promotes relaxation, reduces heart rate and blood pressure, and enhances digestive function (Gerritsen and Band 2018, 5).

Moreover, nasal breathing during sleep has been shown to improve the quality of rest and support the body's natural detoxification processes. As a Chinese medicine practitioner, Edward Neal, notes, "Nasal breathing during sleep allows the body to enter a deeper state of relaxation, enhancing the restorative functions of sleep. It also helps to clear toxins and support the immune system" (Neal 2020, 83).

Step Four - Clear the Space

Consciously remind yourself to bring in the kindness you have experienced and remember the lineage of healers you represent now. Call in their blessings, support, wisdom, and concern for you and your dedication to the work you continue to manifest.

The Memory of Place: How Past Events Shape Present Experiences

Healers typically inhabit spaces infused with powerful and painful emotions in the present moment. Space can also retain the energetic imprints of previous events. For example, the modern hospital has become the container for generations of human suffering and death. One does not have to be in ghosts or evil spirits to acknowledge that revisiting a site where we had previously experienced an adverse event affects us.

One of the most striking examples of how the memory of a place can influence present behavior is the phenomenon of drivers slowing down at the site of a previous accident. A study by the Transport Research Laboratory in the United Kingdom found that drivers consistently reduced their speed when passing a location where they had previously seen or experienced an accident, even if no visible signs of the incident remained (Charlton & Starkey, 2013, p. 371). This finding suggests that a traumatic event's emotional and psychological impact can create a lasting association with a particular place, leading individuals to modify their behavior in response to the memory of that event.

The idea that physical spaces can hold the memory of past traumas is also explored in environmental psychology. Researchers have found that individuals who have experienced a traumatic event in a particular location may develop a heightened sensitivity to that space, experiencing increased anxiety, hypervigilance, or avoidance behaviors when in or near the site of the trauma (Gerson & Rappaport, 2013, p. 143). This concept is particularly relevant in war and conflict, where the physical landscape can become imbued with the memory of violence, loss, and suffering. As author and journalist Christopher Hedges observes, "War is a force that gives us meaning, but it is also a force that can strip us of our humanity. The landscape of war is a landscape of memory, a place where the past is always present" (Hedges, 2002, p. 21).

In traditional Chinese medicine, the concept of ancestor qi, or the energetic imprint left by past generations, is another manifestation of the memory of place. According to this belief, our ancestors' actions, emotions, and experiences can leave a lasting mark on the spaces they inhabit, influencing the health and well-being of future generations (Jarrett, 2013, p. 81). This idea is rooted in the Chinese concept of qi, or life force energy, which is believed to flow through all living things and can be affected by the physical and energetic environment. By acknowledging and working with ancestor qi, traditional Chinese medicine practitioners aim to clear any negative energetic imprints and restore balance and harmony to a space.

The concept of ancestor qi is not unique to Chinese medicine; similar ideas can be found in many other spiritual and cultural traditions worldwide. In African American hoodoo and rootwork traditions, for example, the concept of "laying tricks" involves placing physical objects or performing rituals in a specific location to influence the behavior or experiences of those who come into contact with that space (Chireau, 2003, p. 125). Similarly, in Feng Shui, the ancient Chinese art of geomancy, practitioners work with the energy of a space to clear any negative imprints and promote positive qi flow (Lin, 2000, p. 43). These practices all recognize the powerful influence that past events and energies can have on present experiences and seek to harness that power for healing and transformation.

The memory of the place is not limited to trauma and adverse experiences; positive events and emotions can also leave a lasting imprint on a physical space. A study conducted by researchers at the University of Surrey found that individuals who had experienced a positive life event, such as a wedding or the birth of a child, in a particular location reported increased feelings of happiness, contentment, and nostalgia when revisiting that space (Lewis, 2016, p. 452). This finding suggests that the memory of a place can serve as a powerful trigger for positive emotions and experiences, creating a sense of connection and meaning that endures over time.

Concluding Remarks

Physical places possess a memory that carries powerful cultural, spiritual, and psychological phenomena. From the tangible effects of past traumas on human behavior to the more subtle energetic imprints recognized in traditional healing practices, the memory of place has a powerful influence on our present experiences and perceptions. By acknowledging and working with the memory of place, we can better understand the complex relationship between our environment, history, and well-being and harness that knowledge for personal and collective healing and transformation.

Self-Reflection Questions

1. How aware am I of my healing space's physical and energetic aspects? What steps can I take to enhance my awareness?

2. In what ways does my current work environment support or hinder my ability to provide compassionate care? How might I improve it?

3. How often do I consciously recall my intention as a healer before interacting with patients? What strategies could I use to make this a more consistent practice?

4. How would I describe my current breathing patterns throughout the day? Am I primarily engaging in nasal or mouth breathing, and how might this affect my stress levels and overall well-being?

5. In what ways do I currently incorporate elements of nature, meaningful imagery, or personal artifacts into my healing space? How could I enhance these elements to create a more supportive environment?

6. How do I typically respond to stressful situations in my work? Can I maintain equanimity, or do I find myself easily reactive? What practices could help me cultivate greater balance?

7. To what extent do I consider the "memory of place" in my healing work? How might acknowledging the energetic imprints of past events in my workspace influence my approach to patient care?

8. How often do I take conscious breaths or engage in brief mindfulness practices between patient interactions? What barriers prevent me from doing this more consistently?

9. In what ways do I currently honor or connect with my lineage of healers?

How might strengthening this connection support my work and well-being? 10. How do I currently use non-verbal cues to create a sense of safety and sacred space for my patients? What aspects of my non-verbal communication could I refine or improve?

References

1. Adams, P. (2002). Gesundheit!: Bringing good health to you, the medical system, and society through physician service, complementary therapies, humor, and joy. Rochester, VT: Healing Arts Press. (p. 23)

2. Augenthaler, D. (2018). You are not alone: A heartfelt guide to grief, healing, and hope. New York, NY: Mango Publishing Group. (p. 92)

3. Boyce, P. (2014). Human factors in lighting (3rd ed.). Boca Raton, FL: CRC Press. (p. 213)

4. Chödrön, P. (2010). Taking the Leap: Freeing Ourselves from Old Habits and Fears. Boston: Shambhala. (p. 75)

5. Chödrön, P. (2001). The Places That Scare You: A Guide to Fearlessness in Difficult Times. Boston: Shambhala. (p. 64)

6. Dalai Lama XIV. (2012). The Wisdom of Compassion: Stories of Remarkable Encounters and Timeless Insights. New York: Riverhead Books. (p. 43)

7. Frawley, D. (2018). Ayurveda and the Mind: The Healing of Consciousness. Twin Lakes, WI: Lotus Press. (p. 109)

8. Gerritsen, R. J. S., & Band, G. P. H. (2018). "Breath of Life: The Respiratory Vagal Stimulation Model of Contemplative Activity." Frontiers in Human Neuroscience 12: 397. (p. 5)

9. Halpern, J. (2001). From detached concern to empathy: Humanizing medical practice. New York, NY: Oxford University Press. (p. 67)

10. Kornfield, J. (2010). The Wise Heart: A Guide to the Universal Teachings of Buddhist Psychology. New York: Bantam Books. (p. 67)

11. Lad, V. (1999). The Complete Book of Ayurvedic Home Remedies. New York: Three Rivers Press. (p. 63)

12. Lundberg, J. O., Weitzberg, E., & Gladwin, M. T. (1999). "The Nitrate-Nitrite-Nitric Oxide Pathway in Physiology and Therapeutics." Nature Reviews Drug Discovery 7, no. 2: 156-167. (p. 7121)

13. McKeown, P. (2015). The Oxygen Advantage: Simple, Scientifically Proven Breathing Techniques to Help You Become Healthier, Slimmer, Faster, and Fitter. New York: William Morrow. (p. 28)

14. McKeown, P. (2019). The Breathing Cure: Develop New Habits for a Healthier, Happier, and Longer Life. Palm Beach Gardens, FL: Humanix Books. (p. 42)

15. Mehrabian, A. (1972). Nonverbal communication. Chicago, IL: Aldine-Atherton. (p. 44)

16. Moss, M., Hewitt, S., Moss, L., & Wesnes, K. (2008). Modulation of cognitive performance and mood by aromas of peppermint and ylang-ylang. International Journal of Neuroscience, 118(1), 59-77. (p. 1091)

17. Neal, E. (2015). Ancient Wisdom for Modern Health: Rediscover the Simple, Timeless Secrets of Health and Happiness. Bloomington, IN: Balboa Press. (p. 17)

18. Neal, E. (2020). The Art of Breathing: Restore Your Health and Vitality through the Power of Conscious Breathing. London: Watkins Publishing. (p. 83)

19. Nhất Hạnh, T. (2012). You Are Here: Discovering the Magic of the Present Moment. Boston: Shambhala Publications. (p. 7)

20. Nhất Hạnh, T. (2014). How to Love. Berkeley, CA: Parallax Press. (p. 62)

21. Nichtern, E. (2017). The Dharma of The Princess Bride: What the Coolest Fairy Tale of Our Time Can Teach Us About Buddhism and Relationships. New York: North Point Press. (p. 127)

22. Nightingale, F. (1860). Notes on nursing: What it is, and what it is not. London: Harrison. (p. 34)

23. Osler, W. (2013). The Quotable Osler. Edited by Mark E. Silverman, T. Jock Murray, and Charles S. Bryan. Philadelphia: American College of Physicians. (p. 64)

24. Remen, R. N. (1996). Kitchen table wisdom: Stories that heal. New York, NY: Riverhead Books. (p. 52, 144)

25. Rumi, M. J. M. (2004). The Essential Rumi. Translated by Coleman Barks. New York: HarperOne. (p. 45)

26. Russo, M. A., Santarelli, D. M., & O'Rourke, D. (2017). "The Physiological Effects of Slow Breathing in the Healthy Human." Breathe 13, no. 4: 298-309. (p. 5)

27. Sadhguru, J. V. (2016). Inner Engineering: A Yogi's Guide to Joy. New York: Spiegel & Grau. (p. 117)

28. Sayorwan, W., Siripornpanich, V., Piriyapunyaporn, T., Hongratanaworakit, T., Kotchabhakdi, N., & Ruangrungsi, N. (2012). The effects of lavender oil inhalation on emotional states, autonomic nervous system, and brain electrical activity. Journal of the Medical Association of Thailand, 95(4), 598-606. (p. 667)

29. Suzuki, S. (2011). Zen Mind, Beginner's Mind: Informal Talks on Zen Meditation and Practice. Boston: Shambhala Publications. (p. 21)

30. Trungpa, C. (2002). Cutting Through Spiritual Materialism. Boston: Shambhala Publications. (p. 20)

31. Trungpa, C. (2013). The Bodhisattva Path of Wisdom and Compassion. Vol. 2 of The Profound Treasury of the Ocean of Dharma. Boston: Shambhala. (p. 3, 13)

32. Ulrich, R. S., Simons, R. F., Losito, B. D., Fiorito, E., Miles, M. A., & Zelson,

M. (1991). Stress recovery during exposure to natural and urban environments. Journal of Environmental Psychology, 11(3), 201-230. (p. 224)

33. Wangyal, T. (2011). Tibetan Sound Healing: Seven Guided Practices for Clearing Obstacles, Accessing Positive Qualities, and Uncovering Your Inherent Wisdom. Louisville, CO: Sounds True. (p. 57)

34. Yondong, L., & Wangyal, T. (2012). Tibetan Wisdom for Modern Life. San Francisco: Hay House. (p. 86)

35. Chireau, Y. (2003). Black magic: Religion and the African American conjuring tradition. Berkeley, CA: University of California Press. (p. 125)

36. Gerson, R., & Rappaport, N. (2013). Traumatic stress and posttraumatic stress disorder in youth: Recent research findings on clinical impact, assessment, and treatment. Journal of Adolescent Health, 52(2), 137-143. (p. 143)

37. Hedges, C. (2002). War is a force that gives us meaning. New York, NY: PublicAffairs. (p. 21)

38. Jarrett, L. S. (2013). Nourishing destiny: The inner tradition of Chinese medicine. Stockbridge, MA: Spirit Path Press. (p. 81)

39. Lewis, G. J. (2016). Nostalgia and the regulation of positive and negative affect: An experimental approach. Personality and Individual Differences, 101, 451-456. (p. 452)

40. Lin, H. (2000). The art and science of Feng Shui: The ancient Chinese tradition of shaping fate. St. Paul, MN: Llewellyn Worldwide. (p. 43)

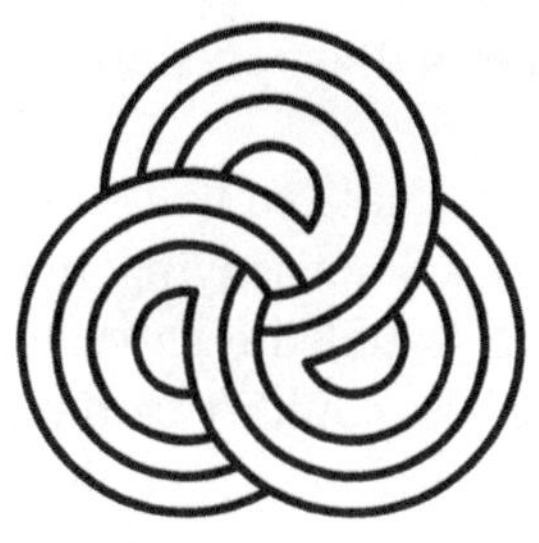

CHAPTER 18

Asana Three: Be Present

Instruction: Wash your hands and become presence.

"The present is holy ground."
Alfred North Whitehead

In the early days of my career as a faculty member at Harvard Medical School, I had the privilege of teaching medical students during their month-long rotations within our department. These bright, enthusiastic students never failed to inspire me with their passion for learning and fresh perspectives. As their teacher, I constantly reflected on my knowledge and perceptions, challenged to grow alongside them.

One particularly poignant experience during this time taught me a profound lesson about the power of presence. A colleague asked me to visit Susan, a middle-aged woman in the intensive care unit who was on a ventilator due to Guillain-Barré syndrome. This autoimmune disorder had caused rapid, progressive paralysis throughout her body, leaving her in excruciating pain and unable to communicate. My colleague hoped I could help alleviate her evident distress, as she would become tearful whenever someone entered her room.

As I walked into Susan's room, I felt an overwhelming sense of helplessness. With no means of verbal or nonverbal communication, I struggled to find a way to connect with her and offer comfort. Sitting beside her, I observed my feelings of inadequacy. I recognized that the only thing I could offer was my presence - a doorway into the experience of her suffering and its potential relief.

While sitting with Susan, I noticed that whenever I made an emotionally charged comment, such as acknowledging my helplessness or imagining her distress, her vital signs would dramatically increase. This observation suggested that even though we couldn't communicate in a typical way, we could work together to help her control her vital signs with her mind. To my surprise, as soon as I made this suggestion, her blood pressure and pulse rate immediately returned to normal.

From that moment on, I committed to visiting Susan daily, spending time in meditation, and observing her vital signs to monitor her response and well-being. Despite my initial discomfort with this unconventional approach, I persisted, and the ICU staff began to rely on my visits, often calling me if I was delayed.

During one of these visits, a medical student accompanying me expressed skepticism about my methods, questioning whether this approach was appropriate for Harvard Medical School, where evidence-based medicine was the norm. He wondered if people might view it as quackery. His concerns mirrored my doubts over the preceding weeks. However, I reminded him that we had no other options to offer Susan and that the nursing staff believed our work together was beneficial. As we sat and practiced breathing and meditation techniques with Susan, the student observed with surprise the favorable changes in her vital signs.

My work with Susan continued for six weeks as she gradually began to recover her neurological function. One day, I received an urgent page from the ICU requesting my immediate presence. Fearing a medical crisis, I rushed to the unit, only to find Susan in a wheelchair, surrounded by her entire treatment team. They informed me that she would be transferring to a rehabilitation program that morning but had insisted on meeting with me and the team before her departure.

Susan expressed her gratitude for the tireless efforts of the ICU staff, acknowledging their crucial role in her survival and recovery. Then, turning to me, she shared a message that would forever change my understanding of the healing process. She explained that while everyone's contributions had been invaluable, it was my willingness to show up repeatedly at her bedside, without any agenda other than to bear witness to her suffering and recognize the power of her mind and spirit, that had made it possible for her to survive the descent into hell. Without this, she declared, she would never have made it through.

That day, Susan gave me an extraordinary gift. She reminded me of the truth in Shantideva's words: "May I be both the doctor and the medicine" (1, p. 98). She illuminated the transformative power of presence, demonstrating that we can always be present even in the most challenging circumstances. Her experience reaffirmed that presence is the foundation of our work as healers.

In the years since I have carried this teaching with me. Whenever I want to flee from a difficult situation, I remember Susan and the profound impact of simply showing up, being authentic, and being fully present. Her story is a constant reminder that presence can transform lives and that by embodying this principle, we can make a meaningful difference in the world.

The concept of presence can be challenging to grasp. We can consider a model encompassing three essential elements: physical, personal, and authentic. Each of these aspects contributes to the overall experience of being fully present and engaged at the moment, whether in a therapeutic setting or our daily lives.

The three types of presence are:

a. *Physical presence*: The embodied, tangible aspect of being present, including posture, gestures, and nonverbal communication.
b. *Personal presence*: The unique qualities and characteristics an individual brings to their interactions, such as confidence, charisma, and self-awareness.
c. *Authentic presence*: The genuine, open-hearted connection that arises when one is fully attuned to the present moment and the needs of others.

What is "Healing Presence" ?

Healing presence is a profound state of being that emerges when a healer can bring their whole, authentic self to the therapeutic relationship. It involves a deep attunement to the patient's experience, a willingness to sit with their pain and suffering, and a compassionate, non-judgmental stance. When healers embody this presence, they create a safe, nurturing space where transformation and healing can occur.

Being Absent

Scientific objectivity shapes our absence from one another
While valuable in many contexts, the pursuit of scientific objectivity can sometimes lead to a sense of disconnection and absence in our

relationships. When we prioritize detached observation and analysis over empathetic engagement, we risk losing sight of the human experience that underlies the data. As Shari Geller notes, "Equanimity is not the same as objective detachment" (2, p. 35). True equanimity involves maintaining an open, compassionate stance while remaining grounded and stable under challenging emotions.

The "near enemies" of equanimity, such as indifference or apathy, can be mistaken for the real thing, leading to a sense of absence and disconnection. Similarly, the "far enemies," such as agitation or overwhelm, can pull us out of the present moment and into reactivity (2, p. 36). By cultivating the Four Immeasurables (loving-kindness, compassion, empathetic joy, and equanimity), we can find a middle path that allows for genuine presence and connection.

The characteristics of "absence" i.e., "ab-sense" versus "pre-sense"
Absence, or "ab-sense," is characterized by a lack of attunement, engagement, and responsiveness. When we are absent, we may be physically present but emotionally or mentally disconnected, unable to take in the experience of the "other" fully. This can manifest in various ways, such as:

1. Preoccupation with our thoughts or agenda
2. Failure to listen actively or empathetically
3. Lack of eye contact or nonverbal attunement
4. Rushedness or impatience
5. Judgment or criticism
6. Emotional reactivity or defensiveness
7. Inability to tolerate silence or discomfort
8. Avoidance of difficult topics or emotions

In contrast, "pre-sense" involves being fully engaged, attuned, and responsive to the present moment and the needs of others. When we embody presence, we bring our whole selves to the interaction, offering our undivided attention, compassion, and support.

Shari Geller describes eight signs of in-session absence (2, p. 40):

1. Feeling anxious, bored, or distracted
2. Thinking about other things
3. Judging the client or oneself
4. Engaging in self-talk or internal chatter
5. Planning what to say or do next
6. Losing energy or feeling drained

7.   Feeling detached or disconnected
8.   Engaging in habitual or scripted responses

Similarly, Geller identifies seven signs of post-session absence (2, p. 41):

1.   Difficulty remembering details of the session
2.   Feeling drained or depleted
3.   Ruminating about the session or the client
4.   Feeling guilty, inadequate, or self-critical
5.   Experiencing somatic symptoms (e.g., tension, headache)
6.   Having a sense of unfinished business
7.   Struggling to transition to other activities or relationships

These signs of absence highlight the connection between burnout and compassion fatigue. When we are consistently unable to be fully present and engaged, we may experience emotional exhaustion, decreased empathy, and a sense of ineffectiveness in our work. Over time, this can lead to disillusionment, cynicism, and a loss of meaning or purpose (2, p. 42).

Being absent essentially blinds us to our inherent vitality and the generative power of intersubjectivity. When trapped in a state of absence, we lose touch with the intrinsic aliveness and creativity that emerges from genuine connection. As Martin Buber writes, "All real living is meeting" (3, p. 11). Through the I-Thou relationship, characterized by presence, openness, and mutuality, we access the transformative power of intersubjectivity.

In contrast, the I-It relationship, marked by objectification and instrumentality, leaves us feeling isolated, disconnected and drained (3, p. 23). When we relate to others as objects to be analyzed, fixed, or controlled, we miss the opportunity for growth, healing, and co-creation that arises from authentic encounters.

The Three Types of Absencing

1.   *Dissociating and depersonalization*: When we become overly identified with a narrow aspect of our identity, such as our professional role or expertise, we risk losing touch with our full humanity. By isolating ourselves in an ego identity, we limit our capacity for empathy, flexibility, and creative problem-solving (2, p. 44).
2.   *Intellectualization*: In pursuing knowledge and mastery, modern healers can become overburdened by facts and theories, neglecting the importance of nonverbal, experiential, and intuitive ways of knowing. As Nietzsche reminds us, "There is more wisdom in your body than in your deepest

philosophy" (4, p. 39). By relying solely on intellectual understanding, we miss the rich, embodied information essential for healing presence.

3. *Habits and routines*: When we become rigidly attached to prescribed protocols and procedures, we lose the ability to respond flexibly to each individual's unique needs. While structure and consistency are important, overemphasizing routines can lead to disconnection and absence (2, p. 46).

The Three Types of Presence

1. Physical presence: The embodied dimension of presence includes factors such as posture, gestures, facial expressions, and vocal qualities. Research has shown that expansive, open postures can communicate confidence and power, while closed, constricted postures convey submissiveness and vulnerability. In the medical context, signals of authority such as white coats and exam tables can reinforce power differentials and hinder authentic connection.

    It's important to recognize that physical presence can be used as an ethological "display behavior" to exert authority and subjugate others to our will. Dominant postures, assertive gestures, and commanding vocal tones can establish hierarchy and control rather than foster genuine connection and understanding. When physical presence is used this way, it is not motivated by compassion but by a desire to impose one's agenda or perspective onto others.

2. Personal presence: Personal presence, also known as "executive presence," refers to the unique qualities and characteristics an individual brings to their interactions, such as charisma, warmth, and self-assurance. Amy Cuddy describes executive presence as a dynamic mix of communication skills, gravitas (confidence and credibility), and appearance (professional demeanor) (5, p. 12). Similarly, Tony Robbins emphasizes cultivating a commanding presence through purposeful body language, vocal tone, and intention (6, p. 56).

    However, like physical presence, personal or executive presence can be used to assert dominance and control over others. Charisma and confidence can be wielded as tools of manipulation, designed to sway opinions and decisions in one's favor. When personal presence is driven by self-interest rather than a genuine desire to serve and connect, it becomes another display behavior that ultimately undermines authentic relationships and trust.

3. Authentic presence: While physical and personal presence can be co-opted for self-serving purposes, authentic presence holds the most

significant potential for healing and transformation. Shari Geller writes,
4.   "Therapeutic presence involves being fully in the moment on many levels: physically, emotionally, cognitively, and spiritually" (2, p. 18). This type of presence requires a willingness to be vulnerable, transparent, and open-hearted, meeting the other person with curiosity, acceptance, and compassion.

To cultivate authentic presence, Geller offers the acronym PRESENCE as a guide (2, pp. 19-24):

- *PAUSE*: Take a moment to stop and collect yourself before engaging with another person. This pause allows you to let go of distractions and bring your full attention to the present moment.
- *RELAX*: Soften your facial muscles and release tension in your body. This physical relaxation helps create a sense of ease and openness for yourself and the person you are connecting with.
- *ENHANCE*: Focus on deepening and lengthening your exhalations. This conscious breathing helps to calm your nervous system and bring you into a more grounded, centered state.
- *SENSE*: Be aware of what you feel in your body and emotions. Notice any sensations, thoughts, or feelings that arise without judgment or resistance. This self-awareness is essential for attuning to another person's experience.
- *EXPAND*: Open your sensory awareness to take in the fullness of the moment—notice details about the other person's nonverbal cues, tone of voice, and overall energy. Allow yourself to be curious and receptive to whatever unfolds in the interaction.
- *NOTICE*: Observe what is true now without getting caught up in stories or interpretations. Stay present with what is actually happening, rather than getting lost in thoughts about the past or future.
- *CENTER* and GROUND yourself: Connect with a sense of inner stability and resilience. Feel your feet on the ground and your body supported by the chair or floor. This centering helps you remain steady and present, even in difficult emotions or challenging situations.
- EXTEND: yourself to make contact.Reach out to the other person with your full attention and care. Make eye contact, if appropriate, and convey your openness and willingness to connect. This extension of yourself is an invitation to genuine engagement and dialogue.

Geller further describes the process of developing authentic presence as involving three key components (2, p. 18):

1. Being open and receptive to the client's experience
2. Inwardly attending to one's bodily resonance with the client's experience
3. Extending and making contact with the client from this place of receptivity and inward contact

These components create a deep, empathetic connection between therapist and client, facilitating healing and growth.

Geller also identifies four aspects of the experience of presence (2, p. 20):

1. Immersion: Being fully engaged and absorbed in the moment without distraction or preoccupation.
2. Expansion: A sense of openness, spaciousness, and connection beyond the boundaries of the self.
3. Grounding: Feeling centered, stable, and rooted in one's body and the present moment.
4. Being with and for the client: A deep sense of attunement, empathy, and commitment to the client's well-being.

The neurophysiology of presence is closely linked to the functioning of the autonomic nervous system, particularly the ventral vagal complex. Stephen Porges' Polyvagal Theory (7) suggests that the ventral vagal pathway, when activated, promotes feelings of safety, connection, and social engagement. This "social engagement system" is critical for establishing an authentic, empathetic presence that fosters healing relationships.

Similarly, Dan Siegel's concept of "mindsight" (8) emphasizes the importance of attuned, compassionate presence in promoting the integration of neural networks associated with self-awareness, emotional regulation, and interpersonal connection. By cultivating mindsight and activating the social engagement system, therapists can create the optimal conditions for healing and transformation.

Geller encapsulates the essence of therapeutic presence as follows:

"Therapeutic presence is a way of being with the client that optimizes the doing of therapy. It involves therapists bringing their whole selves to the encounter and being present on multiple levels, physically, emotionally, cognitively, relationally, and spiritually. TP involves being grounded in one's self, while receptively attuning to the verbal and non-verbal expression of client's moment-to-moment experience" (2, p. 17).

Thomas Hübl, a contemporary spiritual teacher and trauma expert, further illuminates the role of presence in healing trauma. He writes:

"Trauma is an experience of overwhelming energy that cannot be processed and integrated at the moment. It is a rupture in our capacity to be present... The healing of trauma requires us to build the capacity to stay present with what is, even if it feels uncomfortable or painful. It invites us to develop a new relationship with the energy of life that moves through us, to befriend it and allow it to find its natural flow and expression" (9, p. 45).

Hübl emphasizes that presence is not just a state of being but a skill that can be developed through practice. He offers a three-step process for cultivating presence in the face of trauma (9, pp. 87-92):

1. Grounding: Establishing a sense of safety and stability in the body through practices such as mindful breathing, sensing the feet on the ground, and feeling the support of the earth.
2. Attunement: Bringing a kind, curious attention to the felt sense of the body, emotions, and mind without judgment or resistance. This allows us to build the capacity to be with challenging experiences without becoming overwhelmed.
3. Integration: Allowing the energy of the trauma to be processed and released through the body while staying connected to the ground of presence. This may involve gentle movement, sound, or expressive arts.

    By developing the capacity for presence in the face of trauma, we can begin to heal the fragmentation and disconnection that often result from overwhelming experiences. As Hübl notes, "Presence is the key to integrating trauma. It is the light that illuminates the frozen places within us, allowing them to thaw and come back to life" (9, p. 87).

4. Ultimate Presence: Beyond authentic presence, we can conceive of an even deeper, more expansive state of being—ultimate Presence. This is the limitless manifestation of the enlivened, interdependent, compassionate universe. When we tap into Ultimate Presence, we recognize our fundamental oneness with all of life and experience a profound sense of love, wisdom, and interconnectedness.

The thirteen characteristics of Ultimate Presence are (2, p. 25):

1. Humble: A deep recognition of our smallness and the vastness of the universe.
2. Reflective: The capacity to witness and learn from our own experience.
3. Caring: A genuine concern for the well-being of all beings.
4. Compassionate: The ability to empathize with and alleviate the suffering of others.
5. Luminous: A radiant, light-filled quality that emanates from within.
6. Non-dual: Transcending the perception of separation and experiencing unity.

7. Boundless: A sense of expansiveness and freedom from limitations.
8. Enlivening: An invigorating, vitalizing force that awakens us to our full potential.
9. Confident: A deep trust in the inherent wisdom and goodness of life.
10. Creative: The capacity to bring forth new possibilities and solutions.
11. Joyful: A state of contentment, appreciation, and delight in the present moment.
12. Beautiful: Recognizing the inherent beauty and perfection in all things.
13. Autotelic: Engaging in activities for their own sake, without attachment to outcomes.

By cultivating these qualities and opening ourselves to the experience of Ultimate Presence, we can access a profound source of healing, wisdom, and transformation, both for ourselves and those we serve.

Cultivating Presence: A Path to Healing and Connection

Developing the capacity for authentic presence is a lifelong journey that requires dedication, self-reflection, and a willingness to step outside our comfort zones. Committing to this path enhances our ability to support others and deepens our sense of wholeness, resilience, and connection.

One of the foundational practices for cultivating presence is mindfulness. As Jon Kabat-Zinn defines it, mindfulness is "paying attention in a particular way: on purpose, in the present moment, and non-judgmentally" (10, p. 4). Regular mindfulness practice teaches us to observe our thoughts, feelings, and sensations with greater clarity and stability, reducing the grip of habitual patterns and reactivity.

In addition to formal meditation practice, we can bring mindfulness into our daily lives by engaging in activities with full attention and care. Thich Nhat Hanh, the renowned Buddhist teacher, speaks of the power of "washing the dishes to wash the dishes" – that is, bringing our complete presence to even the most mundane tasks (11, p. 3). By approaching life with this sense of reverence and appreciation, we cultivate a deeper understanding of connection and aliveness.

Another critical aspect of cultivating presence is self-compassion. As Kristin Neff explains, self-compassion involves treating ourselves with the same kindness, care, and understanding that we would offer to a good friend (12, p. 41). When we can meet our struggles and imperfections with gentleness and acceptance, we create a foundation of inner safety and stability that allows us to be more fully present with others.

Cultivating self-compassion also involves setting healthy boundaries and practicing self-care. As Rachel Naomi Remen notes, "The expectation that we can be immersed in suffering and loss daily and not be touched by it is as unrealistic as expecting to be able to walk through water without getting wet" (13, p. 52). By attending to our own needs for rest, nourishment, and renewal, we prevent burnout and maintain our capacity for compassionate presence.

Cultivating presence in healing also requires a willingness to confront power, privilege, and oppression issues. As Camara Phyllis Jones reminds us, "Racism is a system of structuring opportunity and assigning value based on the social interpretation of how one looks" (14, p. 1212). By examining our own biases and working to dismantle systemic inequities, we create the conditions for genuine, healing connections across differences.

Ultimately, the path of presence is one of continual learning, growth, and transformation. As we deepen our capacity for presence, our sense of identity shifts from a narrow, isolated self to a more expansive, interconnected sense of being. As Ram Dass writes, "We're all just walking each other home" (15, p. 324).

By walking this path with courage, compassion, and humility, we can support others in their healing journeys while finding our way home – to a place of wholeness, connection, and abiding presence. As Rumi, the great Sufi mystic, reminds us:

"Out beyond ideas of wrongdoing and rightdoing,
there is a field. I'll meet you there.
When the soul lies down in that grass,
the world is too full to talk about." (16, p. 36)

May we have the grace and the strength to meet each other in that field, again and again, with open hearts and loving presence.

The Integration of Presence: Bringing It All Together

As we explore the various facets of presence – physical, personal, and authentic – it becomes clear that true presence is not a compartmentalized skill but a holistic way of being. When we cultivate presence in one area of our lives, it naturally infuses and transforms other areas.

For example, as we develop greater mindfulness and self-awareness, our physical presence becomes more grounded, centered, and attuned. As we practice self-compassion and set healthy boundaries, we may notice our presence becoming more confident, authentic, and resilient. And as we engage in the ongoing work of self-reflection and growth, we may discover that our capacity for authentic presence deepens and expands.

This integration of presence is beautifully captured in the concept of "presencing" articulated by Otto Scharmer and his colleagues at the Presencing Institute. Presencing, a blend of the words "presence" and "sensing," refers to the ability to sense and actualize one's highest future potential. It involves letting go of habitual patterns and assumptions, opening oneself to new possibilities, and acting from a place of deep alignment with one's values and purpose (17, p. 8).

As Scharmer writes, "The key to presencing is to get out of the echo chamber of our own mind and to connect with the surrounding world in a more open and intentional way. It's about shifting the inner place from which we operate" (17, p. 12).

This shifting of our inner place is the essence of the transformative power of presence. When we can meet the present moment with openness, curiosity, and compassion, we create the conditions for profound healing, connection, and growth – both for ourselves and those we serve.

Of course, this is not always easy or comfortable. Cultivating presence requires us to confront our fears, doubts, and limitations and lean into the discomfort of not knowing, not fixing, and not controlling. It asks us to relinquish our attachment to outcomes and trust in the inherent wisdom and resilience of the human spirit.

Yet, as challenging as this work can be, it is gratifying and nourishing. As Rachel Naomi Remen writes, "When you listen generously to people, they can hear the truth in themselves, often for the first time" (13, p. 219). By offering our presence as a sacred gift, we create space for others to connect with their inner knowing and access their healing and wholeness capacity.

Ultimately, the integration of presence is a journey of coming home to ourselves and our interconnectedness with life. As Thich Nhat Hanh puts it, it is a recognition that "We are here to awaken from the illusion of our separateness" (11, p. 35). By cultivating presence in all its dimensions, we dissolve the barriers that keep us feeling isolated and alone and open ourselves to the boundless love, wisdom, and creativity that is our true nature.

As we walk this path of presence, let us remember the words of Parker Palmer: "The soul is like a wild animal – tough, resilient, savvy, self-sufficient and yet exceedingly shy. If we will walk quietly into the woods and sit silently for an hour or two at the base of a tree, the creature we are waiting for may well emerge" (18, p. 58).

May we have the patience, courage, and trust to keep showing up, moment by moment, breath by breath, until we, too, can meet the wild and tender presence that lives within us all. May we bring that presence forth in service of healing, connection, and the greater good, knowing that our very being is a gift to the world.

The Ripple Effect of Presence: Transforming Our World One Encounter at a Time

As we deepen our understanding and embodiment of presence, it becomes clear that the impact of this practice extends far beyond our individual lives and relationships. When we show up fully in each moment, with an open heart and a compassionate presence, we set in motion a ripple effect that has the power to transform our families, our communities, and our world.

This ripple effect begins with recognizing that every encounter, whether brief or seemingly insignificant, holds the potential for profound connection and healing. As Rachel Naomi Remen writes, "The most important questions don't seem to have ready answers, but the questions themselves have a healing power when they are shared. An answer is an invitation to stop thinking about something, to stop wondering. Life has no such stopping places; life is a process whose every event is connected to the moment that just went by. An unanswered question is a fine traveling companion. It sharpens your eye for the road" (13, p. 296).

By approaching each interaction with the spirit of an unanswered question—with curiosity, humility, and presence—we create the conditions for genuine meeting and discovery. We open ourselves to the possibility of being changed by the encounter, having our assumptions challenged and our perspectives expanded. In doing so, we invite others into a space of mutual exploration and growth.

This way of being in relationship can transform not only our personal lives but also our professional and societal contexts. For example, a growing body of research demonstrates the importance of presence and empathy in promoting positive outcomes and patient satisfaction. As Jodi Halpern notes in her book "From Detached Concern to Empathy: Humanizing Medical Practice," "Empathy is not detached concern, but engaged curiosity about another's particular emotional perspective" (19, p. 17).

By bringing this engaged curiosity and presence to our work as healers, we create a context in which patients feel seen, heard, and valued – not just as a collection of symptoms or diagnoses, but as whole persons with unique stories, strengths, and challenges. This kind of care can activate the body's innate healing capacities, alleviate suffering, and restore a sense of meaning and purpose in the face of illness and adversity.

Similarly, in education, presence can transform how we teach and learn. As Parker Palmer writes in "The Courage to Teach," "Good teaching cannot be reduced to technique; good teaching comes from the identity and integrity of the teacher" (18, p. 10). When we show up fully in the classroom, committed to our ongoing growth and self-discovery, we create a space where students feel inspired, challenged, and supported to bring forth their unique gifts and contributions.

At a societal level, the cultivation of presence and compassion is essential for addressing the complex challenges of our time – from social and economic inequities to environmental degradation and political polarization. By approaching these issues with a willingness to listen deeply, to hold multiple perspectives, and to work collaboratively towards solutions, we can begin to heal the divisions that threaten to tear us apart and create a more just, sustainable, and thriving world for all.

Ultimately, the ripple effect of presence begins with our willingness to show up fully in this moment, the next, and the next. As Rumi reminds us: "Yesterday I was clever, so I wanted to change the world. Today I am wise, so I am changing myself." (16, p. 125)

By changing ourselves—by cultivating presence, compassion, and wisdom in our hearts and minds—we become agents of transformation in the world around us. May we have the courage and dedication to keep showing up, to keep opening, and to keep letting our light shine forth for the benefit of all beings.

The Power of Presence: A Call to Awakening

As we come to the end of our exploration of presence and its transformative potential, let us take a moment to reflect on the journey we have undertaken together. We have delved into what it means to be truly present—to show up fully in each moment with an open heart and a curious mind. We have examined the obstacles that can prevent us from embodying presence and explored practices and perspectives that can help us cultivate this essential quality in our lives.

Along the way, we have discovered that presence is not just a nice idea or a fleeting experience but a powerful force for healing, connection, and transformation. When we are present, we tap into a source of wisdom, compassion, and creativity beyond ourselves. We become conduits for the energy of life itself, and we participate in the great unfolding of the universe.

This realization can be both humbling and empowering. It reminds us that we are not separate from the world around us but intimately interconnected with all of life. It challenges us to let go of our attachment to our minor, ego-driven concerns and to align ourselves with a greater purpose. At the same time, it affirms our inherent worth and potential and invites us to step fully into our power as agents of change.

As we contemplate the call to presence that echoes throughout the ages, let us remember the words of the great spiritual teacher Ramana Maharshi: "Your own Self-realization is the greatest service you can render the world"

(20, p. 77). By awakening to our true nature and embodying presence in our lives, we transform ourselves and contribute to the healing and awakening of all beings.

We cannot accomplish this task alone, nor will it be completed in a single lifetime. It is a collective journey that requires the participation and support of all who feel called to walk the path of presence. At times, the challenges of this path may feel overwhelming, and we may be tempted to give up or turn back. In these moments, let us remember the words of the Sufi poet Rumi: "The wound is the place where the Light enters you" (16, p. 142). Let us trust that our struggles and failures are not obstacles to presence but opportunities for more profound healing and growth.

Ultimately, the call to presence is to love ourselves, one another, and the world in all its beauty and brokenness. As we cultivate presence in our lives, we discover that love is not just an emotion but a way of being – a radiant expression of our deepest nature.

May we have the courage and the compassion to answer this call, to show up fully in each moment, and to let our lives be a testament to the power of presence. May we support and inspire one another on this journey and trust in the unfolding of life's great mystery.

May we remember that, in the end, the path of presence is not a destination but a way of being – a moment-to-moment choice to embrace our humanity's fullness and live in alignment with our most profound truth. As we walk this path together, let us celebrate the beauty and wonder of this precious life and be the presence that we wish to see in the world.

In this way, we will transform ourselves and leave a legacy of love and awakening that will ripple through the ages, touching countless lives and contributing to our world's healing. May we rise to this great calling and find joy, meaning, and purpose in the journey. May we always remember that the power of presence is within us, waiting to be discovered and expressed in every moment of our lives.

Self-Reflection Questions

1. How do I demonstrate physical presence in my interactions with others? Do I maintain eye contact, use open body language, and offer nonverbal cues of attentiveness and engagement?

2. How would I describe my personal presence? Do I bring a sense of authenticity, warmth, and self-assurance to my relationships, or do I sometimes hide behind a façade or persona?

3. When I think about authentic presence, how fully do I allow myself to be vulnerable, transparent, and open-hearted with others? What fears or defenses might be holding me back from deeper levels of connection and intimacy?

4. how well do I maintain a grounded, centered presence in challenging or emotionally charged situations? Do I have practices or techniques that help me stay present and regulated in the face of difficulty or discomfort?

5. How attuned am I to the subtleties of my own inner experience – my thoughts, feelings, sensations, and intuitions? Do I have a regular practice of self-reflection or contemplation that helps me deepen my self-awareness?

6. How attentive and responsive am I to their verbal and nonverbal cues when communicating with others? Do I listen with curiosity and empathy, seeking to understand their unique perspective and experience?

7. In my role as a healer or helper, how consistently do I embody therapeutic presence? Do I bring my whole self to the encounter, with a commitment to being with and for the client in their moment-to-moment experience?

8. How comfortable am I with silence, stillness, and spaciousness in my interactions? Do I allow room for pauses, reflection, and emergence, or do I tend to fill the space with words and activity?

9. In what ways might my presence be shaped by power dynamics, cultural conditioning, or unconscious biases? How willing am I to examine and take responsibility for my impact on others, even when unintentional?

10. How do I cultivate presence in my relationship with myself? Do I offer myself the same qualities of attention, compassion, and acceptance that I strive to offer others?

References

1. Shantideva. (1997). The Way of the Bodhisattva (Padmakara Translation Group, Trans.). Shambhala Publications.

2. Geller, S. M. (2017). A Practical Guide to Cultivating Therapeutic Presence. American Psychological Association.

3. Buber, M. (1971). I and Thou (W. Kaufmann, Trans.). Charles Scribner's Sons.

4. Nietzsche, F. (1954). Thus Spoke Zarathustra (W. Kaufmann, Trans.). Penguin Books.

5. Cuddy, A. (2015). Presence: Bringing Your Boldest Self to Your Biggest Challenges. Little, Brown and Company.

6. Robbins, T. (1992). Awaken the Giant Within: How to Take Immediate Control of Your Mental, Emotional, Physical and Financial Destiny. Free Press.

7. Porges, S. W. (2011). The Polyvagal Theory: Neurophysiological Foundations of Emotions, Attachment, Communication, and Self-regulation. W. W. Norton & Company.

8. Siegel, D. J. (2010). Mindsight: The New Science of Personal Transformation. Bantam Books.

9. Hübl, T. (2020). Healing Collective Trauma: A Process for Integrating Our

Intergenerational and Cultural Wounds. Sounds True.

10. Kabat-Zinn, J. (2013). Full Catastrophe Living: Using the Wisdom of Your Body and Mind to Face Stress, Pain, and Illness. Bantam Books.

11. Hanh, T. N. (2015). The Heart of the Buddha's Teaching: Transforming Suffering into Peace, Joy, and Liberation. Harmony Books.

12. Neff, K. (2011). Self-Compassion: The Proven Power of Being Kind to Yourself. William Morrow.

13. Remen, R. N. (1996). Kitchen Table Wisdom: Stories that Heal. Riverhead Books.

14. Jones, C. P. (2000). Levels of racism: a theoretic framework and a gardener's tale. American Journal of Public Health, 90(8), 1212-1215.

15. Dass, R. (1979). Be Here Now. Lama Foundation.

16. Rumi. (2004). The Essential Rumi (C. Barks, Trans.). HarperOne.

17. Scharmer, O. (2016). Theory U: Leading from the Future as It Emerges. Berrett-Koehler Publishers.

18. Palmer, P. J. (2007). The Courage to Teach: Exploring the Inner Landscape of a Teacher's Life. Jossey-Bass.

19. Halpern, J. (2001). From Detached Concern to Empathy: Humanizing Medical Practice. Oxford University Press.

20. Maharshi, R. (1985). The Spiritual Teaching of Ramana Maharshi. Shambhala Publications.

CHAPTER 19

Asana Four: Make Connection

Instruction: Take a seat.

*"Empathy is the ability to feel yourself as part of a larger whole.
It's the recognition that we are all interconnected, that we are all
part of the same human family. When we can feel that connection,
that's when true healing becomes possible."*
Thomas Hübl [23]

In the realm of healthcare, the ability to connect with patients on a deep, empathic level is a critical skill that can have a profound impact on the quality of care, patient satisfaction, and health outcomes. However, in the fast-paced, technology-driven environment of modern healthcare, establishing genuine empathy can be a challenging task. This chapter explores the concept of empathy, its various components, and the factors that influence empathic accuracy. It also examines how the modern healthcare system's focus on scientific materialism can hinder empathic connection, and discusses strategies for cultivating deep listening, appreciative inquiry, and empathic communication in clinical settings.

Compassion and Empathy: Understanding the Distinct Yet Interconnected Qualities

Compassion and empathy are two closely related yet distinct qualities that play crucial roles in our emotional lives and social interactions. While often used interchangeably, understanding the nuances between these two concepts can help us cultivate more meaningful connections with others and respond to suffering in a more effective and authentic manner.

Empathy, at its core, is the ability to understand and share the feelings of another person. It involves stepping into someone else's shoes, imagining their perspective, and vicariously experiencing their emotions. When we empathize with someone, we resonate with their joy, pain, or confusion, gaining a deeper appreciation for their subjective experience. Empathy allows us to establish an emotional bond with others, creating a sense of connection and understanding that transcends differences in background, beliefs, or circumstances.

Compassion, on the other hand, goes beyond the realm of emotional resonance. While empathy is feeling with someone, compassion is feeling for them and being moved to help. Compassion arises when we encounter suffering and feel a deep desire to alleviate that suffering. It is a heart-centered response that combines the emotional attunement of empathy with a strong motivation to take action and provide support, comfort, or relief. Compassion is not just about sharing someone's pain, but actively seeking to ease it.

One way to understand the difference between empathy and compassion is through the lens of personal distress versus empathic concern. When we empathize with someone who is suffering, we may experience a degree of personal distress, feeling overwhelmed or upset by their pain. This emotional contagion can sometimes lead to empathic overarousal, where we become so engrossed in another's suffering that we lose sight of our own well-being and ability to help. Compassion, in contrast, involves a more balanced and grounded response. It allows us to maintain a sense of equanimity and perspective, even in the face of intense suffering, so that we can offer our presence and support in a more sustainable and effective way.

Another key distinction between empathy and compassion is their universality. Empathy is often easier to feel towards those who are similar to us or with whom we have a personal connection. We may struggle to empathize with people whose experiences, beliefs, or identities are very different from our own. Compassion, however, extends beyond the boundaries of familiarity or affinity. It is a more inclusive and impartial response, rooted in the fundamental recognition of our shared humanity and the inherent worth of all beings. Compassion allows us to feel concern and care for strangers, adversaries, and even those who have caused harm, recognizing that all individuals, regardless of their actions or circumstances, deserve to be free from suffering.

While distinct, empathy and compassion are deeply interconnected and mutually reinforcing. Empathy lays the foundation for compassion by allowing us to understand and connect with the emotional realities of others. It opens our hearts to the presence of suffering and invites us to respond with care and concern. Compassion, in turn, builds upon the emotional resonance of empathy, channeling it into a more focused and action-oriented response. It moves us beyond the realm of shared feeling into the realm of shared responsibility and active engagement.

Cultivating both empathy and compassion is essential for creating a more just, caring, and connected world. By developing our capacity for empathy, we can bridge divides, challenge stereotypes, and foster a deeper sense of understanding and solidarity with others. By nurturing compassion, we can transform our empathic insights into a powerful force for healing, service, and social change. Together, empathy and compassion form a potent combination that can uplift individuals, strengthen communities, and contribute to a more loving and inclusive human family.

In our daily lives, we can practice empathy by actively listening to others, seeking to understand their perspectives and experiences, and validating their emotions. We can cultivate compassion by regularly reflecting on the suffering of others, engaging in acts of kindness and generosity, and supporting causes and organizations that work to alleviate suffering on a larger scale. By consciously integrating empathy and compassion into our thoughts, words, and actions, we can create a more nurturing and resilient world, one interaction at a time.

DEFINING EMPATHY AND RELATED TERMS

Empathy (Cognitive and Emotional)

Empathy is a multifaceted concept that involves both cognitive and emotional components. Cognitive empathy refers to the ability to understand and perceive another person's perspective, thoughts, and feelings. As psychologist Daniel Goleman explains, "Cognitive empathy, simply put, is the ability to understand another person's perspective. It's literally the ability to put yourself in someone else's shoes" [1]. Emotional empathy, on the other hand, involves actually feeling and sharing the emotions of another person. According to researcher Brené Brown, "Empathy is a choice, and it's a vulnerable choice. In order to connect with you, I have to connect with something in myself that knows that feeling" [2].

Empathic Accuracy

Empathic accuracy refers to the degree to which one's understanding of another person's thoughts and feelings aligns with that person's actual experience. As psychologist William Ickes defines it, "Empathic accuracy is the extent to which one person accurately understands the specific content of another person's thoughts and feelings" [3]. Empathic accuracy is a key component of effective empathic communication and is influenced by various factors, which will be discussed later in this chapter.

Sympathy (versus Empathy)

While empathy and sympathy are often used interchangeably, they represent distinct concepts. Sympathy involves feeling concern or compassion for another person's suffering, while empathy involves a deeper understanding and sharing of that person's emotional experience. As nursing scholar Theresa Wiseman clarifies, "Sympathy is feeling sorry for someone; empathy is feeling with someone" [4]. In healthcare settings, both sympathy and empathy can play important roles in providing compassionate care, but empathy is often seen as a more powerful tool for building trust and rapport with patients.

Spontaneous Communication

Spontaneous communication, as described by psychologist Ross Buck, refers to the nonverbal, often unconscious transmission of emotional states between individuals. Buck explains that "spontaneous communication is the display of emotional states that are not necessarily intended to be communicated, but which are expressed in facial expressions, vocalizations, postures, and movements" [5]. This type of communication plays a crucial role in empathic understanding, as it allows individuals to pick up on subtle emotional cues and respond accordingly.

Emotional Contagion

Emotional contagion is a phenomenon in which an individual's emotions and related behaviors directly trigger similar emotions and behaviors in other people. As psychologist Elaine Hatfield and her colleagues define it, "Emotional contagion is the tendency to automatically mimic and synchronize expressions, vocalizations, postures, and movements with those of another person's and, consequently, to converge emotionally" [24]. This process often occurs unconsciously and can play a significant role in shaping the emotional tone of interpersonal interactions, including those between healthcare providers and patients.

Factors Influencing Empathic Accuracy

Empathic accuracy, or the ability to accurately understand another person's thoughts and feelings, is influenced by a range of factors. Some of these factors can enhance empathic accuracy, while others may inhibit it. In the context of modern healthcare, several aspects of the clinical environment can make it particularly challenging to establish empathy.

One key factor that enhances empathic accuracy is the quality of the relationship between the empathizer and the target. As psychologist Daniel Siegel notes, "The more we feel connected to someone, the more we attune to their internal world, and the more accurate our empathy becomes" [6]. Building rapport and trust with patients is essential for fostering empathic understanding in healthcare settings.

However, the fast-paced, time-pressured nature of modern healthcare can make it difficult for clinicians to devote sufficient time and attention to building relationships with patients. As physician David Rakel observes, "In the current healthcare system, where time is money and efficiency is paramount, it can be challenging for clinicians to slow down and truly listen to their patients' stories" [7].

Another factor that can inhibit empathic accuracy is the presence of distractions or competing demands on attention. In the healthcare setting, clinicians are often juggling multiple tasks and responsibilities, which can make it difficult to fully focus on individual patient interactions. As nursing scholar Jean Watson points out, "In the busyness of the clinical environment, it can be easy to lose sight of the human being in front of us and fall into a task-oriented mode of care" [8].

Additionally, the emotional intensity of healthcare work can sometimes lead clinicians to distance themselves emotionally from patients as a coping mechanism. As I have written elsewhere, "Constantly bearing witness to suffering can take a toll on clinicians' emotional well-being. In order to protect themselves, some may unconsciously pull back from fully engaging empathically with patients" [9].

Scientific Materialism and Objectification in Modern Healthcare

The modern healthcare system is heavily influenced by the paradigm of scientific materialism, which emphasizes objective, quantifiable data and tends to view patients as collections of symptoms and biological processes rather than as whole persons with unique subjective experiences. This perspective can lead to the objectification of patients and a devaluing of their first-person narratives.

As medical anthropologist Arthur Kleinman argues, "The biomedical model, with its focus on pathophysiology and treatment of disease, often fails to address the illness experience – the way the sick person and the members of the family or wider social network perceive, live with, and respond to symptoms and disability" [10]. When clinicians are trained to prioritize objective data over subjective experience, it can create a barrier to empathic understanding.

Moreover, the objectification of patients can serve a defensive function for clinicians, allowing them to maintain emotional distance and avoid the discomfort of fully engaging with suffering. As physician and scholar Rita Charon observes, "By keeping patients at arm's length, we may be protecting ourselves from the pain of empathy, but we are also missing out on the joy and meaning that come from genuine human connection" [11].

However, this emotional distancing can come at a cost, both to clinicians' own well-being and to the quality of care they provide. As Brené Brown notes, "Empathy is the antidote to shame. It's the only balm that can heal the pain of disconnection. But it requires vulnerability. It requires us to show up and be seen, even when it's uncomfortable" [2].

Deep Listening and Empathy

One of the most powerful tools for cultivating empathy in healthcare settings is the practice of deep listening. Deep listening involves fully focusing one's attention on the speaker, suspending judgment, and seeking to understand their perspective and experience. As Buddhist scholar and philosopher Thich Nhat Hanh explains, "Deep listening is the kind of listening that can help relieve the suffering of another person. You can call it compassionate listening. You listen with only one purpose: to help him or her to empty his heart" [12].

In the context of healthcare, deep listening can help clinicians to move beyond surface-level communication and connect with patients on a more profound level. As physician and author Rachel Naomi Remen suggests, "Listening is the oldest and perhaps the most powerful tool of healing. It is often through the quality of our listening and not the wisdom of our words that we are able to effect the most profound changes in the people around us" [13].

Deep listening involves not only attending to the content of the patient's words but also to the emotional layers beneath them. As psychologist Carl Rogers, a pioneer of humanistic psychology, notes, "Active listening is an important way to bring about changes in people. If you can really understand how another person feels, if you can see things from their perspective, it can radically change the way you interact with them" [14].

Appreciative Inquiry and Empathy

Appreciative inquiry is a strengths-based approach to communication and organizational change that focuses on identifying and amplifying what works well rather than on problems and deficits. In healthcare settings, appreciative inquiry can be valuable for building empathy and fostering positive, collaborative relationships with patients.

Organizational psychologist David Cooperrider, one of the originators of appreciative inquiry, explains, "Appreciative inquiry is about the coevolutionary search for the best in people, their organizations, and the relevant world around them. In its broadest focus, it involves systematic discovery of what gives 'life' to a living system when it is most alive, most effective, and most constructively capable in economic, ecological, and human terms" [15].

In healthcare, appreciative inquiry can involve asking patients questions that elicit their strengths, resources, and hopes, rather than solely focusing on their symptoms and challenges. As physician and scholar William Miller notes, "Appreciative inquiry invites us to look for and nurture the seeds of health and resilience in our patients, even in the midst of illness and suffering" [16].

By approaching patients with curiosity and appreciation, clinicians can create a space for empathic understanding to emerge. As psychologist and meditation teacher Tara Brach suggests, "The more we can appreciate the goodness in others, the more we can see that same goodness in ourselves. And the more we can appreciate the goodness in ourselves, the more we can appreciate it in others. It's a powerful reciprocal process" [17].

Strategies for Enhancing Empathic Connection

There are many simple, concrete steps that clinicians can take to enhance empathic connection and accuracy in their interactions with patients. Some of these strategies involve verbal communication techniques, while others focus on nonverbal cues and physical presence.

One of the most basic yet powerful strategies is simply to sit down with patients at eye level, rather than standing over them or talking from across the room. As physician and author Abraham Verghese advises, "Pull up a chair. Sit close. Make eye contact. Take your time. Be present" [18]. This simple act of physical proximity can help to create a sense of equality and partnership in the clinical encounter.

Another key strategy is to attend to nonverbal communication, both the patient's and one's own. As psychologist and author Judith Orloff suggests, "Empathy involves tuning in to another person's emotional state through careful observation of their facial expressions, body language, and tone of voice. It also involves being aware of your own nonverbal cues and how they might be impacting the interaction" [19].

Active listening techniques, such as reflecting back what the patient has said, asking open-ended questions, and allowing for moments of silence, can also help to deepen empathic understanding. As physician and scholar Joel Bennett notes, "Active listening is not just about hearing the words the patient is saying, but also listening for the meaning and emotion behind those words" [20].

Clinicians can also cultivate empathy by practicing mindfulness and self-awareness. As psychiatrist and author Daniel Siegel explains, "Mindfulness is the foundation of empathy. By observing our thoughts, feelings, and sensations with curiosity and acceptance, we develop the capacity to attune to others' internal worlds with greater clarity and compassion" [21].

Finally, clinicians must prioritize self-care and establish healthy boundaries to sustain their capacity for empathy over time. As physician and scholar Jodi Halpern emphasizes, "Empathy is not about taking on the suffering of others as one's own, but rather about maintaining a clear sense of self while still connecting deeply with another's experience. This requires clinicians to have a strong foundation of self-awareness and self-compassion" [22].

Concluding Remarks

Empathy is a vital yet often overlooked aspect of healthcare that can transform the quality of clinical interactions and improve patient outcomes. By understanding the nuances of empathy, the factors that influence empathic accuracy, and the strategies for cultivating empathic connection, clinicians can bring greater humanity and healing to their work.

As healthcare systems continue to evolve and adapt to new challenges, it is crucial that empathy remains at the forefront of clinical training and practice. By prioritizing deep listening, appreciative inquiry, and empathic communication, clinicians can create a healthcare environment that honors the inherent dignity and worth of every patient.

Ultimately, empathy is not just a clinical skill but a way of being in the world that recognizes our fundamental interconnectedness as human beings. As author and spiritual teacher, Thomas Hübl reminds us, "Empathy is the ability to feel as part of a larger whole. It's the recognition that we are all interconnected, that we are all part of the same human family. When we can feel that connection, that's when true healing becomes possible" [23].

Self-Reflection Questions

1. How would I rate my own empathic abilities as a healthcare provider? In which areas do I excel, and where do I have room for improvement?

2. What factors in my work environment might be inhibiting my ability to establish deep, empathic connections with patients? How can I mitigate these factors?

3. Do I find myself falling into the trap of objectifying patients or prioritizing objective data over subjective experiences? How might this be impacting my capacity for empathy?

4. How often do I practice deep listening with my patients? What strategies can I implement to enhance my active listening skills and create a space for genuine understanding?

5. In what ways might I be unconsciously distancing myself emotionally from patients as a coping mechanism? How can I strike a balance between empathy and self-care?

6. How can I incorporate the principles of appreciative inquiry into my patient interactions? What questions can I ask to elicit patients' strengths, resources, and hopes?

7. Am I fully present and attuned to nonverbal cues during patient encounters? How can I enhance my awareness of both my own and my patients' nonverbal communication?

8. How often do I engage in self-reflection and mindfulness practices to cultivate self-awareness and emotional regulation? What steps can I take to prioritize these practices in my daily routine?

9. In what ways might my own biases, assumptions, or personal experiences be influencing my ability to empathize with certain patients? How can I work to identify and challenge these barriers?

10. How can I foster a culture of empathy and compassion within my healthcare team or organization? What role can I play in advocating for practices and policies that prioritize empathic care?

References

[1] Goleman, D. (2017). What is empathy? Emotional Intelligence. Retrieved from https://www.danielgoleman.info/what-is-empathy/

[2] Brown, B. (2013). RSA Short: Empathy. Retrieved from https://www.youtube.com/watch?v=1Evwgu369Jw

[3] Ickes, W. (1993). Empathic accuracy. Journal of Personality, 61(4), 587-610.

[4] Wiseman, T. (1996). A concept analysis of empathy. Journal of Advanced Nursing, 23(6), 1162-1167.

[5] Buck, R. (1984). The communication of emotion. Guilford Press.

[6] Siegel, D. J. (2010). Mindsight: The new science of personal transformation. Bantam Books.

[7] Rakel, D. (2018). The compassionate connection: Enhancing the power of clinical empathy. The Permanente Journal, 22.

[8] Watson, J. (2008). Nursing: The philosophy and science of caring (Rev. ed.). University Press of Colorado.

[9] Duffy, J. (2016). Empathy, compassion fatigue, and self-care for clinicians. In Gawande, A. (Ed.), Being mortal: Medicine and what matters in the end (pp. 219-238). Metropolitan Books.

[10] Kleinman, A. (1988). The illness narratives: Suffering, healing, and the human condition. Basic Books.

[11] Charon, R. (2001). Narrative medicine: A model for empathy, reflection, profession, and trust. JAMA, 286(15), 1897-1902.

[12] Nhat Hanh, T. (2011). The art of communicating. Parallax Press.

[13] Remen, R. N. (2006). Kitchen table wisdom: Stories that heal. Riverhead Books.

[14] Rogers, C. R. (1995). A way of being. Houghton Mifflin Harcourt.

[15] Cooperrider, D. L., & Whitney, D. K. (2005). Appreciative inquiry: A positive revolution in change. Berrett-Koehler Publishers.

[16] Miller, W. R., & Rollnick, S. (2013). Motivational interviewing: Helping people change (3rd ed.). The Guilford Press.

[17] Brach, T. (2003). Radical acceptance: Embracing your life with the heart of a Buddha. Bantam Books.

[18] Verghese, A. (2010). Cutting for stone. Vintage Books.

[19] Orloff, J. (2017). The empath's survival guide: Life strategies for sensitive people. Sounds True.

[20] Bennett, J. (2016). Empathy and presence: Attentional foundations of compassionate care. In Wallis, S. E., & Callahan, J. M. (Eds.), Healthcare performance and organizational culture (pp. 37-56). Oxford University Press.

[21] Siegel, D. J. (2007). The mindful brain: Reflection and attunement in the cultivation of well-being. W.W. Norton & Company.

[22] Halpern, J. (2011). From detached concern to empathy: Humanizing medical practice. Oxford University Press.

[23] Hübl, T. (2019). The power of we: Awakening in the relational field [Video]. Sounds True. https://product.soundstrue.com/power-of-we/free-video-series/

[24] Hatfield, E., Cacioppo, J. T., & Rapson, R. L. (1993). Emotional contagion. Current Directions in Psychological Science, 2(3), 96-100.

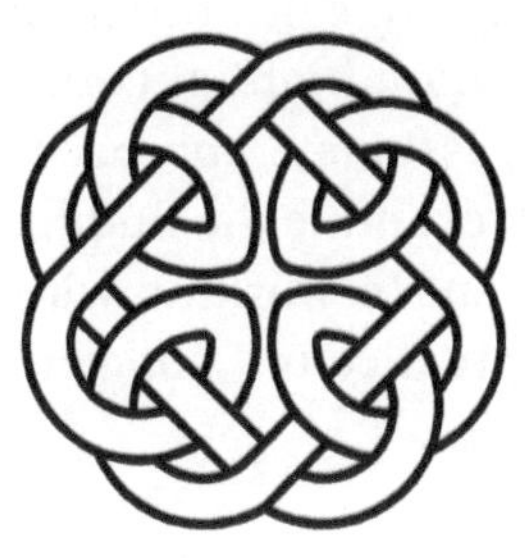

CHAPTER 20

Asana Five: Be Courageous

Instruction: Hold your seat and ask the suffering question.

"Courage is what it takes to stand up and speak;
courage is also what it takes to sit down and listen".
Winston Churchill

I often refer to palliative medicine as the "suffering specialty." The specialty within the broad range of medical practice that makes the recognition, acknowledgment, and response to suffering its central goal. This takes great courage and wisdom. In the early days of the emergence of palliative medicine, we often discussed the importance of avoiding the development of another medical specialty. Our goal was to provide a role model for physicians to work with suffering and always pursue caring, even if caring was not an option. Simply stated, our goal was to model the importance of showing up.

Encountering and responding to human suffering is the most fundamental aspect of the healer's work. Yet, this is the most challenging experience for modern healers. In a previous chapter, I explored the concept of suffering and made suggestions for an integral understanding of human suffering. This chapter delves into the multifaceted nature of this challenge by exploring the psychological, ethical, and practical dimensions that healthcare providers must navigate when confronting the suffering of others. We will examine the limitations of allopathic scientific medical paradigms and the strategies often employed to avoid engaging with suffering. This exploration highlights the importance of developing a more nuanced and compassionate approach to addressing suffering in healthcare settings. We will examine the Buddhist concept of "Taking Your Seat" and how this is relevant to working with suffering. Finally, we will learn about the Buddhist practice of "Tonglen" and discuss how this can effectively transform suffering.

Factors Promoting the Avoidance of Suffering
The human tendency to avoid or flee from the suffering of others is deeply rooted in our evolutionary history and psychological makeup. This avoidance response, known as empathic distress, is a complex phenomenon involving innate and learned components.

1. *Evolutionary Factors*
    From an evolutionary standpoint, recognizing and responding to signs of distress in others was crucial for survival. Our ancestors needed to quickly identify potential environmental threats, including signs of pain or suffering in-group members that might indicate danger. While essential for survival, this rapid threat detection system can also lead to an automatic avoidance response when confronted with others' suffering.

    As evolutionary psychologist Robert Trivers explains: "Natural selection has built into us a tendency to avoid situations that might harm us, including the suffering of others which may signal danger or the risk of emotional contagion." [1]

2. *Neurobiological Factors*
    Recent neuroscientific research has provided insights into the biological underpinnings of empathic distress. When we witness someone in pain, our brain activates regions associated with our own experience of pain, a phenomenon known as "mirror neurons." This neurological mirroring can trigger a stress response in the observer, leading to a desire to escape the situation to alleviate one's own discomfort.

    Neuroscientist Tania Singer elaborates: "The shared neural activations between self and other in empathy for pain can lead to personal distress, which may result in a self-oriented, aversive response that can lead to withdrawal rather than helping behavior." [2]

3. *Psychological Factors*
    In addition to these innate responses, individuals often develop psychological defenses to protect themselves from the emotional impact of others' suffering. These defenses can include:

a. Rationalization: Explaining away suffering to make it seem less severe or meaningful.
b. Denial: Refusing to acknowledge the reality or severity of someone's suffering.
c. Projection: Attributing one's uncomfortable feelings about suffering to others.
d. Intellectualization: Focusing on abstract or technical aspects of suffering to avoid emotional engagement.

In her work on ego defense mechanisms, psychologist Anna Freud noted: "The ego's defenses against unpleasurable or unmanageable feelings and thoughts are not just occasional reactions to difficulty but are a constant and essential part of its functioning." [3]

Cultural Factors
Anthropologist Arthur Kleinman observes, "How we respond to the suffering of others is deeply influenced by cultural models of what constitutes appropriate emotional expression and social interaction" [4]. Cultural norms and societal expectations also shape individuals' responses to suffering. In many Western cultures, a strong emphasis is on maintaining a positive outlook and avoiding displays of negative emotions. This cultural context can reinforce the tendency to avoid or minimize suffering.

Dysfunctional Empathy: Emotional vs. Cognitive Empathy vs. Sympathy
Unfortunately, most healers receive very little formal education on the structure and function of the neural systems underlying empathy. All too often, healers believe that empathy is simply an inherent trait of all effective healers that merely needs to be expressed in all clinical situations. This naivete inevitably frequently results in both the healer and their patient experiencing emotional distress. Therefore, all healers must understand how to interpret and modulate their empathic response to any clinical encounter.

The Importance of Balancing Emotional and Cognitive Empathy
Understanding the difference between emotional and cognitive empathy is crucial for healthcare providers seeking to engage with patients suffering effectively while maintaining their well-being. As discussed in the previous

chapter, empathy, the ability to understand and share the feelings of another, is a crucial skill for building strong relationships and creating a more compassionate society. However, empathy is not a monolithic concept; it can be divided into two distinct types: emotional and cognitive empathy. If we are to recognize and respond to our patients' suffering, we must develop and balance both cognitive and emotional empathy.

The Challenge of Understanding Suffering Within Scientific Materialism

The dominant paradigm of scientific materialism in modern medicine presents significant challenges to effectively understanding and addressing suffering. As discussed in a previous chapter, scientific materialism is a philosophical stance that posits that all phenomena, including consciousness and subjective experiences, can be explained solely through physical processes and matter. This translates to a focus on measurable, biological aspects of health and disease in medicine.

Philosopher and psychiatrist Iain McGilchrist critiques the limitations of scientific materialism: "The problem with the materialist view is not that it's wrong, but that it's partial. It leaves out everything that makes life worth living, everything that makes us human." [22]

In his writings on the nature of suffering, Eric Cassell points out: "The failure to understand the nature of suffering can result in medical intervention that (though technically adequate) not only fails to relieve suffering but becomes a source of suffering itself." [23]

Experiencing Suffering Through the Lens of Scientific Materialism

Assuming a scientific materialist perspective as a healer will very significantly impede our capacity to recognize and respond to our patients' suffering through:

a. Reductionism: Scientific materialism tends to reduce complex experiences like suffering to their simplest components, often neglecting the holistic nature of human experience.
b. Neglect of Subjective Experience: The emphasis on objective, measurable data can lead to disregarding the subjective, lived experience of suffering.
c. Mind-Body Dualism: Despite attempts to overcome it, scientific materialism often reinforces a separation between mind and body, making it challenging to address psychosomatic aspects of suffering.
d. Lack of Meaning: The materialist approach struggles to account for the existential and spiritual dimensions of suffering that often concern patients.
e. Overemphasis on Physical Symptoms: This paradigm can lead to a focus

on treating physical symptoms while neglecting psychological, social, and spiritual aspects of suffering.

Consequences of the Materialist Approach

a.   Fragmented Care: Treating symptoms in isolation without addressing the whole person's experience.
b.   Overreliance on Pharmacological Solutions: Tendency to prescribe medications for complex psychosocial issues.
c.   Neglect of Narrative: Failing to consider the patient's story and the meaning they attribute to their suffering.
d.   Dehumanization: Viewing patients as collections of symptoms rather than whole persons.
e.   Burnout Among Providers: The disconnect between the materialist approach and the reality of patient suffering can contribute to healthcare provider burnout.

Avoidance Strategies in Modern Medicine

Modern medicine has developed various strategies to avoid direct engagement with suffering. While these strategies may serve protective functions in the short term, they often lead to a disconnection from the core purpose of healing and a diminished capacity to address patients' suffering effectively. Common avoidance strategies employed by modern medicine include:

a.   *Depersonalization:*
Depersonalization involves viewing patients as cases or diagnoses rather than as whole persons. This strategy creates emotional distance but can lead to dehumanizing care.

Sociologist Erving Goffman observed: "The medical gaze tends to objectify patients, turning them into a collection of symptoms and test results rather than complex human beings." [25]
b.   *Emotional Detachment:*
Many healthcare providers are trained to maintain professional distance to avoid emotional involvement. While some emotional boundaries are necessary, extreme detachment can hinder empathetic care. Physician Danielle Ofri writes: "We're taught to be detached, but the reality is that connection is at the heart of medical care. Without it, we risk becoming mere technicians." [26]
c.   *Overreliance on Technology:*
Advanced medical technology can serve as a buffer between healthcare providers and patients' suffering. While technology is crucial for diagnosis

and treatment, overreliance can lead to a neglect of human interaction. Medical ethicist Daniel Callahan warns: "The danger is that we become so enamored with what technology can do that we lose sight of the human needs of our patients." [27]

d.   *Time Constraints*:

The pressure to see many patients in limited time frames can lead to brief, symptom-focused encounters that avoid deeper engagement with suffering. Healthcare researcher Victor Montori notes: "The industrialization of healthcare has led to a system where there's often no time for the kind of careful, attentive care that addressing suffering requires." [28]

e.   *Medicalization of Suffering*:

By framing all suffering as medical problems, healthcare providers can avoid engaging with the complex existential and social dimensions of distress. Psychiatrist and philosopher Carl Erik Fisher observes: "There's a tendency in modern medicine to pathologize normal human responses to difficulty, turning existential struggles into medical disorders." [29]

f.   *Defensive Medicine*:

The fear of malpractice litigation can lead to a focus on defensive practices rather than holistic patient care. Legal scholar Michelle Mello explains: "Defensive medicine practices, while intended to protect against liability, can create a barrier to meaningful engagement with patients and their suffering." [30]

The Consequences of Avoidance Strategies

a.   Reduced Quality of Care: Avoiding engagement with suffering can lead to missed diagnoses, ineffective treatments, and poor patient outcomes.

b.   Patient Dissatisfaction: Patients may feel unheard or dismissed when their suffering is not fully acknowledged.

c.   Provider Burnout: Paradoxically, strategies intended to protect providers from emotional distress can contribute to burnout by disconnecting them from the meaningful aspects of their work.

d.   Erosion of Trust: Avoidance strategies can damage the crucial trust between healthcare providers and patients.

e.   Missed Opportunities for Healing: Engaging with suffering often provides insights that can lead to more effective, holistic care.

Alternatives to Avoidance

Physician and author Rachel Naomi Remen advises: "The way to grow strong in the broken places is not to avoid them but to embrace them with compassion and skill." [31] To address these issues, healthcare providers and systems can:

a.   *Cultivate Mindfulness*: Develop present-moment awareness to engage more fully with patients.
b.   *Practice Narrative Medicine*: Incorporate patients' stories and perspectives into care.
c.   *Implement Team-Based Care*: Share the emotional burden of caring for suffering patients among a diverse team.
d.   *Provide Emotional Support for Providers*: Offer resources like counseling and support groups for healthcare workers.
e.   *Restructure Healthcare Delivery*: Advocate for systemic changes that allow more time and resources for meaningful patient interactions.
f.   *Emphasize Holistic Education*: Train healthcare providers in approaches that address the full spectrum of human suffering.

Psychotropic Medications and Analgesics as Avoidance

The prescription of psychotropic medications and analgesics can sometimes serve as a means to avoid engaging with the deeper, existential aspects of a person's suffering. While these medications are valuable tools in managing symptoms, their overuse or misuse can mask underlying issues without addressing root causes.

Psychotropic medications and analgesics have revolutionized the treatment of mental health disorders and pain management. They can provide significant relief and improve the quality of life for many patients. However, the ease of prescribing these medications can sometimes lead to their use as a first-line response.

Cultural Influence on the Experience of Suffering

Western Cultures

The American expectation of a pain-free existence has led to a culture where the use of analgesics is not just accepted but often expected," notes medical anthropologist Arthur Kleinman. [4] In many Western cultures, particularly in the United States and Western Europe, there is usually a low tolerance for pain and a strong emphasis on its immediate alleviation. This approach is reflected in the high consumption of analgesics, both over-the-counter and prescription.

This cultural attitude stems from several factors:

a.   Technological optimism: A belief that modern medicine should be able to eliminate most forms of suffering.

b.   Individualism: An emphasis on personal comfort and well-being.
c.   Productivity focus: The view that suffering is the same as pain and is an obstacle to be overcome for the sake of efficiency and productivity.

Key Consequences of this cultural perspective include:

a.   Emphasis on mechanical and physical etiology of subjective distress.
b.   External locus of control around relief (i.e., medications, surgery, technology).
c.   Limited reliance on social support

East Asian Cultures

"In traditional Chinese medicine, pain is seen as an imbalance in the body's energy flow. The goal is not to mask the pain but to restore balance," explains Dr. Ted Kaptchuk, professor of medicine at Harvard Medical School. [32] In many East Asian cultures, influenced by philosophies like Buddhism and Taoism, there's often a greater acceptance of pain as a natural part of life. This perspective can lead to a more restrained use of analgesics.

Key Consequences of this cultural perspective include:

a.   Holistic view: Pain is experienced as part of a larger pattern of disharmony in the body and mind.
b.   Emphasis on endurance: Bearing pain can be viewed as a form of character building.
c.   Non-pharmacological approaches: Greater reliance on practices like acupuncture, herbal medicine, and qigong for pain management.

Latin American Cultures

"In many Latin American contexts, suffering can be imbued with spiritual meaning, sometimes seen as a form of penance or a way to connect with the divine," observes medical anthropologist Nancy Scheper-Hughes. [33] Many Latin American cultures exhibit a complex relationship with pain and analgesics, influenced by a mixture of indigenous traditions, Catholicism, and modern medical practices.

Key Consequences of this cultural perspective include:

a.   Religious significance: Pain may be viewed as a test of faith or a means of spiritual purification.
b.   Social bonding: Sharing in suffering can be seen as a way to strengthen community ties.
c.   Machismo culture: In some contexts, enduring pain without medication

may be seen as a sign of strength, particularly among men.

African Cultures
"In many African societies, pain is often contextualized within a broader social and spiritual framework, rather than being seen purely as a medical issue," notes medical anthropologist John M. Janzen. [34] The approach to pain and analgesic use in various African cultures is diverse, reflecting the continent's vast cultural heterogeneity. However, some common themes emerge:
Key Consequences of this cultural perspective include:

a.   Communal approach: Pain and suffering are often addressed within the context of family and community support.
b.   Traditional healing practices: Many rely on herbal and spiritual healing alongside or instead of Western analgesics.
c.   Stoicism: In some cultures, there's a value placed on enduring pain without complaint.

Middle Eastern Cultures
"Islamic bioethics emphasizes the sanctity of life and the importance of seeking treatment but also recognizes suffering as potentially having spiritual value," explains Dr. Aasim Padela, Director of the Initiative on Islam and Medicine at the University of Chicago. [35] In many Middle Eastern cultures, attitudes towards pain and analgesic use are influenced by Islamic teachings and traditional medical practices.
Key Consequences of this cultural perspective include:

a.   Religious framing: Pain may be seen as a test from God or a means of cleansing sins.
b.   Gender differences: In some contexts, there may be different expectations for pain tolerance between men and women.
c.   Blend of approaches: Traditional remedies are often used alongside modern analgesics.

Implications for Healthcare of Cultural Differences on Suffering
Understanding these cultural differences is crucial for providing culturally competent healthcare. It affects how pain is perceived and reported and how analgesics should be prescribed and administered.
"Cultural competence in pain management isn't just about knowing cultural facts; it's about developing the skills to explore each patient's unique cultural context and beliefs about pain," advises Dr. Carla Boutin-Foster, a specialist in cross-cultural medicine. [36]

Key considerations when working with different cultures include:

a. Avoiding stereotypes: While cultural trends exist, individual variation is significant.
b. Communication: Developing skills to discuss pain and treatment options across cultural boundaries.
c. Flexible treatment plans: Incorporating culturally appropriate pain management strategies.
d. Education: Helping patients understand the benefits and risks of analgesics within their cultural framework.

Cultural differences reflect profound differences in how societies conceptualize suffering, resilience, and medical care goals. By recognizing and respecting these differences, healthcare providers can offer more effective, culturally sensitive care while gaining insight into the diverse ways humans relate to and find meaning in the universal experience of suffering.

Taking Your Seat and Holding the Space

In Buddhist teachings, "taking your seat" is a powerful metaphor for meditation and cultivating mindfulness and presence. It refers to the act of physically sitting down to meditate and the mental and emotional process of fully engaging with the present moment. By taking our seat, we commit to being present with whatever arises in our experience without judgment or avoidance. As Chögyam Trungpa Rinpoche explains, "Taking your seat means taking your place in life. It means accepting the truth of who you are, as you are, without deception" [37].

The practice of taking one's seat is not always easy, as it requires us to confront the full range of our thoughts, emotions, and sensations, including those that may be uncomfortable or painful. However, by learning to sit with these experiences, we cultivate a deeper sense of acceptance, compassion, and resilience. Suzuki Roshi, the founder of the San Francisco Zen Center, emphasizes the importance of this practice: "Take your seat, take your position, and trust your life just the way it is. This is the most important thing to do" [38].

One key challenge in taking our seat is the tendency of the mind to wander and get caught up in distractions, a phenomenon that is particularly prevalent in our modern, fast-paced world. Ethan Nichtern, a contemporary Buddhist teacher, describes this challenge: "In a culture of constant distraction, taking your seat is a revolutionary act. It means choosing to be present, even when everything around you is pulling you away from the moment" [39, p. 17].

To help practitioners navigate the challenges of taking their seat, Buddhist teachings often refer to the concept of the "Eight Worldly Winds." These are the eight fundamental forces that can blow us off course in our practice and our lives:

1. Pleasure and pain
2. Gain and loss
3. Praise and blame
4. Fame and disgrace

These winds are called "worldly" because they are part of the fabric of human experience, and everyone, including modern healers, is subject to their influence. Pema Chödrön, a beloved Buddhist teacher and author, explains: "The eight worldly winds are the forces that keep us confused and trapped in cycles of suffering. They are the ways we grasp at pleasure and try to avoid pain, the ways we seek approval and validation from others, and the ways we try to protect our ego and our sense of self" [40, p. 64].

For modern healers, the eight worldly winds can be particularly challenging as they navigate the demands of their profession and the needs of their patients. The desire for success, recognition, and validation can be strong, as can the fear of failure, criticism, or loss. Joan Halifax, a Buddhist teacher and pioneer in end-of-life care, speaks to this challenge: "As healers, we are constantly confronted with the eight worldly winds. We may feel great satisfaction when we are able to help a patient, but we may also feel deep sadness or frustration when we cannot. We may be praised for our skills and compassion, but we may also face criticism or blame when things do not go as hoped" [41].

The key to working with the eight worldly winds is to develop a sense of equanimity, or balance, in the face of these forces. This means recognizing when we are being pulled or pushed by these winds and cultivating the ability to respond with presence, compassion, and wisdom. Chögyam Trungpa Rinpoche offers this guidance: "The way to work with the eight worldly winds is not to try to escape them or to conquer them, but to befriend them. This means learning to stay present and grounded in the midst of their turbulence, and to use their energy to deepen our understanding and compassion" [37].

In the context of modern healing, taking one's seat and working with the eight worldly winds can be a powerful practice for cultivating resilience, compassion, and presence in the face of the many challenges and demands of the profession. By learning to sit with the full range of our pleasant and unpleasant experiences and by developing a sense of equanimity in the face of the eight worldly winds, healers can cultivate a deeper understanding of connection, empathy, and wisdom in their work.

Ultimately, taking one's seat is a practice of radical acceptance and presence. It is a way of saying yes to the fullness of our experience and cultivating the courage and compassion to be with whatever arises. As Suzuki Roshi reminds us, "The most important thing is to find your seat, to find your place in the world, and to accept it fully, with all its joys and sorrows. This is the path of true healing and liberation" [38].

Tonglen: Exchanging Ourself with Other

Tonglen is a meditation practice that originated in Tibetan Buddhism, particularly within the Mahayana tradition. The word "tonglen" is Tibetan for "giving and taking" or "sending and receiving." This practice involves visualizing taking in the suffering of others with the in-breath and sending out relief and happiness to them with the out-breath. It's considered a powerful method for developing compassion and bodhicitta; the altruistic wish to attain enlightenment for the benefit of all sentient beings. Tonglen challenges practitioners to reverse their usual tendency of avoiding pain and grasping at pleasure, instead cultivating a sense of openness and compassion towards the suffering of others. This practice is often taught as part of the lojong (mind training) teachings and is seen as a way to transform adverse circumstances into the path of awakening.

Pema Chödrön, an American Tibetan Buddhist nun and renowned teacher, has written extensively about Tonglen in her books and teachings. She describes the practice: "In the practice of Tonglen, we visualize taking in the pain of others with every in-breath and sending out whatever will benefit them on the out-breath. In the process, we become liberated from age-old patterns of selfishness. We begin to feel love for both ourselves and others; we begin to take care of ourselves and others" [40]

The practice of Tonglen unfolds in several steps. First, practitioners consider a person or situation causing distress or suffering. This could be a loved one who is ill, a community affected by violence or disaster, or even their own painful emotions or experiences. Next, they visualize breathing in the suffering of this person or situation, imagining it as a dark, heavy smoke that enters their body with each inhalation.

As Chödrön explains, "We breathe in with the wish to take away all the pain and suffering of others. We breathe out with the wish to give them all our happiness and well-being. We breathe in with the desire to take on the suffering, and we breathe out with the desire to give joy and happiness" [40].

With each exhalation, practitioners visualize sending out relief, compassion, healing, and joy to the person or situation they have in mind.

They may imagine this as a bright, warm light radiating from their body and touching all suffering. This process of breathing in pain and breathing out relief is repeated for several minutes, with the practitioner focusing on their profound wish to alleviate suffering and bring comfort to others.

One of the unique aspects of Tonglen is that it does not shy away from the reality of suffering but instead invites practitioners to confront it directly. As Chödrön notes, "In Tonglen practice, we use the breath to ingest, accept, and embrace what we usually are very afraid of—and we send out what we usually hold on to quite fixedly" [40]. By breathing in the pain of others, practitioners learn to overcome their aversion to suffering and cultivate a more profound sense of empathy and connection.

However, engaging in Tonglen is not without its challenges and potential risks. One common obstacle is the fear that breathing in the suffering of others will be overwhelming or harmful to oneself. Chödrön addresses this concern: "Tonglen does not increase our suffering. It gives us a way to transform our suffering into compassion and love. It gives us a way to use our personal sorrows as a stepping stone to understanding the sorrows of all beings" [40].

Another challenge is the tendency to get caught up in the story or details of the suffering being contemplated rather than focusing on the pure wish to alleviate pain. Chödrön advises practitioners to keep the practice simple and direct, noting, "Tonglen practice is not about the details but about the underlying dynamic: breathing in pain and breathing out relief" [40].

It is also essential to recognize that Tonglen is not a substitute for taking practical action to address suffering in the world. While the practice can help cultivate compassion and resilience, it must be balanced with engaged, compassionate activity in one's daily life. As Chödrön emphasizes, "Tonglen is a practice of creating space, breathing in pain, and sending out relief. But it's not meant to substitute for taking action" [40].

Despite these challenges, Tonglen's benefits are significant. By regularly engaging in this practice, individuals can develop greater emotional resilience, empathy, and compassion. They may be less reactive to difficult situations and more able to respond with kindness and understanding. Over time, Tonglen can help practitioners cultivate a more open and inclusive heart that is willing to embrace the full spectrum of human experience.

As Chödrön beautifully expresses, "Tonglen reverses the usual logic of avoiding suffering and seeking pleasure. In the process, we become liberated from a very ancient prison of selfishness. We begin to feel love for ourselves and others, and we also begin to take care of ourselves and others. It awakens our compassion and it also introduces us to a far larger view of reality" [40].

In conclusion, Tonglen is a transformative practice that challenges us to turn towards suffering rather than away from it. By breathing in pain and breathing out relief, we cultivate a heart that is both courageous and compassionate, able to hold the sorrow and joy of the world with equanimity and grace. This practice invites us to recognize our fundamental interconnectedness and extend our care circle to all beings without exception. As we engage in Tonglen, we not only alleviate the suffering of others but also discover a deeper sense of meaning, purpose, and resilience in our own lives. In this way, Tonglen serves as a powerful catalyst for personal and collective transformation, helping us to build a more loving and inclusive world, one breath at a time.

Concluding Remarks

The journey of a healer requires courage, compassion, and a deep commitment to engaging with the suffering of others. As we have explored in this chapter, the challenges of confronting suffering are multifaceted and rooted in our evolutionary history, neurobiological makeup, and cultural conditioning. While providing invaluable advancements, the dominant paradigm of scientific materialism in modern medicine has also limited our ability to fully understand and address the complex nature of human suffering.

We have examined the importance of balancing emotional and cognitive empathy, the pitfalls of sympathy, and the necessity of establishing and maintaining energetic boundaries. We've also explored various avoidance strategies commonly employed in modern medicine, their consequences, and the cultural influences on the experience and treatment of suffering.

The practices of "taking your seat" and Tonglen offer powerful tools for healers to cultivate presence, resilience, and compassion in the face of suffering. These practices invite us to turn towards pain rather than away from it, transforming our relationship with suffering and expanding our capacity to be with the full spectrum of human experience.

As healers, our task is not to eliminate suffering—an impossible goal— but to meet it with wisdom, compassion, and skill. By developing a more nuanced and holistic approach to suffering, we can provide care that addresses the whole person's needs. This involves not only treating physical symptoms but also engaging with the psychological, social, and spiritual dimensions of a person's experience.

The path forward requires a shift in medical education and healthcare systems to prioritize these more comprehensive approaches to healing. It calls for a balance between the precision of scientific knowledge and the wisdom of contemplative practices, between the power of modern technology and the irreplaceable value of human connection.

Ultimately, the healer's courageous heart remains open in the face of suffering, dares to be vulnerable, and recognizes the shared humanity in every patient encounter. Through practices like Tonglen, it learns to transform suffering into compassion, fear into courage, and isolation into connection.

As we continue on this path, our ability to heal others is intimately connected to our own journey of healing and growth. By cultivating our capacity to be with suffering—our own and others—we become more effective healers and contribute to a more compassionate and resilient world.

Self-Reflection Questions

1. How do I typically respond to suffering in my professional role? Can I identify any avoidance strategies I tend to use?

2. In what ways does my cultural background influence my approach to pain and suffering, both personally and professionally?

3. How do I balance emotional and cognitive empathy in patient interactions? Are there areas where I could improve this balance?

4. Can I recall a time when I confused sympathy with empathy? How did this impact my interaction with the patient?

5. How do I establish and maintain energetic boundaries in my work? Are there areas where I struggle with this?

6. In what ways has the scientific materialist paradigm shaped my understanding of and approach to suffering? How might I expand this perspective?

7. How comfortable am I with "taking my seat" and being present with difficult emotions or situations? What practices could help me develop this skill further?

8. How might incorporating the practice of Tonglen affect my ability to engage with suffering in my professional role?

9. In what ways do I see the "Eight Worldly Winds" affecting my work as a healer? How might I cultivate more stability in the face of these forces?

10. How can I integrate the insights from this chapter into my daily practice as a healer? What specific changes or practices am I inspired to implement?

References

1] Trivers, R. L. (1971). The evolution of reciprocal altruism. The Quarterly Review of Biology, 46(1), 35-57.

[2] Singer, T., & Klimecki, O. M. (2014). Empathy and compassion. Current Biology, 24(18), R875-R878.

[3] Freud, A. (1936). The ego and the mechanisms of defense. International Universities Press.

[4] Kleinman, A. (1988). The illness narratives: Suffering, healing, and the human condition. Basic Books.

[5] Hodges, S.D., & Myers, M.W. (2007). Empathy. In R.F. Baumeister & K.D. Vohs (Eds.), Encyclopedia of Social Psychology (Vol. 1, pp. 297-298). Sage.

[6] Smith, A. (2006). Cognitive empathy and emotional empathy in human behavior and evolution. The Psychological Record, 56(1), 3-21.

[7] Hatfield, E., Rapson, R.L., & Le, Y.L. (2009). Emotional contagion and empathy. In J. Decety & W. Ickes (Eds.), The Social Neuroscience of Empathy (pp. 19-30). MIT Press.

[8] Figley, C.R. (2002). Compassion fatigue: Psychotherapists' chronic lack of self care. Journal of Clinical Psychology, 58(11), 1433-1441.

[9] Oakley, B. (2013). Pathological Altruism. Oxford University Press.

[10] Bloom, P. (2017). Against Empathy: The Case for Rational Compassion. Random House.

[11] Tone, E.B., & Tully, E.C. (2014). Empathy as a "risky strength": A multilevel examination of empathy and risk for internalizing disorders. Development and Psychopathology, 26(4pt2), 1547-1565.

[12] Zaki, J. (2019). The War for Kindness: Building Empathy in a Fractured World. Crown.

[13] Bird, G., & Viding, E. (2014). The self to other model of empathy: Providing a new framework for understanding empathy impairments in psychopathy, autism, and alexithymia. Neuroscience & Biobehavioral Reviews, 47, 520-532.

[14] Krznaric, R. (2014). Empathy: Why It Matters, and How to Get It. Penguin.

[15] Brown, B. (2012). Daring Greatly: How the Courage to Be Vulnerable Transforms the Way We Live, Love, Parent, and Lead. Gotham Books.

[16] Neff, K. (2011). Self-Compassion: The Proven Power of Being Kind to Yourself. William Morrow.

[17] Zuckerman, D. (2014). Your Sacred Anatomy: An Owner's Guide to the Human Energy Structure. Desdaimona Publications.

[18] Hübl, T. (2020). Healing Collective Trauma: A Process for Integrating Our Intergenerational and Cultural Wounds. Sounds True.

[19] Vaillant, G. E. (2008). Spiritual Evolution: A Scientific Defense of Faith. Broadway Books.

[20] Rogers, C. R. (1995). On Becoming a Person: A Therapist's View of Psychotherapy. Houghton Mifflin Harcourt.

[21] Levine, P. A. (2010). In an Unspoken Voice: How the Body Releases Trauma and Restores Goodness. North Atlantic Books.

[22] McGilchrist, I. (2009). The Master and His Emissary: The Divided Brain and the Making of the Western World. Yale University Press.

[23] Cassell, E. J. (2004). The Nature of Suffering and the Goals of Medicine. Oxford University Press.

[24] Brody, H. (2003). Stories of Sickness. Oxford University Press.

[25] Goffman, E. (1961). Asylums: Essays on the Social Situation of Mental Patients and Other Inmates. Anchor Books.

[26] Ofri, D. (2013). What Doctors Feel: How Emotions Affect the Practice of

Medicine. Beacon Press.

[27] Callahan, D. (2009). Taming the Beloved Beast: How Medical Technology Costs Are Destroying Our Health Care System. Princeton University Press.

[28] Montori, V. M. (2017). Why We Revolt: A Patient Revolution for Careful and Kind Care. The Patient Revolution.

[29] Fisher, C. E. (2020). The Urge: Our History of Addiction. Penguin Press.

[30] Mello, M. M., & Brennan, T. A. (2002). Deterrence of medical errors: theory and evidence for malpractice reform. Texas Law Review, 80(7), 1595-1637.

[31] Remen, R. N. (2000). My Grandfather's Blessings: Stories of Strength, Refuge, and Belonging. Riverhead Books.

[32] Kaptchuk, T. J. (2000). The Web That Has No Weaver: Understanding Chinese Medicine. Contemporary Books.

[33] Scheper-Hughes, N. (1992). Death Without Weeping: The Violence of Everyday Life in Brazil. University of California Press.

[34] Janzen, J. M. (1978). The Quest for Therapy in Lower Zaire. University of California Press.

[35] Padela, A. I. (2007). Islamic medical ethics: a primer. Bioethics, 21(3), 169-178.

[36] Boutin-Foster, C., Foster, J. C., & Konopasek, L. (2008). Physician, know thyself: the professional culture of medicine as a framework for teaching cultural competence. Academic Medicine, 83(1), 106-111.

[37] Trungpa, C. (2009). The Profound Treasury of the Ocean of Dharma: The Bodhisattva Path of Wisdom and Compassion. Shambhala Publications.

[38] Suzuki, S. (2011). Zen Mind, Beginner's Mind: Informal Talks on Zen Meditation and Practice. Shambhala Publications.

[39] Nichtern, E. (2015). The Road Home: A Contemporary Exploration of the Buddhist Path. North Point Press.

[40] Chödrön, P. (2001). The Places That Scare You: A Guide to Fearlessness in Difficult Times. Shambhala Publications.

[41] Halifax, J. (2008). Being with Dying: Cultivating Compassion and Fearlessness in the Presence of Death. Shambhala Publications.

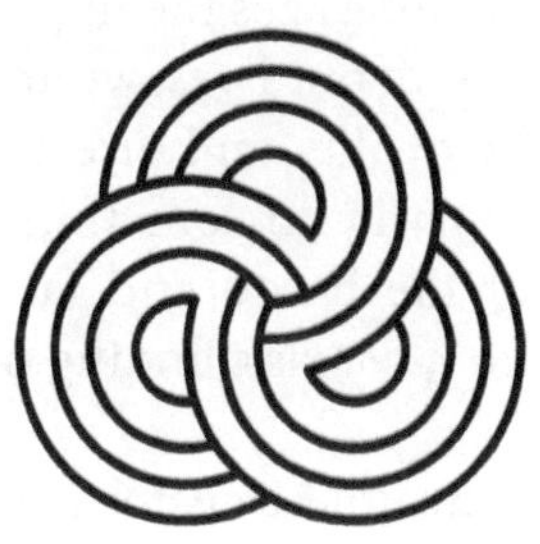

Chapter 21

Asana Six: Closing and Dedicating the Space
Recognizing and Dedicating Each Moment

Instruction: Consciously close and dedicate each encounter.

"Each night, when I go to sleep, I die.
And the next morning, when I wake up, I am reborn."
Mahatma Gandhi

The crucial importance of mindfully concluding each interaction cannot be overstated. As practitioners, we must recognize the significance of taking a moment to consciously review the characteristics of each engagement before moving on to the next patient. This process allows us to digest the emotional energy generated during the session and maintain a state of presence, enabling us to approach each new interaction with a fresh perspective and creative potential.

Recognizing the Bardos: The Space Between Each Moment
In Buddhist philosophy, the concept of bardos refers to the "intermediate state" between experiences, not just the stages of dying [2]. Chögyam Trungpa explains, "Bardo is a Tibetan word that simply means a 'transition' or a gap

between the completion of one situation and the onset of another" [3]. As healthcare practitioners, we can envisage the space between each patient engagement as a bardo.

Dr. Nida Chenagtsang emphasizes the importance of recognizing these transitions: "In every moment of our lives, we are in a bardo. How we live in these bardos determines the quality and direction of our next experience" [4]. Each bardo opens a doorway to something new, for better or worse. If we are not cognizant of the bardo and fail to process the emotional residue from each interaction, we risk finding ourselves trapped in a cycle of compounded distress.

Robert Thurman elucidates the transformative potential of the bardos: "The key to the bardo experiences is that they are all opportunities for liberation, if one can only recognize them and act appropriately" [5]. By mindfully navigating the space between patient interactions, we can release the "karmic residue" of challenging encounters and open ourselves to the healing potential of the present moment.

Consciously Reviewing the Interaction

When concluding each engagement with a patient, it is crucial to take a moment to consciously review the characteristics of that interaction. This includes reflecting on what overtly occurred, the energy of the interaction, the emotion that pervaded the end of the session, and the emotional energy we are carrying from this interaction. As Thomas Hübl states, "The more we are able to be present with what is happening in the moment, the more we can respond to life from a place of clarity and wisdom" [6].

It is essential to consider how we choose to digest this emotional energy. Lonny Jarrett emphasizes the importance of not remaining attached to the previous experience, stating, "Our history lies behind us" [7]. While it is healthy to have a memory of the interaction, we must not allow this memory to trap us in old patterns. Dr. Dan Siegel highlights the significance of integration in the healing process, explaining that "integration is the linkage of differentiated elements of a system" [8].

The Danger of Undigested Experiences

Undigested experiences can keep us trapped and destined to repeat patterns. In the context of Chinese medicine, these unprocessed experiences are known as "samskaras". Christopher Wallis explains that "samskaras are the impressions left by our experiences, which then influence our future responses and behaviors" [9].

Dr. Gabor Maté emphasizes the impact of unresolved emotional experiences on our well-being, stating, "The attempt to escape from pain, is what creates more pain" [10].

Thomas Hübl underscores the importance of addressing unprocessed traumatic experiences in healthcare settings: "Every clinical interaction is potentially traumatic, for both the patient and the healer. If we do not consciously process and integrate these experiences, they can become stuck in our system, leading to burnout, compassion fatigue, and secondary traumatic stress" [6].

Hübl further explains that "trauma is not just a personal experience, but a collective one. As healthcare providers, we are constantly exposed to the collective trauma of our patients and our society. If we do not have practices in place to metabolize this energy, it can accumulate and cause harm" [6].

Expressing Emotions and Avoiding Entrapment

The Daoist principle of "No emotion should be unexpressed" highlights the importance of acknowledging and processing our emotions [7]. As healers, it is crucial that we do not become trapped in the suffering of each clinical interaction. This does not mean that we do not care; in fact, it is quite the opposite.

Lonny Jarrett further elaborates on this concept, stating, "The practitioner who is able to be present with their own experience, without being overwhelmed by it, is able to create a space of healing for their patients" [7].

Dr. Christine Caldwell, a somatic psychotherapist, emphasizes the importance of embodiment in processing emotions, explaining that "the body is the gateway to the present moment" [11].

Thomas Hübl stresses the significance of emotional regulation in preventing traumatic overwhelm: "When we are able to stay present with our emotions without becoming overwhelmed by them, we create a space of healing for ourselves and others. This requires a deep capacity for self-regulation, which can be cultivated through practices like meditation, mindfulness, and somatic experiencing" [6].

Worry and the Trap of Self-Doubt

One of the most significant challenges faced by healthcare practitioners is the trap of self-doubt, which often manifests as ruminative patterns of anxiety. These patterns typically arise from the root of self-doubt, powered by shame. Brené Brown defines shame as "the intensely painful feeling or experience of believing that we are flawed and therefore unworthy of love and belonging" [12].

Self-compassion is a powerful antidote to combat shame. Kristin Neff defines it as "being touched by and open to one's own suffering, not avoiding or disconnecting from it, generating the desire to alleviate one's suffering and to heal oneself with kindness" [13].

Dr. Paul Gilbert, a leading researcher in compassion-focused therapy, emphasizes the importance of cultivating a compassionate inner dialogue, stating, "Compassion is a sensitivity to suffering in self and others, with a commitment to try to alleviate and prevent it" [14].

Take a Breath and Release the Tension

In stressful work environments, it is common to experience a "knot in our stomach" even when we are not in the workplace. This maintains the crisis-driven sympathetic arousal and makes it challenging to relax and restore. The breath can facilitate moving out of sympathetic arousal and into a ventral vagal parasympathetic state where we can "rest and digest" [15].

Dr. Stephen Porges, the originator of the Polyvagal Theory, explains that "the vagus nerve serves as a bidirectional communication pathway between the brain and the body" [16].

Clearing the External Space

Traditional healers have always recognized the importance of clearing negative energies from an environment. In modern times, hospitals have become places where our communities sequester suffering and dying, leading to an accumulation of challenging energies. It is important to note that we are not referring to spirits or ghosts, but rather the energetic traces created by any interaction.

As healers, we inhabit spaces with our patients that include suffering, fear, anger, and many other difficult emotions. Ancient healing traditions have long employed space clearing ceremonies to address these energetic imprints. For example, the Native American tradition of smudging with sage is used to purify a space and promote healing [24]. In Traditional Chinese Medicine, the practice of feng shui is employed to optimize the flow of qi (life force energy) in a given environment [25].

In a modern healthcare setting, we can adapt these practices to clear the energetic space between patient interactions. Simple actions like opening a window, consciously setting an intention to clear the space, or repeating a mantra can help to reset the energetic tone of the environment. Dr. Jean Watson, a nursing theorist and founder of the Watson Caring Science Institute, emphasizes the importance of creating a healing environment, stating, "A caring environment is one that offers the development of potential while allowing the person to choose the best action for himself or herself at a given point in time" [17]. By clering the space, we create an environment that is not constrained by the energetic imprints of past experience.

Close the Space

Developing rituals to close the space after a patient interaction can help us transition from one encounter to the next with greater ease and clarity. It is important to note that closing the space does not mean forgetting the encounter, but rather letting go of the energetic entanglements generated by the interaction. This enables us to see things without distortion and maintain a "wise mind," which means "to see things as they actually are" [26].

In Western culture, the term "closure" is often used to refer to finding a resolution, explaining, or forgetting an event. However, this is not what we are referring to when we suggest "closing the space." In fact, by closing the space and releasing entanglements, we actually open up the space of our heart.

Pema Chödrön speaks to the power of open-heartedness: "The essence of bravery is being without self-deception. However, it takes tremendous fortitude to see ourselves as we are and not flinch. The ground of not being afraid is called enlightened heart, or bodhichitta, or great love, great compassion. It is equated, in part, with complete self-acceptance" [27].

John Welwood elaborates on the concept of the open heart: "An open heart is an inclusive heart. It loves and embraces all parts of us, both the light and the dark, with unconditional friendliness. An open heart has room for our humanness as well as our divinity, for our confusion as well as our clarity" [28].

As Dr. Larry Dossey states, "Rituals are a way of creating order out of chaos, of affirming our connection to the past and the future, and of reminding ourselves of what is truly important" [18]. Dr. Michael Kearney, a palliative care physician and author, emphasizes the importance of creating boundaries and transitions in our work, noting that "the ritual of closure allows us to let go of the emotional residue of one encounter and open ourselves to the next" [19].

Dedicating the Work

The word "dedication" comes from the Latin dedicare, meaning "to consecrate, to devote, to set apart for a deity or for sacred uses" [29]. In the context of our work as healers, dedication is an act of reverence for both the work itself and the transcendent meaning behind the work.

In the Buddhist tradition, the concept of "good in the beginning, good in the middle, good in the end" emphasizes the importance of maintaining a positive and intentional mindset throughout any endeavor [20]. One way to embody this principle is through the practice of dedicating merit.

As Pema Chödrön explains, "Dedicating the merit is like planting a seed in the ground of all beings' consciousness, which will ripen and bear fruit in the future" [21].

Thich Nhat Hanh teaches that "when we practice mindfulness, concentration, and insight, we generate peace and joy in our body and mind. We can then offer this energy of peace and happiness to others" [22].

Developing a dedication statement can help to anchor our intention and infuse our work with a sense of transcendent purpose. This dedication statement may be the same as our intention statement or can be synergistic with it. Here are five examples of dedication statements relevant to being a healer:

1. "May this work be of benefit to all beings, and may it help to alleviate suffering wherever it may be found."
2. "I dedicate the merit of this work to the healing and awakening of all beings, without exception."
3. "May this work be a catalyst for compassion, wisdom, and skillful action in the world."
4. "I offer this work as a prayer for the well-being and flourishing of all life, in all realms and dimensions."
5. "May this work be a humble contribution to the great ocean of healing that is the birthright of all beings."

As Sogyal Rinpoche reminds us, "To dedicate the merit is to offer up the goodness and positive energy created by any virtuous act, so that it may benefit all beings and help them to find their way to their ultimate freedom and peace" [30].

Concluding Remarks

The practice of consciously reviewing and dedicating each session is essential for healers and practitioners. By taking a moment to reflect on the characteristics of each interaction, processing our emotional energy, sealing the experience, clearing the external space, closing the space, and dedicating the merit of our work, we can maintain a state of presence and approach each new engagement with fresh perspective and creative potential.

As Dr. Rachel Naomi Remen reminds us, "The most basic and powerful way to connect to another person is to listen. Just listen. Perhaps the most important thing we ever give each other is our attention" [23].

Self-Reflection Questions

1. How often do I take the time to consciously review the characteristics of each patient interaction? What insights have I gained from this practice?
2. How might undigested experiences from patient interactions influence my thoughts, emotions, and behaviors? How can I work to process and integrate

these experiences more effectively?

3. How do I navigate the potential for traumatic overwhelm in my work as a healthcare provider? What practices do I have to regulate my emotions and maintain a state of presence?

4. Do I allow myself to experience and express my emotions related to patient carefully? What barriers might prevent me from doing so, and how can I overcome them?

5. How do I recognize and address feelings of self-doubt or shame that arise in my work as a healthcare practitioner? In what ways can I cultivate greater self-compassion and resilience?

6. How often do I incorporate breathing exercises or other mindfulness practices into my daily routine, particularly between patient interactions? How have these practices affected my ability to manage stress and maintain presence?

7. How might my workplace's physical environment impact the emotional and energetic well-being of myself and my patients? What steps can I take to create a more positive, nurturing space?

8. How do I understand "closing the space" after a patient interaction? What rituals or practices can I develop to help me transition more seamlessly between encounters?

9. How do I cultivate an open-hearted presence in my work as a healthcare provider? How might this impact my ability to connect with and care for my patients?

10. How can I incorporate the practice of dedicating merit into my work as a healthcare practitioner? In what ways might this practice help me stay connected to the deeper purpose and meaning of my work?

References

1. Gandhi, M. (1953). *Gandhi: An autobiography - The story of my experiments with truth.* Public Affairs Press.

2. Padmasambhava. (2018). *The Tibetan book of the dead.* Shambhala Publications.

3. Trungpa, C. (2009). *The truth of suffering and the path of liberation.* Shambhala Publications.

4. Chenagtsang, N. (2013). *The Tibetan art of dream analysis.* Sky Press.

5. Thurman, R. (1994). *The Tibetan book of the dead: Liberation through understanding in the between.* Bantam Books.

6. Hübl, T. (2019). *Healing collective trauma: A process for integrating our intergenerational and cultural wounds.* Sounds True.

7. Jarrett, L. S. (2004). *Nourishing destiny: The inner tradition of Chinese medicine.* Spirit Path Press.

8. Siegel, D. J. (2010). *Mindsight: The new science of personal transformation.* Bantam Books.

9. Wallis, C. D. (2016). *Tantra illuminated: The philosophy, history, and practice of a timeless tradition.* Mattamayūra Press.

10. Maté, G. (2003). *When the body says no: Understanding the stress-disease connection.* John Wiley & Sons.

11. Caldwell, C. (1996). *Getting our bodies back: Recovery, healing, and transformation through body-centered psychotherapy.* Shambhala Publications.

12. Brown, B. (2012). *Daring greatly: How the courage to be vulnerable transforms the way we live, love, parent, and lead.* Gotham Books.

13. Neff, K. (2011). *Self-compassion: The proven power of being kind to yourself.* William Morrow.

14. Gilbert, P. (2014). The origins and nature of compassion focused therapy. *British Journal of Clinical Psychology, 53*(1), 6-41.

15. Gilbert, P. (2009). *The compassionate mind: A new approach to life's challenges.* New Harbinger Publications.

16. Porges, S. W. (2011). *The polyvagal theory: Neurophysiological foundations of emotions, attachment, communication, and self-regulation.* W. W. Norton & Company.

17. Watson, J. (2008). *Nursing: The philosophy and science of caring* (Revised Edition). University Press of Colorado.

18. Dossey, L. (1993). *Healing words: The power of prayer and the practice of medicine.* HarperSanFrancisco.

19. Kearney, M. (2009). *A place of healing: Working with nature and soul at the end of life.* New World Library.

20. Rinpoche, S. (1992). *The Tibetan book of living and dying.* HarperSanFrancisco.

21. Chödrön, P. (2001). *The wisdom of no escape: And the path of loving-kindness.* Shambhala Publications.

22. Nhat Hanh, T. (2007). *The art of power.* HarperOne.

23. Remen, R. N. (1996). *Kitchen table wisdom: Stories that heal.* Riverhead Books.

24. Foor, D. (2017). *Ancestral medicine: Rituals for personal and family healing.* Bear & Company.

25. Huo, S. (1995). *The essence of feng shui.* Nantien Institute.

26. Beck, J. S. (2011). *Cognitive behavior therapy: Basics and beyond.* Guilford Press.

27. Chödrön, P. (2006). *The places that scare you: A guide to fearlessness in difficult times.* Shambhala Publications.

28. Welwood, J. (2000). *Toward a psychology of awakening: Buddhism,

psychotherapy, and the path of personal and spiritual transformation.* Shambhala Publications.

29. Harper, D. (n.d.). *Dedicate (v.).* In Online Etymology Dictionary. Retrieved from https://www.etymonline.com/word/dedicate
30. Rinpoche, S. (2002). *The future of Buddhism.* Rider.

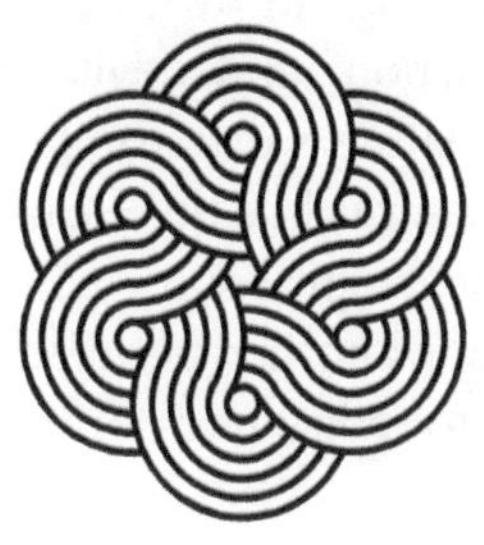

CHAPTER 22

Asana Seven: Experience Joy

Instruction: Be joyful about your work as a healer.

"If you carry joy in your heart, you can heal any moment."
Carlos Santana

$\mathcal{B}$eing a healer, whether a doctor, nurse, therapist, or any other type of healthcare provider, inherently involves physical, emotional, and spiritual challenges. Healers are constantly exposed to their patients' suffering, pain, and struggles. They work long hours, often in high-stress environments, and carry the weight of their patients' well-being on their shoulders. The work can be physically demanding, emotionally draining, and spiritually taxing [1].

Given these challenges, it is absolutely critical that healers find a way to experience enlivenment and vitality in their work rather than exhaustion and depletion. As the spiritual teacher Sadhguru wisely said, "What patients need from their doctor is their vitality" [2]. Patients need caregivers who are energized, present, and deeply connected to the meaning and purpose of their healing work. They need healers who radiate life force [1].

Unfortunately, we are seeing a growing pandemic of burnout among healthcare providers. Studies show that over 50% of doctors and nurses report symptoms of burnout, such as emotional exhaustion, depersonalization, and a reduced sense of personal accomplishment [3]. This burnout crisis is a manifestation of the devitalization of modern medicine. We have come to view ourselves as machines rather than vital beings. We push ourselves to work harder and faster, sacrificing our own wellbeing in the process [1].

The antidote to this burnout and devitalization is not necessarily to spend less time doing our healing work, to play more golf, or to take more vacations. While self-care practices like these can certainly be helpful, they do not address the root cause of the problem - which is our loss of connection. Connection to ourselves, to one another, to the sacredness and meaning of our work. What we need most is to rediscover our innate capacity for joy, wonder, and aliveness [1].

The Power of Joy

The experience of joy opens us to the vitality of the universe. When we are joyful, we feel expansive, energized, and deeply connected to life. We sense our own sacredness and the sacredness of all beings. The boundaries between self and other soften, and we experience a felt sense of unity and belonging [1].

This state of joyful vitality is our birthright. Children come into the world naturally radiating this energy. But over time, we learn to constrict and suppress our life force. We internalize familial and societal messages that we need to be serious, productive, and in control at all times. We cut ourselves off from the wonder and magic of life in the process [1].

Our professional medical education often further divorces us from our capacity for joy and aliveness. We are taught to view the body as a machine, and to focus on pathology rather than the miracle of life. We learn to suppress our emotions, viewing them as a liability rather than a source of wisdom and vitality. We become very skilled at treating disease, but risk losing touch with the deeper art of healing [1].

To reclaim our vitality, we must consciously reconnect to our capacity for joy and wonder. This does not mean that we deny the very real challenges and suffering we encounter in our work as healers. The spiritual path is not about whitewashing reality or pretending everything is okay when it's not. Rather, it's about expanding our field of awareness to include both the joys and the sorrows of life [1].

The great Sufi poet Rumi spoke to this when he wrote:

"Sorrow prepares you for joy. It violently sweeps everything out of your house, so that new joy can find space to enter. It shakes the yellow leaves from the bough of your heart, so that fresh, green leaves can grow in their place. It pulls up the rotten roots, so that new roots hidden beneath have room to grow. Whatever sorrow shakes from your heart, far better things will take their place" [4].

In other words, the way to work with the challenges of our healing work is not to try to suppress our fears and worries, but to acknowledge these realities while also opening to a larger and more abundant experience of ourselves and our world. We must learn to dance with both the sorrows and the joys, letting them transform and enliven us [1].

The Indian goddess Kali provides a powerful metaphor for this dance. Kali is the goddess of time, change, and transformation. She is often depicted dancing in a field of flames, wearing a necklace of skulls and a skirt of dismembered arms. To the Western eye, Kali can appear fearsome and terrifying. But in the yogic tradition, she represents the transformative power of consciousness. She reminds us that joy and terror, life and death, are inseparable parts of the whole. By learning to dance with Kali, to say yes to all that life brings us, we open to vast reservoirs of energy, wisdom and compassion [1].

Mother Teresa, one of the greatest healers of the modern era, understood this well. She used to tell the novice nuns in her charity, "Find joy here or go home" [5]. She knew that it was essential for her caregivers to stay connected to the bliss of selfless service, even amidst the unimaginable poverty, illness and suffering they confronted daily. Their capacity to experience joy not only sustained them personally, it radically enhanced the healing impact they had on those they served. The patients could feel the nuns' authentic delight and presence, and this alone transmitted a profound healing energy [1].

The Five Doorways to Joy

Joy is a fundamental human experience that uplifts and enlivens us. It connects us to the sacred dimension of life and imbues our existence with meaning and purpose. While joy is our birthright, many of us struggle to consistently access this exalted state. The good news is that there are specific pathways - what we might call the five doorways to joy - that can reliably guide us home to our natural vitality and aliveness. These doorways are: 1) Humility, 2) Gratitude, 3) Awe, 4) Beauty, and 5) Channeling Joy. By consciously cultivating these qualities of being, we open ourselves to greater and greater experiences of joyful presence [6].

1. The Doorway of Humility

The first doorway to joy is the practice of humility. Humility has been celebrated as a virtue in all the world's great spiritual traditions. The Christian mystic Thomas Merton wrote, "Pride makes us artificial and humility makes us real" [7]. When we let go of our ego's need to feel separate and superior, we open to the joy of authentic connection - to ourselves, others, and the living web of creation [6].

Humility does not mean thinking less of oneself, but rather thinking of oneself less. It is a shift from self-preoccupation to a more expansive and inclusive state of awareness. Buddhist teacher Jack Kornfield explains, "Humility does not mean you think less of yourself. It means you think of yourself less" [8].

Research confirms that humility is strongly correlated with experiences of joy, contentment, and overall well-being. A 2016 study published in the Journal of Positive Psychology found that "humility predicts greater psychological well-being, more positive affect, and less negative affect" [9]. By releasing our defensive ego structures, we create space for the energies of joy to naturally arise [6].

The quote "Arrogance is the worst form of ignorance" adds another layer to the discussion of humility and joy. Arrogance can be understood as the opposite of humility - a rigid, inflated sense of self-importance that cuts us off from the richness and complexity of reality. When we are arrogant, we assume that we already know everything worth knowing, and we close ourselves off to new information or perspectives that might challenge our preconceptions [6].

Sadly, modern healthcare training often encourages forms of intellectualization and ego-attachment that can foster arrogance. The competitive nature of medical education, the emphasis on specialization and expertise, and the pressure to project an image of unassailable competence can all contribute to a culture of arrogance among healthcare professionals [6].

When we become overly identified with our intellectual knowledge or professional status, we risk losing touch with the humility that is essential for true healing. We may start to see patients as problems to be solved rather than whole persons to be understood and cared for. We may become dismissive of alternative perspectives or approaches that fall outside our narrow domain of expertise [6].

Arrogance has several characteristic features that distinguish it from healthy self-confidence or assertiveness. Arrogant individuals tend to be rigid and inflexible in their thinking, unable to adapt to new situations or information. They may be dismissive or contemptuous of others' opinions, seeing themselves as superior in knowledge or ability. Arrogant people often have difficulty admitting mistakes or acknowledging their own limitations [6].

One of the most damaging consequences of arrogance is that it breeds empathic blindness. When we are so full of ourselves and our own perspectives, we lose the ability to truly see and connect with others. We may become impatient, judgmental, or emotionally tone-deaf in our interactions. This empathic failure is particularly problematic in healthcare, where the ability to understand and attune to the experiences of suffering individuals is paramount [6].

Moreover, arrogance constricts our capacity for openness and flexibility in engaging with the world around us. When we assume we already have all the answers, we lose the ability to be surprised, inspired, or transformed by new experiences. We may miss out on valuable insights or opportunities for growth that fall outside our pre-established frameworks of understanding [6].

"Be like the bamboo, the higher you grow, the lower you bow" (Chinese proverb) [10]. Cultivating humility, on the other hand, allows us to approach each moment with a beginner's mind, open to the freshness and possibility of the present. When we are humble, we are better able to listen deeply, to tolerate uncertainty, and to be moved by the beauty and mystery of life. We are more likely to approach others with empathy, respect, and a genuine desire to understand their unique perspectives and experiences [6].

For healthcare professionals, cultivating humility is not just a nice-to-have, but an essential aspect of effective and compassionate care. By letting go of the need to be right or to have all the answers, we create space for true connection, collaboration, and healing to occur. We become more attuned to the subtle cues and needs of our patients, and more responsive to the ever-changing demands of the healing process [6].

Ultimately, the path of humility is a path of liberation - from the prison of our own egoic constructs, and into the vast, open space of authentic joy and connection. As the Zen master Shunryu Suzuki once said, "In the beginner's mind there are many possibilities, but in the expert's there are few" [11]. By embracing the beginner's mind of humility, we open ourselves to the infinite possibilities for growth, healing, and transformation that each moment presents [6].

2. *The Doorway of Gratitude*

The second doorway to joy is the practice of gratitude. Gratitude is the felt sense of appreciation and thankfulness for the blessings and gifts of our lives. It is a heart-centered state that connects us to the abundance and benevolence of the universe [6].

Pioneering gratitude researcher Robert Emmons defines gratitude as "a felt sense of wonder, thankfulness, and appreciation for life" [12]. He and other researchers have documented the many benefits of gratitude, which include increased happiness, stronger relationships, better sleep, and even a boosted immune system [13].

The practice of gratitude is indeed a powerful doorway to joy, especially for those in the healing professions. As you mentioned, pioneering researcher Robert Emmons defines gratitude as "a felt sense of wonder, thankfulness, and appreciation for life" [12]. His research, along with many others, has documented numerous benefits of gratitude practice, including increased happiness, stronger relationships, better sleep, and even improved immune function [13].

For healers, there are many specific aspects of our work that can inspire deep gratitude. First and foremost, we can feel grateful for the opportunity to engage in such meaningful and impactful work. As author Laurence G. Boldt writes, "Gratitude unlocks the fullness of life. It turns what we have into enough, and more. It turns denial into acceptance, chaos to order, confusion to clarity" [15]. By focusing on the privilege of serving others and making a positive difference in the world, we shift our perspective from one of scarcity to one of abundance [6].

We can also feel gratitude for the remarkable scientific advancements that allow us to effectively treat conditions that were once fatal. The fact that we have access to sophisticated diagnostic tools, targeted therapies, and evidence-based interventions is truly awe-inspiring when considered in the context of medical history [6].

Moreover, we can practice gratitude for our own health and capacity to do this important work. Recognizing the gift of a sound body and mind that enables us to show up in service to others is a profound practice. As Boldt notes, "Gratitude is a vaccine, an antitoxin, and an antiseptic" [15]. By appreciating our own wholeness, we become more resilient in the face of the inevitable challenges and stresses of healthcare [6].

Another important focus of gratitude is the trust and faith that our patients place in us. Being invited into the intimate realm of another's suffering is a sacred honor that deserves our deepest respect and appreciation. When we approach each patient encounter with a sense of humility and thankfulness, we create space for true healing to occur [6].

As you point out, gratitude is a potent antidote to the experience of scarcity and lack. When we are trapped in a mindset of deficiency, we are unable to fully appreciate the abundance that surrounds us. Gratitude shifts our focus from what is missing to what is present, from what we lack to what we have been given. As Boldt eloquently states, "Gratitude turns what we have into enough, and more. It turns denial into acceptance, chaos to order, confusion to clarity. It can turn a meal into a feast, a house into a home, a stranger into a friend" [15].

This shift from scarcity to abundance is crucial for our ability to experience beauty and joy in our lives and work. When we are trapped in the narrow confines of our own limited perspective, we miss out on the awe-inspiring reality that surrounds us. Gratitude helps us step outside of our internal dialogue and into a world of boundless potential and grace. It reminds us, as Boldt puts it, that "the universe is full and complete, and we are recipients of its abundance" [15].

Importantly, gratitude is an autotelic experience, meaning that it is intrinsically rewarding and self-reinforcing. The more we practice gratitude, the more we find to be grateful for. It is a positive feedback loop that keeps opening us to ever-wider experiences of the goodness and beauty of life [6].

In the context of healthcare, gratitude is particularly important as an antidote to the tendency to focus on "bad outcomes" and perceived failures. As physician and author Abraham Verghese notes, "In medicine, we are often so focused on our failures that we forget to celebrate our successes" [16]. By intentionally cultivating gratitude for the many ways in which we positively impact our patients' lives, we counteract the shame and inadequacy that can arise from an unbalanced focus on mistakes or less-than-optimal results [6].

The Japanese practice of Naikan, which means "inside looking," is a structured method of self-reflection that emphasizes gratitude. Naikan involves regularly contemplating three questions: "What have I received from others? What have I given to others? What troubles and difficulties have I caused others?" [17]. By focusing our attention on the myriad ways in which we are supported and cared for by others, Naikan cultivates a deep sense of appreciation and interconnectedness [6].

Research has consistently shown that gratitude practices produce measurable improvements in physical and mental health. Studies have found that gratitude journaling can significantly increase subjective wellbeing, decrease depression, and improve sleep quality and duration [18]. Gratitude has also been linked to reduced inflammation, lower blood pressure, and improved immune function [19].

Importantly, gratitude is a learnable skill that can be cultivated through practice. Some simple ways to enhance gratitude include [6]:

1. Keeping a daily gratitude journal
2. Expressing appreciation directly to others
3. Savoring positive experiences and consciously reflecting on them
4. Engaging in acts of kindness and service
5. Practicing mindfulness and present-moment awareness

By intentionally cultivating gratitude, we open ourselves to the joy, beauty, and abundance that surrounds us. We counteract the natural human tendency towards negativity bias and scarcity thinking, and we align ourselves with the generative and life-giving forces of the universe. As Rumi so beautifully expressed, "Wear gratitude like a cloak and it will feed every corner of your life" [14].

For healers, the practice of gratitude is a powerful tool for staying connected to the meaning and purpose of our work. It helps us maintain perspective in the face of challenges, and it allows us to fully celebrate and appreciate the profound impact we have on the lives of others. By walking through the doorway of gratitude, we open ourselves to the abundant joy and beauty that is our birthright [6].

3. *The Doorway of Awe*

The third doorway to joy is the experience of awe. Awe is apowerful emotional response to the vastness, beauty, and mystery of existence. It is a state of being thunderstruck by the sheer improbability and grandeur of the universe we find ourselves in [6].

Psychologists define awe as a response to things we perceive as vast and that transcend our existing frames of reference in some way [20]. Awe-inducing experiences range from witnessing a magnificent sunrise to holding a newborn child for the first time to having a spiritual epiphany. What these experiences share in common is that they jolt us out of our usual mental patterns and open us to a profound sense of the sacred [6].

Research has shown that experiences of awe have a range of benefits, including increased feelings of connection, greater humility, and enhanced overall well-being [21]. When we tap into the emotion of awe, we remember that we are part of something unfathomably greater than ourselves. This remembrance is a powerful portal to joy. As the astronomer Carl Sagan wrote, "Somewhere, something incredible is waiting to be known" [22].

The experience of awe is indeed a powerful doorway to joy, especially for those in the healing professions. As you mentioned, awe is defined as a response to things we perceive as vast and that transcend our existing frames of reference [20]. For healers, there are numerous aspects of our work that can evoke this sense of awe and wonder [6].

One of the most profound sources of awe in healthcare is the mystery and complexity of the human body itself. The intricate dance of biochemical processes, the delicate balance of homeostatic mechanisms, the remarkable resilience and regenerative capacities of our tissues - all of these inspire a sense of reverence and astonishment. As surgeon and author Sherwin Nuland wrote, "The human body is an endlessly fascinating repository of secrets. The miracle of the skin, the strength and structure of the bones, the dynamic balance of the muscles - your physical being is knit according to a pattern of incredible purpose" [23].

Another source of awe for healers is the profound privilege of witnessing the human journey from birth to death. To be present at the moment a new life enters the world, or to hold the hand of a person as they take their final breaths - these are experiences that transcend our usual understanding of the world and connect us to something much larger than ourselves. As author and physician Rachel Naomi Remen writes, "The practice of medicine is an act of love. So often we act as though it is an act of competence, but it is an act of love" [24].

Healers also have the opportunity to experience awe through the incredible scientific and technological advancements that enable us to diagnose, treat, and cure conditions that were once impossible to manage. The fact that we can peer inside the human body with advanced imaging techniques, that we can target specific molecular pathways with precision therapies, that we can transplant organs and rebuild damaged tissues - these capabilities are truly awe-inspiring when considered in the context of medical history [6].

Moreover, the experience of awe can arise in the context of the deep human connection that is at the heart of the healing relationship. When we are fully present with another person in their suffering, when we bear witness to their story and their struggle, we touch something profound and sacred. As physician and author Abraham Verghese writes, "The secret of the care of the patient is in caring for the patient" [25]. This level of caring presence opens us to the awe and mystery of human existence [6].

Research has shown that experiences of awe have a range of benefits for mental health and well-being. Awe has been linked to increased feelings of connection and common humanity, greater humility and perspective-taking, and enhanced overall life satisfaction [21]. Awe also has the effect of "shrinking the self," as researcher Dacher Keltner puts it - it shifts our focus from our narrow self-concern to a broader appreciation of the world around us [26].

For healers, cultivating a sense of awe can be a powerful antidote to burnout and compassion fatigue. When we are able to step back and marvel at the incredible nature of our work, it helps us maintain a sense of perspective and purpose. It reminds us that, despite the challenges and frustrations we may face, we are participating in something truly extraordinary and meaningful [6].

There are many ways that healers can cultivate a sense of awe in their daily work. Taking a moment to really look at an X-ray or lab result, marveling at the intricacy of a surgical procedure, pausing to appreciate the trust and vulnerability of a patient sharing their story - all of these can be opportunities for awe. We can also seek out awe-inspiring experiences outside of work, whether it's watching a sunset, listening to a moving piece of music, or reading about the latest scientific discoveries [6].

Ultimately, the experience of awe reconnects us to the sense of sacredness and purpose that called many of us to the healing professions in the first place. It reminds us that, as Carl Sagan so eloquently put it, "Somewhere, something incredible is waiting to be known" [22]. By opening ourselves to the awe and wonder of our world, we tap into a powerful source of joy, meaning, and resilience [6].

In the words of Albert Einstein, "The most beautiful thing we can experience is the mysterious. It is the source of all true art and all science. He to whom this emotion is a stranger, who can no longer pause to wonder and stand rapt in awe, is as good as dead: his eyes are closed" [27]. As healers, may we never lose our capacity for awe, for it is the wellspring of our deepest joy and the essence of our sacred work [6].

4. *The Doorway of Beauty*

The fourth doorway to joy is the appreciation of beauty. "The primary goal of the practice of medicine and classical acupuncture is to restore beauty to the body's ecological landscape and liberate the circulation of organizing illumination (shenming) within the body's tissue plains to establish harmonic order. The end result is beauty and thriving." - Edward Neal MD on "ShenMing" [28]

This profound statement by Dr. Edward Neal points to a fundamental truth that has been largely forgotten in modern medicine - that the ultimate aim of healing is not just the absence of disease, but the restoration of beauty and vitality [6].

Modern healthcare environments present significant challenges for healers seeking to connect with the experience of beauty. As the philosopher W.E.B. Du Bois poignantly stated, "The worst thing we can do is teach our children that ugliness is normal" [29]. Yet this is precisely what many modern medical settings do. Healers are immersed in a world of suffering, confronted daily with the unpleasant physical manifestations of human disease [6].

This challenge is compounded by the fact that modern healing environments are designed from the perspective of a laboratory rather than a natural healing space. Sterile white walls, harsh fluorescent lighting, and the pervasive hum of machines create an atmosphere that is more conducive to discomfort than to the experience of beauty and ease [6].

Moreover, the modern healer is trained to view patients through the lens of scientific materialism. An elderly man dying from dementia, for example, is seen primarily in terms of his physical decay rather than as a being who has lived a life of determination, courage, love, and conviction. The scientific materialist approach, while powerful in many ways, is fundamentally blind to the dimension of beauty. It reduces the human being to a collection of parts rather than seeing the whole person in all their sacred uniqueness [6].

To truly experience beauty in the context of healing, it is essential to distinguish between authentic beauty and profane desire. Authentic beauty is an internal experience, a felt sense of resonance, harmony, and connection.

It is a state of consciousness that uplifts and enlivens us. Profane desire, in contrast, is focused on the external. It is the grasping after material objects or experiences in the hopes that they will fill an inner void [6].

Modern consumer culture, with its relentless focus on acquisition and consumption, has greatly exacerbated our collective tendency towards profane desire. We are conditioned from a young age to seek fulfillment through the purchase of products, the attainment of status, and the chase after fleeting pleasures. This conditioning trains us to look for beauty outside ourselves rather than cultivating it within [6].

For healers to truly serve as conduits of beauty, we must learn to disentangle ourselves from the trap of profane desire. We must cultivate the capacity to experience beauty as an internal state, one that is not dependent on external circumstances. This requires a commitment to practices that still the mind, open the heart, and allow us to rest in the beauty of our own being [6].

While the modern scientific worldview has largely dismissed beauty as subjective and irrelevant, the truth is that every culture throughout history has recognized the nature and importance of beauty. Each tradition has its own unique understanding and articulation of this essential quality [6].

In the Hebrew tradition, beauty is closely associated with the concept of yapha, which means "to glow or bloom" [30]. Beauty here is understood as a radiance that emanates from within, a luminosity of spirit that shines through the physical form [6].

The ancient Greeks used the term kalon to describe beauty. For them, beauty was intimately connected to the realm of ideas and ideals. It was a metaphysical principle, an essential aspect of the harmonious ordering of the cosmos [31].

In Sanskrit, the word sundara is used to describe beauty. Sundara literally means "holiness" [32]. In the Vedic understanding, beauty and divinity are inseparable. To experience true beauty is to taste the sacred [6].

The Japanese have several terms to describe beauty. One is shibusa, which connotes a refined elegance, a beauty that is understated and deeply integrated. Another is wabi-sabi, which points to the beauty of humility, simplicity, and imperfection [33].

In the Navajo tradition, beauty is understood as hozho, a state of harmony, balance, and right relationship. The Daoists use the term rong to describe beauty as a "glimmering immanence," [34] a subtle yet ever-present luminosity that pervades all things [6].

What these diverse cultural understandings reveal is that beauty is not a frivolous extra, but an essential aspect of human experience. It is a universal language that speaks to our deepest longings for meaning, connection, and transcendence [6].

One of the most profound and comprehensive articulations of beauty comes from the Navajo tradition in the form of the "Rainbow Path to Beauty." For the Navajo, the purpose of life is to walk in beauty, to cultivate right relationship with all things [6].

The Rainbow Path to Beauty is a holistic framework that encompasses all dimensions of human experience - the physical, emotional, mental, and spiritual. It is a path of balance and harmony, of aligning oneself with the inherent order and beauty of the cosmos [6].

There are four key principles that guide the Rainbow Path to Beauty [35]:

1. Walking in Beauty: This means living in a way that is in harmony with the natural world, cultivating reverence and respect for all life.
2. Thinking in Beauty: This involves training the mind to focus on thoughts that are uplifting, expansive, and aligned with truth.
3. Speaking in Beauty: This means using language that is honest, kind, and imbued with appreciation and gratitude.
4. Acting in Beauty: This involves behaving in a way that is ethical, compassionate, and in service to the greater good.

By consciously aligning oneself with these principles, the Navajo believe that one can experience the essential beauty of existence. This is not a static state, but a dynamic process of ever-deepening attunement and self-actualization [6].

As healers in the modern world, we face significant challenges in staying connected to the experience of beauty. We are immersed in a medical paradigm that often reduces the human being to a material object, and we are conditioned by a culture that equates beauty with superficial appearances and fleeting pleasures [6].

Yet as the diverse wisdom traditions of the world remind us, beauty is not a luxury but an essential nutrient for the soul. It is the very fabric of a life well-lived, a reminder of our inherent wholeness and sacred purpose [6].

By consciously cultivating beauty - in our inner lives, our relationships, our healing spaces, and our ways of seeing and being - we can become conduits for the organizing illumination of shenming. We can help restore the body's ecological landscape to its natural state of radiance and harmony [6].

This is the great gift and calling of the healer's path - to midwife the rebirth of beauty in a world that has grown weary and disillusioned. May we find the courage and compassion to walk this path with grace, remembering always the luminous beauty at the heart of all things [6].

5. *The Doorway of Channeling Joy*

The final doorway to joy is the practice of channeling joy. This means cultivating the capacity to intentionally access and express joyful states of being. When we channel joy, we become embodied conduits for the energies of celebration, laughter, playfulness, and creative self-expression [6].

One of the most powerful ways to channel joy is through communal singing and dancing. There is a reason that these practices are found in every culture throughout history - they have the power to rapidly shift consciousness and induce ecstatic states. The shamanic traditions know this well. As the anthropologist Hilda Kuper wrote, "A society that sings is one that functions well" [36].

Channeling joy is a skill that gets stronger with practice. The more we intentionally cultivate joyful states, the more easily we are able to access them. This is because of the neuroplasticity of the brain - the more we exercise the neural pathways associated with particular states of being, the stronger and more automatic they become [37].

Joy is a fundamental human experience that uplifts, enlivens, and connects us to the sacred dimension of existence. While joy may arise spontaneously, we can also cultivate it intentionally through the practice of channeling joy. Channeling joy means aligning ourselves with the energies of harmony, unity, vitality, transcendence, and freedom that are the hallmarks of authentic joy. In this essay, we will explore these five characteristics of joy in depth, drawing on the wisdom of thinkers like Donella Meadows and Robert A. Johnson. We will also delve into the eight specific qualities of joy described by Archbishop Desmond Tutu in his book "The Book of Joy," which include the mind qualities of perspective, humility, humor, and acceptance, and the heart qualities of forgiveness, gratitude, compassion, and generosity [6].

The Five Characteristics of Joy

1. *Harmony*: The first characteristic of joy is harmony. Harmony refers to a state of inner and outer alignment, a sense of everything being in its right place. As systems thinker Donella Meadows wrote, "The world is a complex, interconnected, finite, ecological–social–psychological–economic system. We treat it as if it were not, as if it were divisible, separable, simple, and infinite. Our persistent, intractable global problems arise directly from this mismatch" [38]. When we experience joy, we feel a sense of harmony with ourselves, others, and the larger web of life. We recognize our intrinsic connectedness and the beauty of the whole [6].

2. *Unity*: The second characteristic of joy is unity. Unity refers to the felt sense of oneness, the recognition that beneath the surface diversity of life,

there is a fundamental interconnectedness. As Meadows put it, "We are not outside the ecology for which we plan—we are always and inevitably a part of it" [38]. Joy arises when we tap into this underlying unity and experience ourselves as part of the larger unfolding of life. This sense of unity does not negate our individuality, but rather puts it in a larger, more meaningful context [6].

3. *Vitality*: The third characteristic of joy is vitality. Vitality refers to the felt sense of aliveness, energy, and flow that characterizes joyful states. As psychologist Mihaly Csikszentmihalyi described in his work on optimal experience, joy arises when we fully engage our skills in the face of meaningful challenges, losing our self-consciousness in the process [39]. This state of vital engagement is characterized by a sense of effortlessness, timelessness, and inner clarity. We feel truly alive and present [6].

4. *Transcendence*: The fourth characteristic of joy is transcendence. Transcendence refers to the sense of being part of something larger than ourselves, of connecting to a reality beyond our limited egoic perspective. As mythologist Joseph Campbell wrote, "Life is without meaning. You bring the meaning to it. The meaning of life is whatever you ascribe it to be" [40]. Joy arises when we align ourselves with a sense of meaning and purpose that goes beyond our narrow self-interest. This could be through connecting to the beauty of nature, engaging in a creative pursuit, or dedicating ourselves to a cause greater than ourselves [6].

5. *Freedom*: The fifth characteristic of joy is freedom. Freedom refers to the liberation from the limiting beliefs, identities, and patterns that constrain our authentic self-expression. As psychologist Robert A. Johnson wrote, "Our psyche is set up in accord with the structure of the universe, and what happens in the macrocosm likewise happens in the infinitesimal and most subjective reaches of the psyche" [41]. Joy arises when we free ourselves from the conditioned patterns that keep us stuck and align ourselves with the larger unfolding of our soul's journey [6].The Eight Qualities of Joy**

In his book "The Book of Joy," Archbishop Desmond Tutu, in dialogue with the Dalai Lama, identified eight specific qualities that characterize a joyful life. These include four mind qualities and four heart qualities.

The 4 Mind Qualities of Joy

1. *Perspective:* The ability to see the bigger picture, to recognize the impermanence and change that characterize all life. As Tutu wrote, "We

are fragile creatures, and it is from this weakness, not despite it, that we discover the possibility of true joy" [42].

2.   *Humility*: Recognizing our shared humanity and our interconnectedness with all beings. Desmond Tutu noted, "It is when we see ourselves as part of a greater whole that we find our truest joy" [42].

3.   *Humor*: The capacity to find lightness and laughter despite life's challenges. In Tutu's words, "It is humor that allows us to see the irony in our human condition and to find delight in the midst of our struggles" [42].

4.   *Acceptance*: The willingness to embrace life as it is, to say yes to the full range of human experience. Tutu wrote, "We must be willing to accept the reality of our lives, to accept the losses and disappointments as well as the joys and victories" [42].

The 4 Heart Qualities of Joy

1.   *Forgiveness*: The practice of releasing grievances and resentments, of offering compassion to ourselves and others. As Tutu put it, "Without forgiveness, we remain tethered to the person who harmed us" [42].

2.   *Gratitude*: The practice of appreciating the gifts and blessings of our lives, of saying thank you for what we have been given. Tutu wrote, "It is not happiness that makes us grateful. It is gratefulness that makes us happy" [42].

3.   *Compassion*: The capacity to feel with and for others, to recognize our shared vulnerability and aspirations. In Tutu's words, "Compassion is the keen awareness of the interdependence of all things" [42].

4.   *Generosity*: The willingness to give of ourselves, to share our time, energy, and resources with others. Tutu noted, "In the end, generosity is the best way of becoming more, more, and more joyful" [42].

Concluding Remarks

Ultimately, channeling joy is about aligning ourselves with our deepest identity and purpose in the universe. As the poet Kahlil Gibran wrote, "Your joy is your sorrow unmasked. And the selfsame well from which your laughter rises was often filled with your tears" [43]. Our joy is the song of our soul's journey from earth to heaven, from separation to unity, from fear to love. By cultivating the mind and heart qualities that allow us to channel joy, we participate in the great work of healing and transformation that is the essence of the human path [6].

In the words of Archbishop Tutu, "We are made for goodness. We are made for love. We are made for friendliness. We are made for togetherness. We are made for all of the beautiful things that you and I know. We are made to tell the world that there are no outsiders. All are welcome: black, white, red, yellow, rich, poor, educated, not educated, male, female, gay, straight, all, all, all. We all belong to this family, this human family, God's family" [44]. May we each find our unique way of channeling joy and thereby add to the light of the world [6].

As healers, we have the capacity to be conduits for immense vitality, compassion and joy. This potential lies within each of us, but it gets obscured by the challenges of our work and the limitations of our professional conditioning. To step into our full potential, we must commit ourselves to the practice of reconnecting with our innate aliveness and joy. We must learn to dance in the flames, welcoming all that life brings us with wonder, gratitude and an open heart [1].

This is the path of the awakened healer, the one who knows how to draw from the wellspring of Spirit to serve and uplift others. When we anchor ourselves in joy, we become a field of energetic abundance and aliveness. Our presence alone becomes healing [1].

Ultimately, this is the greatest gift we can offer our patients and our world - not just our knowledge and skills, but our full, vital, awakened presence. Our joy becomes their joy; our aliveness enlivens them. By learning how to dance in the flames, we become partners with the evolutionary force of healing and wholeness. We become agents of the sacred transformations that our world urgently calls for. So, let us never forget the words of the great sage Rumi: "Let the beauty we love be what we do. There are hundreds of ways to kneel and kiss the ground" [45]. Let us embrace the path of awakened, joyful service for the benefit of all beings [1].

Humility, gratitude, awe, beauty, and channeling joy are the five doorways that reliably guide us home to our natural state of joyful aliveness. By consciously cultivating these qualities of being, we nourish and enrich our lives in unimaginable ways [6].

The experience of joy is not a frivolous luxury but an existential necessity. Cultivating joy is an essential act of service and healing in a world that is too often filled with cynicism, apathy, and despair. When we learn how to embody joy, we become beacons of hope and transformation. In the words of the spiritual teacher Marianne Williamson, "Joy is what happens to us when we allow ourselves to recognize how good things really are" [46].

May we all find the courage and grace to walk through these five sacred doorways. May we remember, again and again, the beauty and miracle of our existence. And may our joy ripple out and bless all beings everywhere [6].

Self-Reflection Questions

1. In what ways have I experienced burnout or devitalization in my work as a healer? How might reconnecting with my innate capacity for joy and aliveness help to address these challenges?

2. What does it mean to me to "dance in the flames" of life's joys and sorrows? How can I embrace both the light and the shadow aspects of my healing work with greater grace and resilience?

3. How do I understand the relationship between humility and joy? In what ways might cultivating greater humility open me to more authentic experiences of connection and aliveness?

4. What are the specific aspects of my work as a healer that inspire feelings of gratitude? How can I more consistently attune to and appreciate these gifts?

5. When have I experienced a sense of awe in my healing work? What was the impact of this experience on my perspective and well-being?

6. How do I define beauty, and in what ways do I encounter beauty in my work as a healer? How might I more intentionally cultivate an appreciation for beauty in my life and work?

7. What practices or experiences allow me to access and channel joyful states most effectively? How can I prioritize these practices as an essential aspect of my self-care and professional development?

8. In what ways do I see the five characteristics of joy (harmony, unity, vitality, transcendence, and freedom) reflected in my own experiences of joyfulness? How might I consciously cultivate these qualities in my daily life and work?

9. Of the eight qualities of joy identified by Archbishop Tutu (perspective, humility, humor, acceptance, forgiveness, gratitude, compassion, and generosity), which do I most naturally embody, and which could I focus on developing further?

10. What is my deepest aspiration for myself as a healer and human being? How might anchoring myself in the joy experience help me realize this aspiration more fully?

References

1. Original text, "Dancing in the Flames: Experience Joy and Beauty".

2. Sadhguru, J.V. (2016). *Inner Engineering: A Yogi's Guide to Joy.* Spiegel & Grau.

3. Shanafelt, T.D., et al. (2012). Burnout and satisfaction with work-life balance among US physicians relative to the general US population. *Archives of Internal Medicine*, 172(18), 1377-1385.

4. Barks, C. (2004). *The Essential Rumi*. HarperOne.

5. Kolodiejchuk, B. (2007). *Mother Teresa: Come Be My Light: The Private Writings of the Saint of Calcutta*. Image.

6. Original text, "The Five Doorways to Joy".

7. Merton, T. (2007). *New Seeds of Contemplation*. New Directions.

8. Kornfield, J. (2008). *The Wise Heart: A Guide to the Universal Teachings of Buddhist Psychology*. Bantam.

9. Kruse, E., Chancellor, J., Ruberton, P. M., & Lyubomirsky, S. (2014). An upward spiral between gratitude and humility. *Social Psychological and Personality Science*, 5(7), 805-814.

10. Chinese Proverb

11. Suzuki, S. (2020). *Zen Mind, Beginner's Mind*. Shambhala.

12. Emmons, R. A. (2007). *Thanks!: How the new science of gratitude can make you happier*. Houghton Mifflin Harcourt.

13. Emmons, R. A., & McCullough, M. E. (2003). Counting blessings versus burdens: an experimental investigation of gratitude and subjective well-being in daily life. *Journal of personality and social psychology*, 84(2), 377.

14. Barks, C. (2005). *Rumi: The Book of Love: Poems of Ecstasy and Longing*. HarperOne.

15. Boldt, L. G. (1999). *Zen and the Art of Making a Living: A Practical Guide to Creative Career Design*. Penguin.

16. Verghese, A. (2009). The Importance of Being. *Health Affairs*, 28(Suppl1), w596-w598.

17. Krech, G. (2002). *Naikan: Gratitude, grace, and the Japanese art of self-reflection*. Stone Bridge Press.

18. Sansone, R. A., & Sansone, L. A. (2010). Gratitude and well being: The benefits of appreciation. *Psychiatry (Edgmont)*, 7(11), 18.

19. Wood, A. M., Froh, J. J., & Geraghty, A. W. (2010). Gratitude and well-being: A review and theoretical integration. *Clinical psychology review*, 30(7), 890-905.

20. Keltner, D., & Haidt, J. (2003). Approaching awe, a moral, spiritual, and aesthetic emotion. *Cognition and emotion*, 17(2), 297-314.

21. Bai, Y., Maruskin, L. A., Chen, S., Gordon, A. M., Stellar, J. E., McNeil, G. D., ... & Keltner, D. (2017). Awe, the diminished self, and collective engagement: Universals and cultural variations in the small self. *Journal of personality and social psychology*, 113(2), 185.

22. Sagan, C. (2011). *Pale blue dot: A vision of the human future in space*. Ballantine Books.

23. Nuland, S. B. (2011). *How we live.* Vintage.

24. Remen, R. N. (2010). *Kitchen table wisdom: Stories that heal*. Penguin.

25. Verghese, A. (2011). *Cutting for stone*. Vintage.

26. Stellar, J. E., Gordon, A., Anderson, C. L., Piff, P. K., McNeil, G. D., & Keltner, D. (2018). Awe and humility. *Journal of personality and social psychology*, 114(2), 258.

27. Einstein, A. (1931). *Living Philosophies: The Reflections of Some Eminent Men and Women of Our Time*. Simon and Schuster.

28. Neal, E. (2012). *The art of classical acupuncture: The standard textbook*. Singing Dragon.

29. Du Bois, W. E. B. (2015). *The souls of black folk*. Yale University Press.

30. Brown, F., Driver, S. R., & Briggs, C. A. (2000). *Enhanced Brown-Driver-Briggs Hebrew and English Lexicon*. Oak Harbor, WA: Logos Research Systems.

31. Scarry, E. (2001). *On beauty and being just*. Princeton University Press.

32. Apte, V. S. (1965). *The practical Sanskrit-English dictionary: Containing appendices on Sanskrit prosody important literary & geographical names in the ancient history of India*. Motilal Banarsidass Publication.

33. Koren, L. (2008). *Wabi-sabi for artists, designers, poets & philosophers*. Imperfect Publishing.

34. Hinton, D. (2016). *Existence: A Story*. Shambhala Publications.

35. Farella, J. R. (1993). *The wind in a jar*. University of New Mexico Press.

36. Kuper, H. (1947). *An African aristocracy: rank among the Swazi*. Published for the International African Institute by the Oxford University Press.

37. Hanson, R., & Mendius, R. (2009). *Buddha's brain: The practical neuroscience of happiness, love, and wisdom*. New Harbinger Publications.

38. Meadows, D. H. (2008). *Thinking in systems: A primer*. chelsea green publishing.

39. Csikszentmihalyi, M. (1990). *Flow: The psychology of optimal experience*. Harper & Row.

40. Campbell, J. (1991). *The power of myth*. Anchor.

41. Johnson, R. A. (2009). *Inner work: Using dreams and active imagination for personal growth*. Harper Collins.

42. Lama, D., Tutu, D., & Abrams, D. (2016). *The book of joy: Lasting happiness in a changing world*. Avery.

43. Gibran, K. (2019). *The prophet*. Vintage.

44. Tutu, D. (2011). *God has a dream: A vision of hope for our time*. Image.

45. Barks, C. (2010). *Rumi: The big red book: The great masterpiece celebrating mystical love and friendship*. Harper Collins.

46. Williamson, M. (1996). *A return to love: Reflections on the principles of a course in miracles*. Harper Paperbacks.

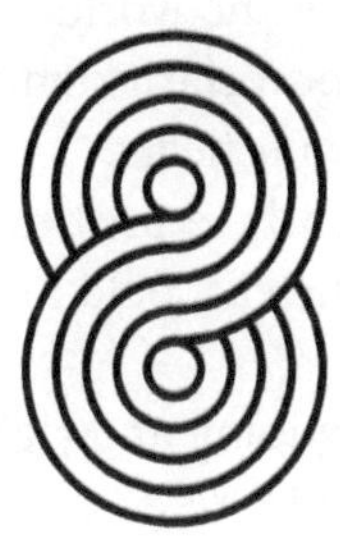

AFTERWORD

$\mathcal{D}$ear Fellow Pilgrim on The Path of the Good-Hearted Physician:

We have explored the foundations for rediscovering our hearts as healers. We have delved into the importance of healers supporting each other, the wisdom of ancient healing traditions, the transformative power of vulnerability and shame, resilience, and the key pillars of thriving healing communities. We have envisioned what it means to be an integral healing community and explored practical strategies for cultivating connection, collaboration, and mutual care in the midst of our challenging work.

It is essential to acknowledge that we are living in difficult times. The work of healers has never been more demanding or more crucial. We face a world grappling with a pandemic, economic upheaval, social injustice, and ecological crisis. We are confronted daily with suffering, uncertainty, and complex ethical dilemmas. The toll on our mental, emotional, and spiritual well-being is significant.

Yet in these times of darkness, the light of compassion and the power of healing are most needed. As the Tibetan sage Padmasambhava reminds us:

"The dark times will naturally pass because soon the sun will shine. Then the time of light will come and all the positive things that you have done during the difficult times will bear fruit. Everything will turn out to your benefit... Do not be discouraged when darkness sets in because, eventually, a new dawn will come. Trust in this." [1]

The path of the good-hearted physician is, at its core, the path of discovering the spaciousness that lies beyond the limitations of our thoughts and emotions. It is the path of learning to rest in the vast and open sky of our true nature, even as the storms of the world rage around us. In that spacious freedom, we can find the resilience, clarity, and compassion to meet whatever arises with an open and courageous heart.

The Sufi poet Rumi eloquently expresses this invitation to step beyond our limited identities and into the vast field of our shared being:

"Out beyond ideas of wrongdoing and rightdoing,
 there is a field. I'll meet you there.
 When the soul lies down in that grass,
the world is too full to talk about.
Ideas, language, even the phrase 'each other'
doesn't make any sense." [2]

As healers, we are called to meet each other in that field beyond right and wrong, beyond healer and patient, beyond self and other. We are called to recognize our fundamental interconnectedness, our shared vulnerability, and strength, our common humanity. From that recognition, we can begin to build healing communities rooted in compassion, trust, and mutual care.

This is a challenging path. It requires us to confront our own shadows, to lean into discomfort and uncertainty, and to let go of the illusion of control. It asks us to keep our hearts open even when the world feels overwhelming and to keep showing up for ourselves and each other even when we feel exhausted and dispirited. But as the Vietnamese Buddhist teacher Thich Nhat Hanh reminds us, this path of compassion and community is also the path of joy and freedom:

"Take my hand.
We will walk.
We will only walk.
We will enjoy our walk
without thinking of arriving anywhere.
Walk peacefully.
Walk happily.
Our walk is a peace walk.
Our walk is a happiness walk." [3]

Dear healer, as you step forward on this path, remember the words that opened this book: Never give up. No matter what is going on around you, never give up. When you feel lost or overwhelmed, come back to your breath, to your heart, to the presence of your fellow healers walking beside you. Trust in the resilience of your spirit, the power of compassion, and the wisdom of your community. of healers

You are not alone on this journey. You are part of a lineage of healers stretching back through time, part of a global community dedicated to the alleviation of suffering. Draw strength from those who have walked this path before you, and those who walk it alongside you now.

Together, with each step, each act of courage and care, we are weaving a new world—a world where the heart of healing is restored to its rightful place at the center of medicine, where healers are nourished and sustained by communities of shared purpose and mutual care, and where compassion and connection are the guiding lights in the darkness.

May you trust in the power of your good heart. May you find refuge in the spaciousness of your true nature. May you always remember the sacred privilege of walking alongside your fellow beings in their journeys of healing and wholeness.

With deep respect and appreciation for your commitment to the path of healing,

References

1. Padmasambhava, & Bays, J. C. (2008). The Tibetan Book of the Dead: The Great Book of Natural Liberation Through Understanding in the Between (Kindle ed.). Dorling Kindersley Ltd.
2. Barks, C. (2003). Rumi: The Book of Love: Poems of Ecstasy and Longing (Kindle ed.). HarperOne.
3. Hanh, T. N. (2014). Peace Is Every Step: The Path of Mindfulness in Everyday Life (p. 104). Random House.

The Oath of the Good-Hearted Physician

As a healer committed to the path of transformative healing practice, I make this sacred oath:

I vow to approach my work with presence, bringing my full attention and awareness to each moment, each encounter, and each opportunity to serve.

I vow to cultivate compassion and kindness, to listen deeply, and to respond with empathy and understanding to the suffering of those in my care.

I vow to pursue my practice with dedication, devotion, and joy and prioritize my growth and development as a foundation for serving others.

I vow to embrace humility, recognizing that I am always a learner, always a beginner, in the face of life's vast complexity and mystery.

I vow to remain flexible and adaptable, meet each challenge with creativity and resilience, and find opportunity in adversity.

I vow to cultivate patience and trust in the healing process and honor each individual's journey towards healing.

I vow to engage my work with discernment and intelligence, refine my skills, expand my understanding continuously, and make wise choices to support health and wholeness.

I vow to embody tenacity and perseverance, remain steadfast in my commitment to healing, and push through obstacles and setbacks with determination and grace.

I vow to summon courage, to face my fears and limitations, to stand in compassionate witness to the suffering of others, and to be a beacon of hope and strength.

I vow to support and nurture my community of healers as we walk this challenging path together.

Above all, I vow to remember that my work is a sacred trust, a privilege, and a responsibility.

I dedicate myself to healing as a way of life, a journey of transformation and service.

Through this oath, I align myself with the highest principles of my calling and commit to the ongoing practice of becoming an instrument of healing and a channel for the innate wisdom and compassion that nourishes the birthright of all beings to flourish.

- The developmental journey of the good-hearted healer, as represented by the story of Chiron, the Greek mythological "wounded healer."
- Exploring the "lexicon" of healing as a doorway to understanding and manifesting the deeper meaning of our work as healers.
- The "Four Immeasurable" attributes of a "good-hearted" healer.